Advanced Trauma Operative Management

Editor
Lenworth M. Jacobs, MD, MPH, FACS
Professor of Surgery
Professor and Chairman
Department of Traumatology
University of Connecticut
Hartford Hospital
Director Trauma Program
Hartford, CT

Associate Editors
Ronald I. Gross, MD, FACS
Assistant Professor of Surgery
University of Connecticut
Hartford Hospital
Associate Director, Trauma Program
Hartford, CT

Stephen S. Luk, MD, FACS
Assistant Professor of Surgery
University of Connecticut
Hartford Hospital
Trauma Program
Hartford, CT

Chapter Contributors
Lenworth M. Jacobs, MD, MPH, FACS
Robert T. Brautigam, MD, FACS
Karyl Burns, RN, PhD
Vicente Cortes, MD, FACS
Ronald I. Gross, MD, FACS
Orlando Kirton, MD, FACS
Stephen S. Luk, MD, FACS
George A. Perdrizet, MD, PhD, FACS

Published by: Ciné-Med, Inc.
                 127 Main Street North
                 Woodbury, CT 06798

Copyright © 2004

All rights reserved. No part of this publication may be reproduced, stored in a retrieval system or transmitted in any form or by any means electronic, mechanical, photocopying, recording or otherwise, without prior written permission of the publisher.

ISBN: 0-9749358-0-8

Preface

The ATOM Course was developed to respond to the challenge of providing excellent care for injured patients. The classic time honored method of teaching operative surgery has been the experiential model. The surgeon is presented with a patient who has sustained a penetrating injury. A diagnosis, a treatment plan, and an appropriate operative intervention are then developed. It has been a sound practice to have a more experienced surgeon expose and assist the operating surgeon with the operating procedure.

The repetitive nature of operative surgery ensures that technical competence is monitored and assured as experience is gained by the operating surgeon. The patient was assured of excellent operative care by the mentoring and preceptorship of the experienced senior surgeon of the inexperienced surgeon.

A decreasing incidence of penetrating trauma, a decreased exposure of surgeons to operative penetrating injuries and the attenuated time available to train surgical residents has mandated a change in the approach to educating surgeons to be expert in the management of penetrating trauma.

The ATOM course is a prototype for simulated operative surgical education. It provides a reproducible method for educating surgeons in complex infrequent penetrating injuries. The course provides for predictable elective management of severe injuries in the exact environment that the surgeon is expected to manage these injuries. This education is also scheduled for when the surgeon and the surgical instructor are alert and maximally prepared to manage challenging penetrating injuries.

The wisdom of master trauma surgeons has been captured and their method, techniques, and tricks of successfully navigating through very difficult operative procedures are found at the end of each chapter. This wisdom represents a safe effective method of dealing with a specific injury. It is hoped that the text will be of benefit to the surgeon who is faced with a challenging penetrating injury in the military or civilian arena. The goal of ATOM is to provide effective education to the surgeon and excellent care to the patient.

It is all worthwhile if even one injured patient's outcome is positively enhanced.

Lenworth M. Jacobs, MD, MPH, FACS

Acknowledgements

This book would not have been possible without continuous review and modification of the ATOM Course and course material by a panel of expert master trauma surgeons. These surgeons have also provided their wisdom in the "Tips from Master Surgeons" contributions. The educational rationale and rigor of the evaluation of the course was provided by Dr. Karyl Burns. Without her the course would not have been properly evaluated. Florence Leishman provided editorial assistance and technical excellence in collecting, collating, and producing the manuscripts. The editorial publishing expertise of Janelle Berthel, Alvaro Cucuta, Brooks Hart, Michael Cohen, and Michael Missett at Ciné-Med as well as the unfailing support of Kevin McGovern and Dr. Paul Zimnik were essential to publishing this book. Finally, to the numerous surgeons who have enthusiastically provided cognitive as well as technical, surgical expertise as ATOM instructors we are most appreciative.

Contributors

Jameel Ali, MD, FACS
Professor of Surgery
University of Toronto
St. Michael's Hospital
Toronto, Ontario, Canada

Juan Asensio, MD, FACS
Associate Professor of Surgery
University of Southern California
Los Angeles, CA

Kenneth Boffard, MB, BCh, FACS
Professor of Surgery
Johannesburg Hospital
Johannesburg, South Africa

Robert Brautigam, MD, FACS
Assistant Professor of Surgery
University of Connecticut
Hartford Hospital
Trauma Program
Director, Resident Education Section
Hartford, CT

Susan Briggs, MD, FACS
Associate Professor of Surgery
Harvard Medical School
Massachusetts General Hospital
Boston, MA

L.D. Britt, MD, FACS
Brickhouse Professor and Chairman
Department of Surgery
Eastern Virginia Medical School
Norfolk, VA

Bruce D. Browner, MD, FACS
Harry Gray Professor and Chairman
Department of Surgery
University of Connecticut
Director, Orthopedics
Hartford Hospital
Hartford, CT

Karyl Burns, RN, PhD
Assistant Professor
University of Connecticut
Hartford Hospital
Trauma Program
Director, Research Section
Hartford, CT

David Burris, MD, FACS, DMCC
COL, MC, USA
Associate Professor
Interim Chairman,
Norman M. Rich Dept of Surgery
Military Region Chief, ACS, COT
Uniformed Services University
Walter Reed Army Medical Center
Bethesda, MD

Patricia Byers, MD, FACS
Associate Clinical Professor
University of Miami
Miami, FL

David L. Ciraulo, DO, FACS
Associate Professor
University of Tennessee
Director, Surgical Research
Chattanooga, TN

Paul E. Collicott, MD, FACS
Director, Member Services
American College of Surgeons
Director of Trauma
Chicago, IL

Alasdair Conn, MD, FACS
Assistant Professor of surgery
Harvard University
Massachusetts General Hospital
Chief, Emergency Medicine
Boston, MA

Edward Cornwell, MD, FACS
Associate Professor of Surgery
Johns Hopkins University
Chief, Adult Trauma Service
Baltimore, MD

Vicente Cortes, MD, FACS
Assistant Professor of Surgery
University of Connecticut
Hartford Hospital
Associate Director
Trauma Program
Hartford, CT

Paul R.G. Cunningham, MD, FACS
Professor and Chairman
Department of Surgery
SUNY Upstate Medical University
Syracuse, NY

Brad Cushing, MD, FACS
Associate Professor of Surgery
Maine Medical Center
Director, Trauma Program
Portland, ME

Demetrios Demetriades, MD, FACS
Professor of Surgery
Director, Trauma/SICU
University of Southern California
Los Angeles County General Hospital
Los Angeles, CA

Blaine L. Enderson, MD, FACS
Professor of Surgery
University of Tennessee
Chief, Trauma Services
Knoxville, TN

William F. Fallon, MD, FACS
Associate Professor
Case Western Reserve University
Department of Surgery Metro Health
Director, Trauma and Critical Care
Medical Center
Cleveland, OH

David Feliciano, MD, FACS
Professor of Surgery
Emory University
Grady Memorial Hospital
Chief of Surgery
Atlanta, GA

Eric R. Frykberg, MD, FACS
Professor of Surgery
University of Florida Health Science Center
Chief, Division of General Surgery
Jacksonville, FL

Ronald I. Gross, MD, FACS
Assistant Professor of Surgery
University of Connecticut
Hartford Hospital
Associate Director, Trauma Program
Hartford, CT

Erwin F. Hirsch, MD, FACS
Professor of Surgery
Boston University
Director of Trauma
Boston Medical Center
Boston, MA

David B. Hoyt, MD, FACS
Monroe E. Trout Professor of Surgery
University of San Diego
Director, Trauma
San Diego, CA

Rao Ivatury, MD, FACS
Professor of Surgery
Virginia Commonwealth University
Chief, Trauma Service
Richmond, VA

Lenworth Jacobs, MD, MPH, FACS
Professor of Surgery
Professor and Chairman
Department of Traumatology
University of Connecticut
Hartford Hospital
Director, Trauma Program
Hartford, CT

Orlando Kirton, MD, FACS
Associate Professor of Surgery
University of Connecticut
Hartford Hospital
Director of Surgery
Hartford, CT

M. Margaret Knudson, MD, FACS
Professor of Surgery
University of California, San Francisco
San Francisco General Hospital
Director, San Francisco Injury Center
San Francisco, CA

Thomas Knuth, MD
Colonel, MC
Directorate of Combat & Doctrine
U.S. Army Trauma Training Center
Fort Sam Houston, TX

Charles E. Lucas, MD, FACS
Professor of Surgery
Wayne State University
Detroit, MI

Fred A. Luchette, MD, FACS
Professor of Surgery
Loyola University Medical Center
Director, Division of Trauma
and Critical Care
Maywood, IL

Stephen S. Luk, MD, FACS
Assistant Professor of Surgery
University of Connecticut
Hartford Hospital
Trauma Program
Hartford, CT

Robert C. Mackersie, MD, FACS
Professor of Surgery
University of California, San Francisco
San Francisco General Hospital
Director, Trauma
San Francisco, CA

Kenneth L. Mattox, MD, FACS
Professor and Vice Chairman
Department of Surgery
Baylor College of Medicine
Chief of Staff
Ben Taub General Hospital
Houston, TX

Kimball L. Maull, MD, FACS
Professor of Surgery
Carraway Methodist Medical Center
Department of Surgery
Director, Residents in Surgery
Birmingham, AL

Norman E. McSwain, Jr., MD, FACS
Professor of Surgery
Tulane University
Director of Surgery
Charity Hospital
New Orleans, LA

J. Wayne Meredith, MD, FACS
Professor and Chairman
Department of Surgery
Wake Forest University Medical Center
Winston-Salem, NC

Rocco Orlando, III, MD, FACS
Associate Professor
University of Connecticut
Hartford Hospital
Hartford, CT

H. Leon Pachter, MD, FACS
Professor of Surgery
New York University
Vice-Chairman, Department of Surgery
New York, NY

Marc D. Palter, MD, FACS
Assistant Professor
University of Connecticut
Hartford Hospital
Director, Neurosurgical ICU
Hartford, CT

George A. Perdrizet, MD, PhD, FACS
Associate Professor of Surgery
University of Connecticut
Hartford Hospital
Director, Hyperbaric and Wound Center
Hartford, CT

Peter Rhee, MD, FACS
Assistant Professor of Surgery
Uniformed Service
University of Health Sciences
Los Angeles, CA

Michael Rhodes, MD, FACS
Professor and Chairman
Department of Surgery
Christiana Care Health System
Wilmington, DE

Aurelio Rodriguez, MD, FACS
Professor of Surgery
Drexel University School of Medicine
Allegheny Medical Center
Pittsburgh, PA

Michael F. Rotondo, MD, FACS
Professor and Vice Chairman
East Carolina University
Department of Surgery
Greenville, NC

Grace Rozycki, MD, FACS
Professor of Surgery
Emory University
Chief, Division of Trauma
and Surgical Critical Care
Atlanta, GA

Thomas M. Scalea, MD, FACS
Professor of Surgery
University of Maryland School of Medicine
R. Adams Cowley Shock Trauma Center
Director of Surgery
Baltimore, MD

C. William Schwab, MD, FACS
Professor of Surgery
Chief of Trauma and Surgical Critical Care
University of Pennsylvania Health Systems
Philadelphia, PA

Glen Tinkoff, MD, FACS
Assistant Professor of Surgery
Christianacare Health Services
Department of Surgery
Newark, DE

Donald D. Trunkey, MD, FACS
Professor of Surgery
Oregon Health Sciences University
Portland, OR

John P. Welch, MD, FACS
Professor of Surgery
University of Connecticut
Hartford Hospital
Department of Surgery
Hartford, CT

Dietmar H. Wittmann, MD, FACS
Professor of Surgery
The Medical College of Wisconsin

Introduction to the Advanced Trauma Operative Management (ATOM) Course

The expectations that any patient has when injured include having a highly skilled surgeon. This expectation is true in urban, rural, wilderness, and military environments, where trauma can range from simple injuries resulting from surface lacerations to complex low and high velocity injuries that affect one or more body systems.

A major expectation of any surgeon is being adequately trained and competent to manage injuries that they may be called to provide emergency care for at any time during their surgical practice. Resident training and continuing education for practicing surgeons have evolved substantially over the last two decades.

In the past, the policy for managing any penetrating injury to the neck and abdomen involved operative exploration of the area. This was thought to be more effective and safe, missing fewer injuries than not exploring the anatomic region that was injured. These policies resulted in a high frequency of abdominal and neck explorations for all surgical trainees. At the completion of a surgical residency, particularly in urban inner-city teaching hospitals, most residents had successfully completed hundreds of explorations and had repaired numerous injured organs, structures, and vessels. Young surgeons in practice were comfortable with these skills in the operating room and were confident that they could manage most injuries. In addition, the Vietnam War, which resulted in hundreds of thousands of casualties, provided vast experience for hundreds of surgeons.

There have been substantial changes in the evaluation and management of injured patients in the last two decades. Policies that have been implemented have resulted in less operative exposure for surgeons. These policies have degraded the confidence and competence of surgeons in their ability to respond to and operate upon penetrating injuries to the neck, chest, and abdomen. In addition, modern diagnostic modalities such as CT scan, angiography enhanced CT, and MRI angiography, along with selective angioembolization, have dramatically improved the diagnosis and nonoperative management of injuries in the chest, abdomen, and pelvis.

The decrease in resident work hours has also had a negative impact on the exposure of residents to trauma and operative repair of penetrating injuries. Penetrating trauma frequently occurs at night and on weekends. Therefore, decreased continuous work periods have resulted in less exposure of surgical residents to trauma.

A decrease in the incidence of penetrating trauma and an increase in more accurate diagnostic investigations and nonoperative management philosophies have mandated a change in the method of educating surgeons on operative management techniques in penetrating trauma. The ATOM course has been designed to provide operative education for the surgeon using a CD-ROM to demonstrate operative management procedures. Surgeons become familiar with the types of injuries that they would be expected to manage in the operating room.

Before participating in the course, surgeons are given a pre-test to determine their knowledge and familiarity with the management of penetrating injuries to solid organs, hollow viscera, and vascular structures in the chest and abdomen. The surgeon's self-confidence in identifying, exposing, and repairing penetrating injuries to multiple structures in the chest and abdomen is also measured using a pre-test, which must be completed prior to the course.

The one day ATOM course is comprised of two sections. The first is a didactic lecture series covering the anatomy, principles of evaluation, and details of operative management of injuries in the chest and abdomen. The second part of the course takes place in an operating suite, where large 50 kg swine are used for the operating experience. The animals are anesthetized, and the operating room is prepared in exactly the same manner that it would be for a human patient. This recreates the same environment, including visual and auditory cues, for the surgeon. The instruments are the same as those used for human operations.

A clinical situation taken from an actual penetrating trauma event is presented to the surgeon. The surgeon is asked to leave the room while the instructor creates the injuries to specific organs and structures. The surgeon is then invited to the operating table, where all of the injuries must be identified. An appropriate operative management plan must be presented to the instructors, and then the injuries must be successfully repaired.

The instruments, stapling devices, sutures, and back table are the same as the ones used in an actual operating environment. The surgeon can request and use the instruments, equipment, and sutures that they feel are appropriate to safely and effectively perform the operative procedure of choice. The instructors are familiar with numerous safe and effective ways to successfully complete repairs of the injuries that are presented to the student surgeons.

At the end of the day, a post-test is used to evaluate the cognitive ability of the surgeon, and a test measuring self-confidence is also administered.

The ATOM course is an intense operative surgical experience that focuses on operative management of penetrating injuries. Its objectives are to educate surgeons on the surgical management of penetrating injuries, improve their self-confidence in managing these injuries, and promote their technical competence in the surgical repair of penetrating injuries. Experienced trauma surgical instructors teach the course, and the intended audience includes senior surgical residents, trauma fellows, military surgeons, and fully trained general surgeons who are not frequently called on to treat penetrating injuries. The ATOM course is a tightly structured educational experience with a rigorous evaluative component. It is designed to be completely reproducible.

The ATOM course is an effective method of increasing surgical competence and confidence in the operative management of penetrating injuries to the chest and abdomen.

Table of Contents

Preface iii
Acknowlegements iv
Contributors v
Introduction ix

Chapter One
Trauma Laparotomy 1
Tips From the Masters 26

Chapter Two
Spleen 69
Tips From the Masters 94

Chapter Three
Liver 107
Tips From the Masters 135

Chapter Four
Pancreas and Duodenum 157
Tips From the Masters 186

Chapter Five
Genitourinary 226
Tips From the Masters 249

Chapter Six
Cardiac 275
Tips From the Masters 300

Chapter Seven
Evaluation 363

Index 381

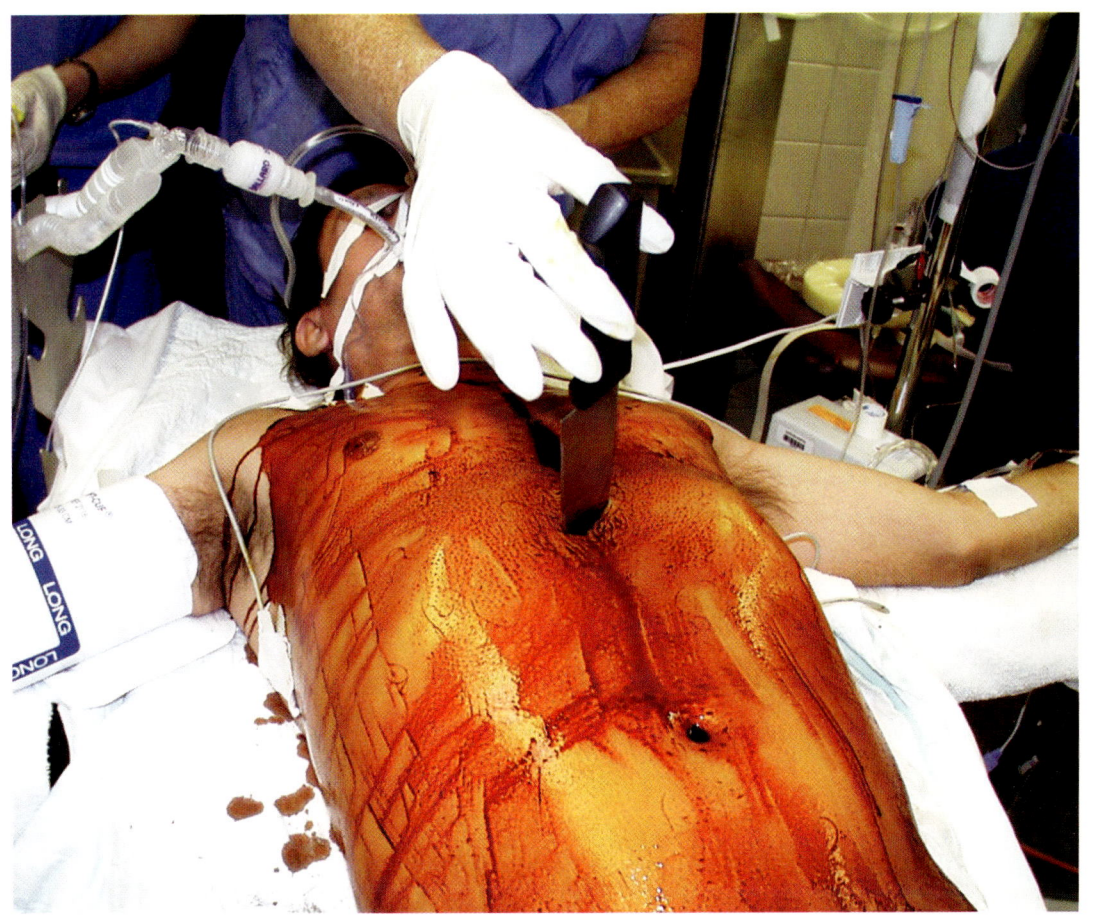

Trauma Laparotomy

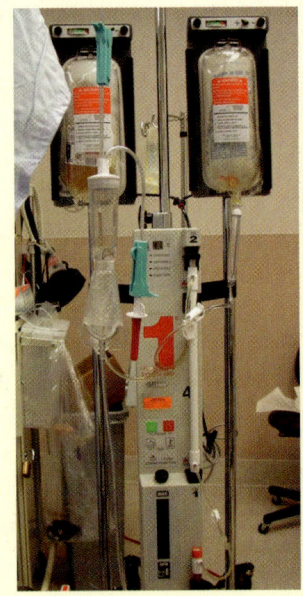
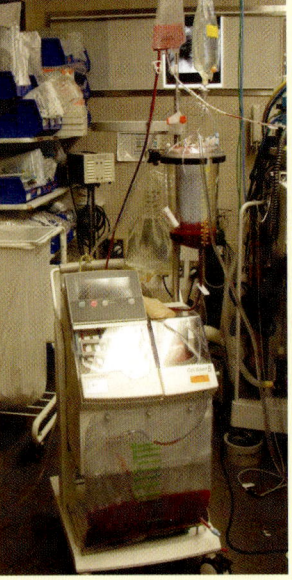

Operating Room

- Warm room

- Level One transfuser

- Autotransfuser

- Prep from neck to mid-thigh and to table laterally

Operating Room

The physical aspects of the operating room environment are a priority in the management of a severely injured hypovolemic patient. The room should be large enough to support multiple operating teams and all of the attendant equipment necessary for a major trauma laparotomy. In addition, the room temperature should be set to the upper 70°F range or the lower 80°F range. A warm room is essential to avoid hypothermia. Patients who are in shock and have been resuscitated with a combination of crystalloid and colloid, which is below body temperature, and have had their clothes removed in order to perform a complete inspection are at risk for hypothermia. The room temperature to maintain an optimal normothermic temperature for the patient is likely to be uncomfortable for the surgeons and support teams.

A rapid transfusion device is an essential piece of equipment. In addition to delivering large volumes of fluid, it can also warm the fluid up to body temperature. Before the incision, the patient should be given blankets or warming devices to prevent further hypothermia. It is essential to be able to collect blood from the peritoneal or pleural cavities. This blood is the optimal resuscitating fluid because it is warm and already typed and cross-matched and has no infectious diseases. It also has an optimal 2, 3 diphosphoglycerate (2, 3 DPG) level. The blood should be washed and centrifuged before autotransfusing the packed red blood cells back to the patient.

The shed blood will be rapidly lost to the laparotomy pads and spilled outside of the abdominal cavity upon opening a tense hemoperitoneum. Therefore, it is critical to have the appropriate equipment and suction devices in place prior to the first incision. The suction devices must be ready and available at the beginning of the exploratory laparotomy.

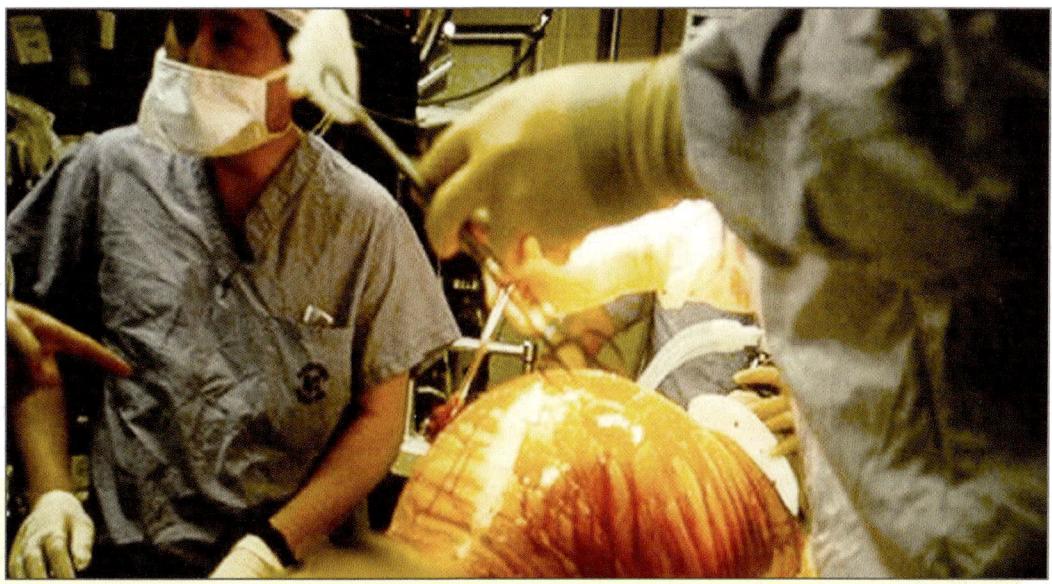

Operating Room

- Incision from xyphoid to symphysis pubis

- Release of tamponade

- Pack all four quadrants

- Allows quick control of hemorrhage, removal of accumulated blood, and anesthesia catch-up time

Preparation of the abdomen, which must be widely prepared and draped, includes the suprasternal notch and continues inferiorly to the mid-thigh. Extensive preparation allows access to the groin if the patient needs further resuscitating with large-bore intravenous lines. It also gives access to the saphenous vein if an autologous vascular conduit is needed. The prep extends down to the operating table on both sides laterally. This allows access to the chest cavities for the placement of a thoracotomy tube or for a thoracotomy. A wide lateral prep on the abdomen allows for the placement of drains or a colostomy.

The large incision provides excellent exposure of the solid organs in the superior abdomen, the entire retroperitoneum, and the pelvis. It also allows the surgeon to have a wide field for control of major hemorrhage. With an adequate number of surgical assistants, the use of handheld abdominal retractors can selectively enhance visualization of organs in the upper quadrants. Self-retaining, multiple–bladed, retractor systems can also be used to enhance exposure. These systems have the advantage of minimizing the need for assistants who only provide handheld exposure.

Once life-threatening hemorrhage has been controlled, the anesthesiologist rapidly resuscitates the patient. At this point, it is important to assess the severity of the patient's injuries, determine if the appropriate personnel are available, and put out a call for surgical assistance, as well as additional anesthesia assistance. The blood bank should be notified of the likelihood of significant blood loss requiring initiation of the massive transfusion protocol. This is the time to assess the situation and assemble the appropriate team, equipment, and supplies in preparation for a major operative intervention.

The trauma laparotomy consists of four essential parts. First, major hemorrhage is controlled. Second, all of the injuries are identified. Third, any contamination from the small or large bowel or the biliary tree is controlled. Finally, the injuries are repaired.

It may not be possible to definitively repair all of the injuries because of the unstable nature of the patient. In these cases, damage control serves to correct life-threatening injuries before moving to the intensive care unit to continue resuscitation. The goals are to return the patient

Four Essential Parts To Trauma Laparotomy

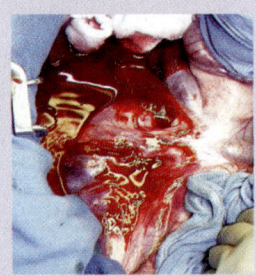

1. Control of bleeding

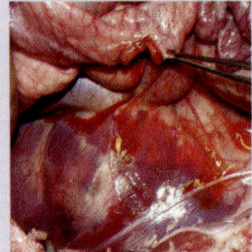

2. Identification of injury

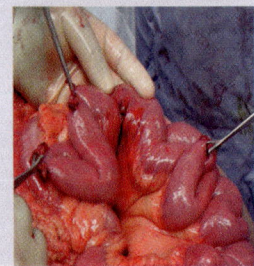

3. Control of contamination

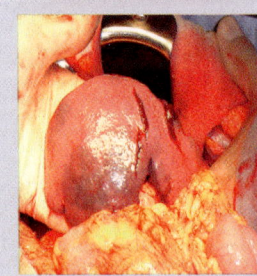

4. Reconstruction (if possible)

Control Hemorrhage

- Central or peripheral vascular control

- Sites of major hemorrhage identified and immediately addressed

- Another chance for anesthesia to catch up

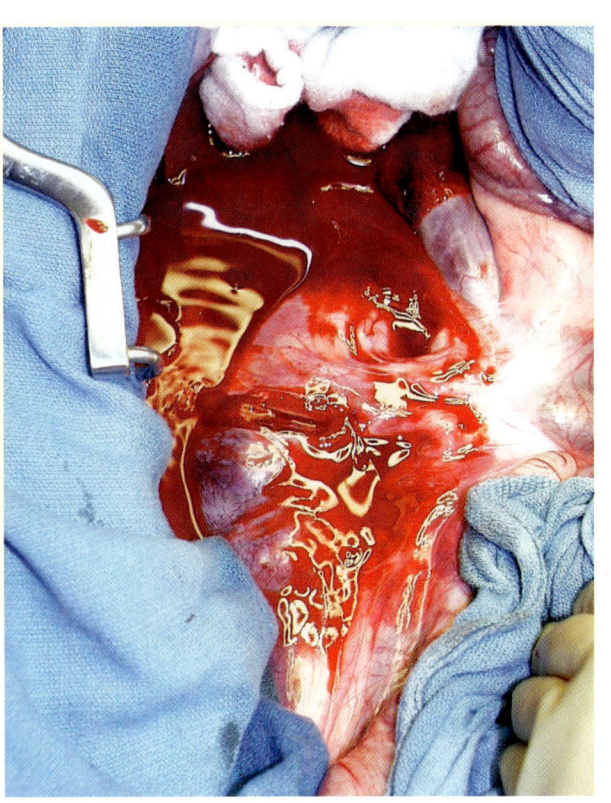

to a stable metabolic state and to correct hypothermia, hypovolemia, acidosis, and coagulopathy. Once these goals have been achieved, the patient is moved back to the operating room for definitive management of any remaining injuries.

Control Hemorrhage

The control of massive exsanguinating hemorrhage is essential. Audible hemorrhage usually results from a large venous laceration on an area such as the inferior vena cava (IVC). A severe vena cava laceration is characterized by a large amount of dark blood welling up from the peritoneum. This must be controlled immediately.

Pulsatile hemorrhage must also be controlled immediately. This control can be achieved either directly on the vessel itself or by gaining proximal vascular control. For example, the hilum of the kidney or spleen can be controlled to stop all arterial inflow to the organ. Once hemorrhage is controlled, more definitive distal vascular control can be achieved, allowing preservation of the organ.

When major hemorrhage is under control, it is again time to reassess the general condition of the patient, assemble appropriate additional personnel, and make sure that the blood and blood products are being transported from the blood bank to the operating room for immediate use. This is now the time to begin autotransfusion of the shed blood collected from the abdominal and pleural cavities. It is essential to warm any transfused fluid to normothermic levels before delivery.

Techniques in Packing

The use of abdominal packs to tamponade bleeding and aid in the identification of ongoing bleeding is an important concept. The technique used is designed to protect the solid organs from iatrogenic injury, as well as allow for the placement of the packs in the most dependent parts of the abdomen.

The abdominal wall is retracted away from the spleen, and a hand is placed over the spleen for protection. Blood and clots are removed from the posterior aspect of the abdomen, and a dry pack is carefully introduced into the deepest recess of the left upper quadrant. More packs are then placed on top of the spleen.

The falciform ligament is taken down sharply, providing excellent exposure of the liver. Blood and clots are then removed from the perihepatic areas. The abdominal wall is retracted superiorly, and the liver is retracted inferiorly. Packs are introduced above the liver, and additional packs are placed below the liver. Manual compression of the organ between the packs ensures a tamponading effect.

Techniques In Packing

- Retraction of anterior abdominal wall
- Hand over organ to protect it
- Take down falciform ligament
- Pack above and below liver and spleen

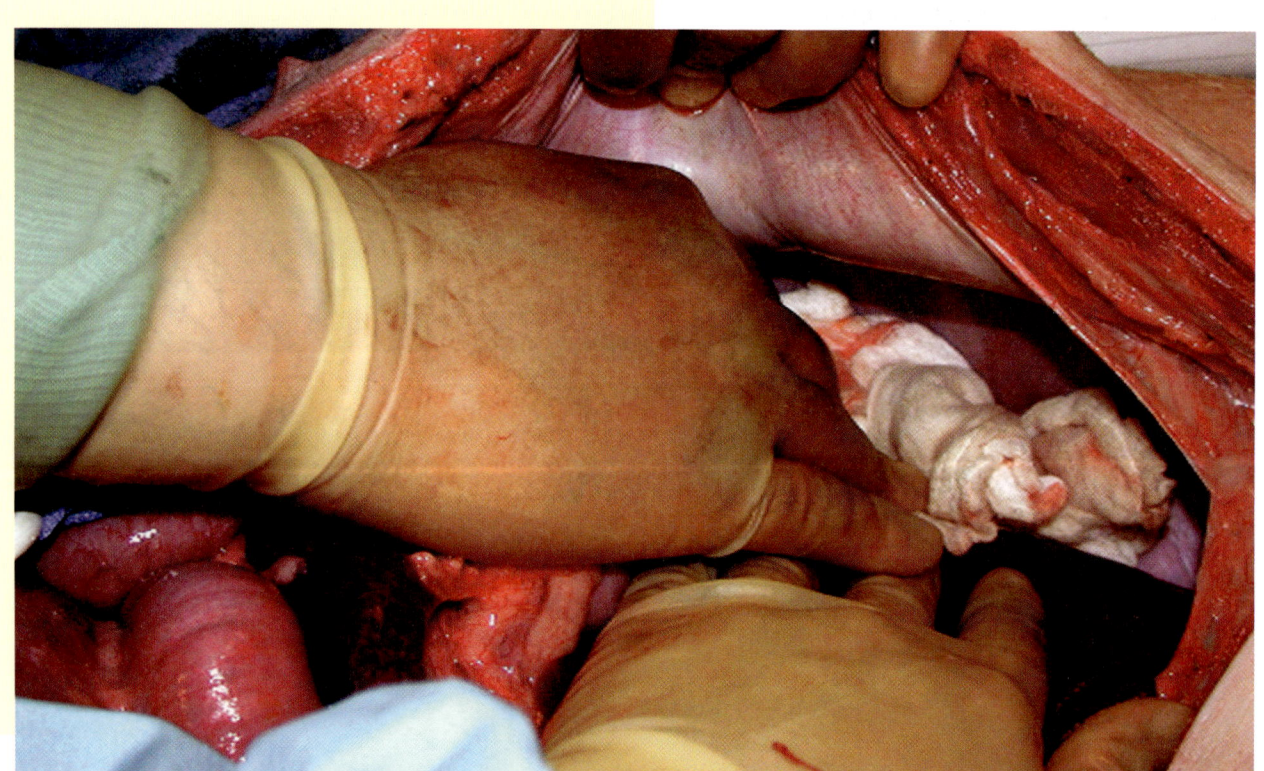

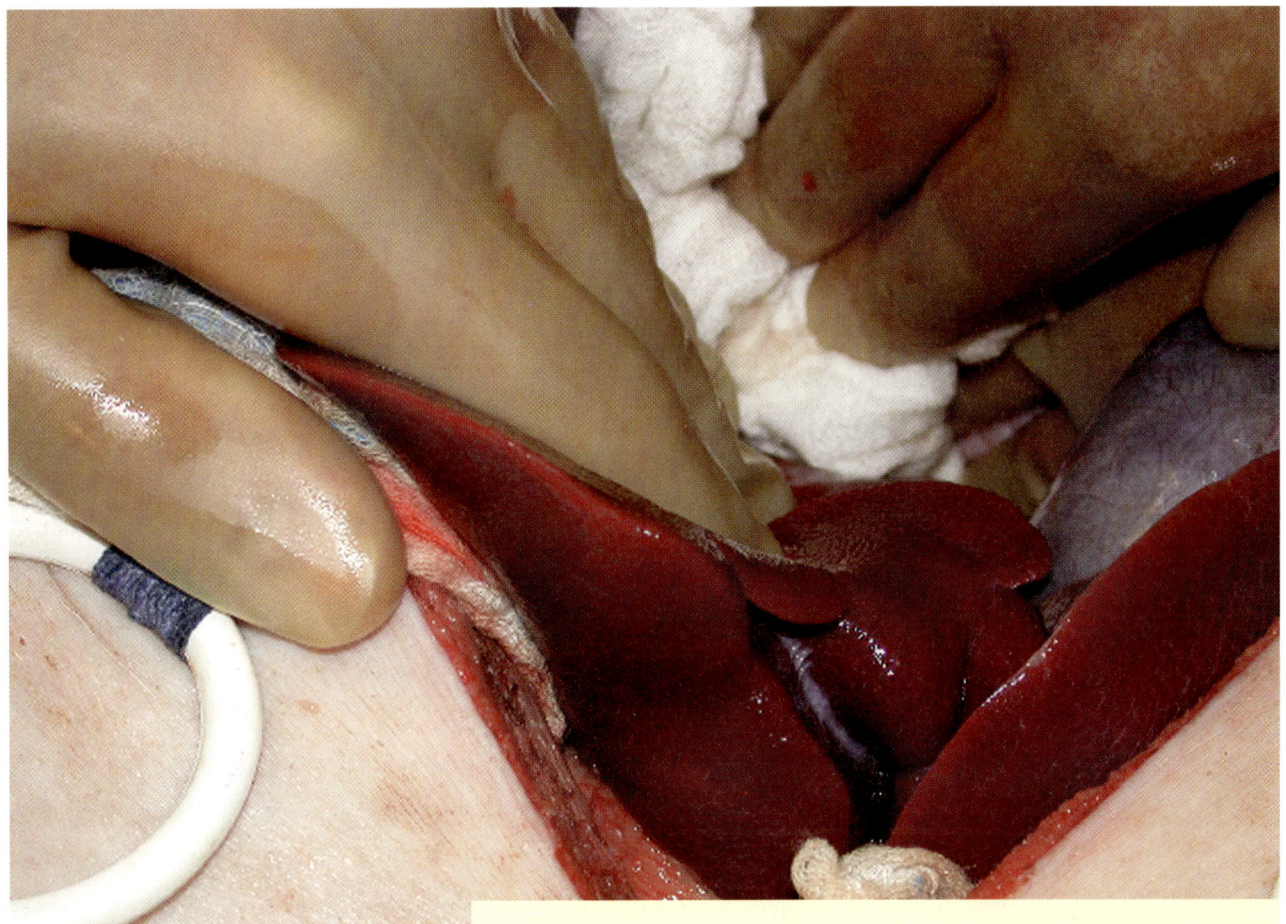

Sweeping the small bowel medially and superiorly allows adequate evaluation of the base of the mesentery and the retroperitoneum. The right colon is retracted medially, and packs are placed in the lateral ascending colic recess of the abdomen. The same

Techniques In Packing

- Sweep small bowel and colon medially to pack paracolic gutters and base of mesentery

- Sweep bowel cephalad to pack pelvis

- Radiopaque pads only with accurate count

procedure is repeated with the descending colon. The sigmoid is drawn out of the pelvis. Blood and clots are removed from the pelvis and packs are placed inside. This process identifies areas of the abdomen without injury and without hematoma. It allows the surgeon to focus on the areas of the abdomen containing injuries.

Only large radiologically marked abdominal packs are used. It is helpful to have packs with radiopaque rings, which are easy to identify digitally and radiographically.

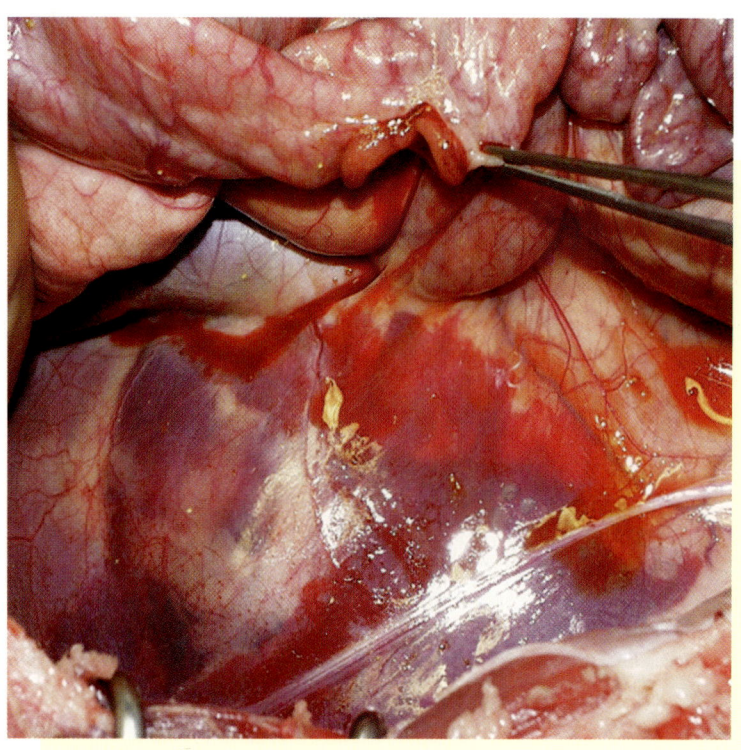

Identify Injury

- Remove packs one quadrant at a time

- Start remote to area of suspected injury

- Inspect for: active bleeding, bowel injury, other non-life threatening injury, i.e. diaphragm, bladder

Identify Injury

A wound in the posterior right upper quadrant can cause injuries in the solid organs and viscera. Free bile in the abdomen or bile staining in the periduodenal and pancreatic tissues raises the possibility of an injury to the duodenum or biliary tree. These organs should be inspected and any injury identified. A large lateral retroperitoneal hematoma indicates an injury to the kidney or renal hilar vessels. The vena cava should also be inspected and a judgment made as to whether the hematoma is arising from the vena cava, the renal pedicle, or the kidney itself.

The laparotomy packs should be removed from one quadrant at a time, starting in the non-injured area and ending in the most seriously injured area. It is critical to determine whether the bleeding has stopped or if there is active ongoing bleeding.

Fresh blood or clots on the laparotomy packs indicate continuing hemorrhage. The active hemorrhage must be controlled and any injury to the small or large bowel identified. Contamination must be controlled immediately. The amount and type of contaminant determines the likelihood of developing sepsis in the future.

The final component of the laparotomy involves identification of other non life-threatening injuries, specifically to the diaphragm and/or the bladder.

Control Contamination

Control of contamination is an important priority. Essential observations to be made include the location of the injury, the number of injuries, the size of the rent, and the location on the mesenteric or antimesenteric border of the bowel. Obvious leakage must be controlled. The entire small bowel, from the ligament of Treitz to the ileocecal valve, and the ascending, transverse, descending, and sigmoid colon need to be inspected. A complete evaluation of the antimesenteric and mesenteric border of the bowel, as well as the mesentery, is essential. Any enterotomy in the bowel can be rapidly controlled with Babcock clamps, skin staples, or sutures. Although this stops ongoing contamination of the operative field, it is not a definitive closure.

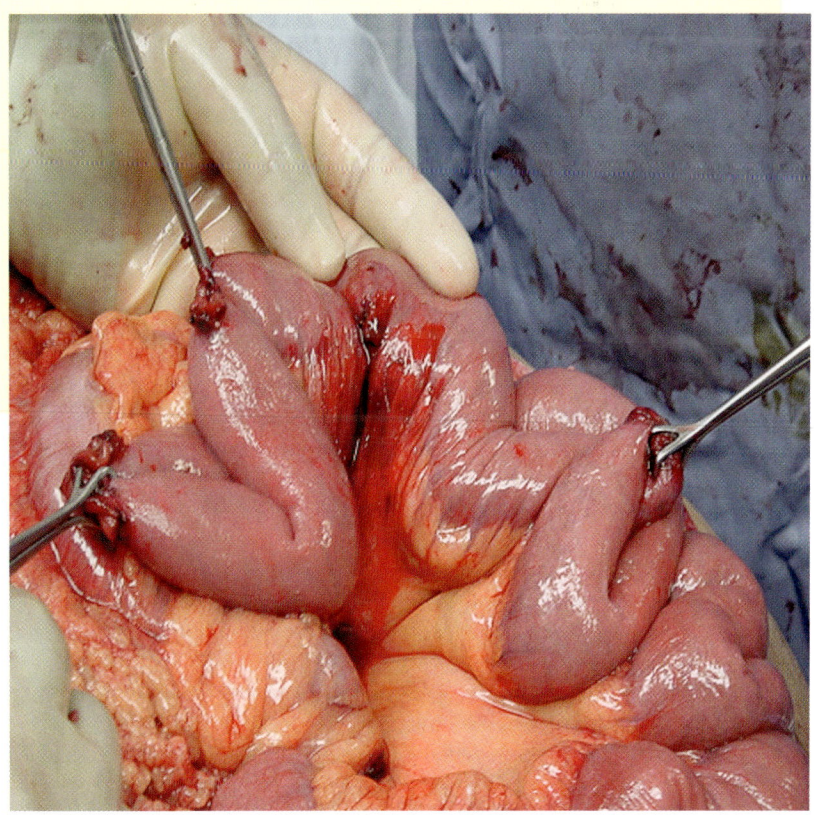

Control Contamination

- Inspect all bowel completely
- Clamps
- Skin staples
- Suture closure
- Resection

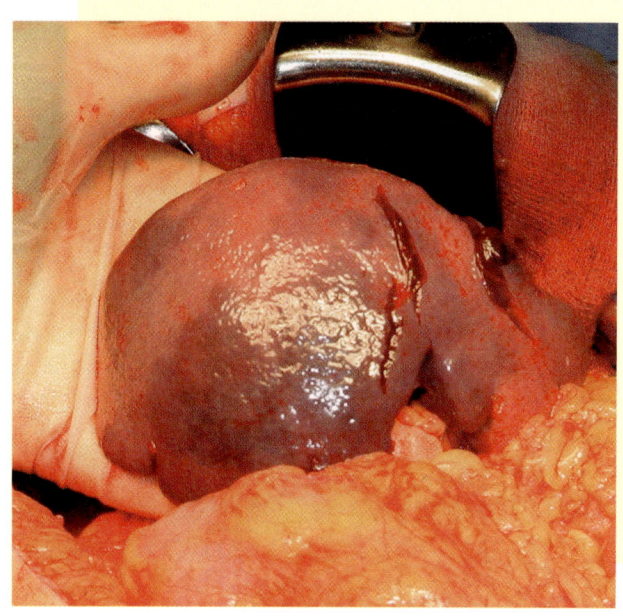

Reconstruction

- Repair/control site(s) of primary injury

- Full mobilization or exposure imperative

- Reassessment of patient condition

- Address other areas of potential injury

Reconstruction

Another major component of the exploratory laparotomy is reconstruction of injured organs and viscera. Definitive repair of significantly damaged organs should fit within the context of the overall patient. Evaluating the injured organ helps to determine whether repairing the injury or removing the organ is a better option. If the organ can be repaired, the next important consideration is whether the organ can be repaired in the presenting patient.

It is essential to evaluate the overall metabolic status of the patient, the amount of additional surgery needed, the extent of acidosis and coagulopathy, and injury to other systems and the impact of these injuries on the patient's overall well-being. A patient with a severe head injury and a splenic injury amenable to splenorrhaphy may not benefit from the extra time spent performing a complex repair. A splenectomy may be more beneficial.

In order to determine if the injured organ can be repaired, the organ must be fully mobilized to evaluate the entire extent of the injury. An injured spleen should be fully mobilized so that the entire organ is brought up to the anterior abdomen. This maneuver allows the convex and concave surfaces of the spleen to be fully inspected to determine the feasibility of a repair.

Zone I: mandatory exploration

Zone II: explore in all penetrating injury and blunt injury with expanding or pulsatile hematoma

Zone III: explore in penetrating injury only

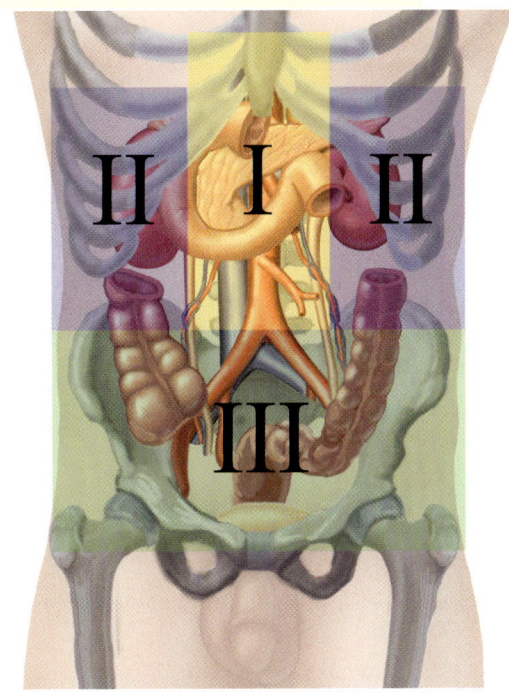

Retroperitoneal Hematoma

The retroperitoneum consists of three zones. Zone I includes the centromedian superior aspect of the retroperitoneum. The centromedian zone extends from the diaphragm to just distal to the bifurcation of the aorta and the IVC. Numerous important vascular structures reside within this zone. They include the celiac trunk, the superior mesenteric artery, the inferior mesenteric artery, the renal pedicle vessels, the aorta, and the vena cava. The pancreas and the second, third, and fourth portions of the duodenum also reside in this area. Any injury in this area requires a mandatory exploration to identify and manage the injury.

Zone II of the retroperitoneum includes the lateral aspects of the superior abdomen. The kidney, adrenal glands, the ureter, and the hilum of the vascular pedicle to the kidney reside in this area. All penetrating injuries in Zone II require an exploration. However, in blunt injury, the area needs to be explored if the hematoma is expanding or pulsating or if there is extravasation of urine. If the hematoma is not expanding or pulsating or if there is no obvious extravasation of urine, the zone needs to be reassessed at the end of the abdominal exploration to see if the injury is stable or if it is getting worse. If the injury is stable, it is prudent to not explore the kidney.

Zone III is the pelvic retroperitoneum. This area is explored only in a penetrating injury such as a transpelvic gunshot wound. It is critical to determine if the vasculature, the ureters, or the intrapelvic colon and rectum have been injured. Exploration of this area is not recommended in blunt trauma. Instead, the appropriate diagnostic maneuver is to control venous pelvic hemorrhage with an external compression device. In addition, an arteriogram can evaluate arterial injury before selectively embolizing the bleeding vessel.

Aortic Control

- Suprarenal through gastrohepatic ligament

- Intrathoracic

- Direct

- Occlusion with:
  Vascular clamp
  Richardson retractor
  Aortic occluder

Although injuries to the aorta can be approached through the left chest, the preferred approach is to gain control of the aorta through the superior abdomen at the hiatus of the diaphragm. The absence of injury in the left chest makes it easy to identify the aorta and gain control of it in the chest with a left thoracotomy. This allows for proximal control of an abdominal aortic injury. However, a significant amount of time is required to make a thoracotomy incision and gain control of the aorta in a situation where the patient is hemorrhaging from an injury to the abdominal aorta.

When approaching injuries through the superior aspect of the abdomen, manual digital occlusion can directly control the aorta, which can then be bluntly dissected. Care should be taken to avoid an injury to the vena cava. Proximal control is achieved by passing a vascular loop around the aorta. Various occluding devices can be applied directly to tamponade the aorta against the vertebral column. Great care should be taken to avoid directly injuring the aorta with the occluding device. In the older population, there is a risk that the occluding device may break off an atherosclerotic plaque and cause it to embolize distally.

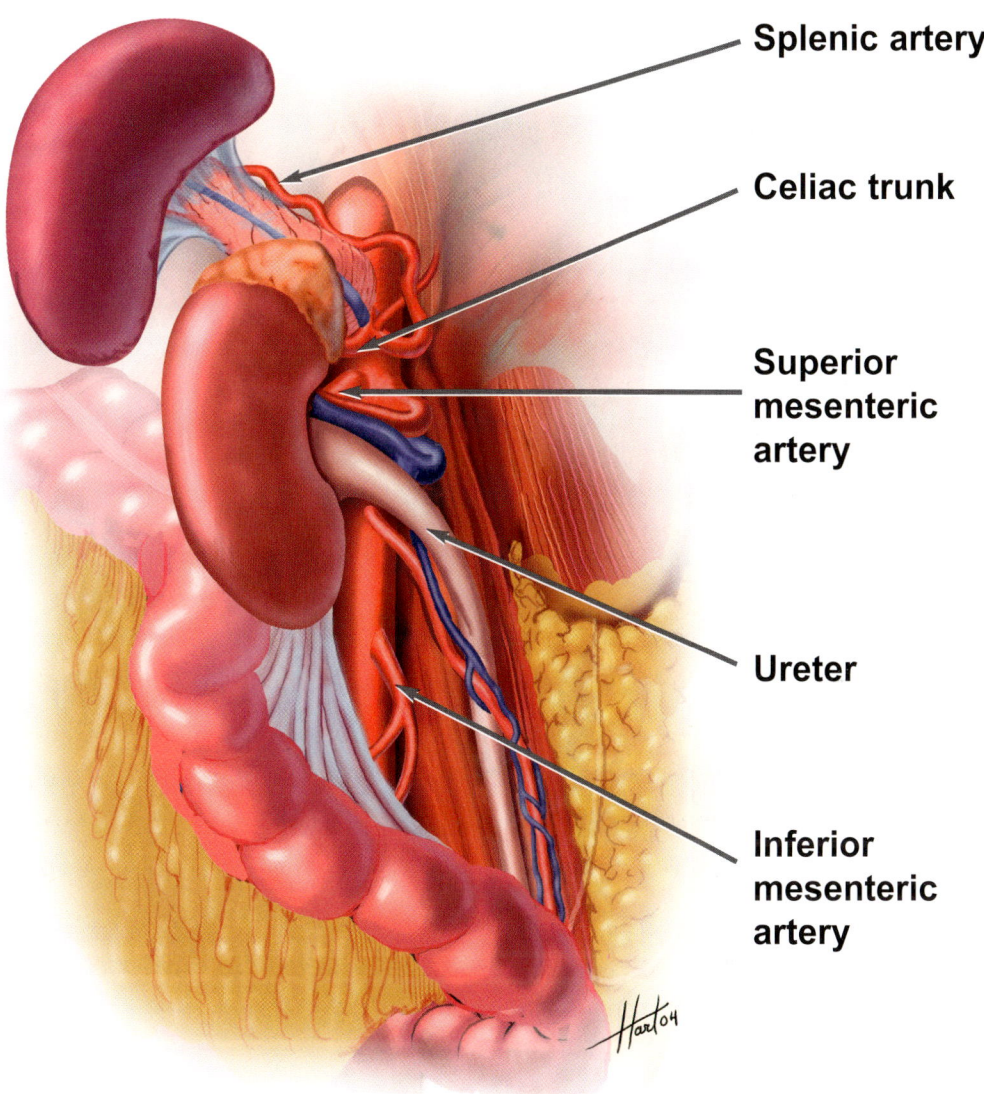

Aortic Exposure: Mattox Maneuver

A number of surgical maneuvers allow identification and control of the proximal abdominal aorta. The left medial rotation, or Mattox maneuver, mobilizes the splenic flexure of the colon inferiorly and medially and then allows mobilization of the kidney, spleen, and pancreas superiorly and medially. This maneuver completely exposes the lateral aspect of the aorta and gives direct access to the celiac trunk, the superior mesenteric artery, and the inferior mesenteric artery. It is possible to place vascular tape or a vascular clamp at the base of the celiac artery or the superior mesenteric artery, where they take off from the aorta. This allows for proximal control of exsanguinating hemorrhage from these vessels.

Aortic Exposure: Modified Mattox Maneuver

The modified left medial rotation is performed by allowing the kidney to remain in Gerota's fascia and selecting a dissection plane that includes the spleen and the pancreas. These organs are then rotated medially and superiorly. This approach helps gain excellent exposure to the celiac trunk and the superior mesenteric artery. The exposure also gives ready access to the left renal pedicle vessels.

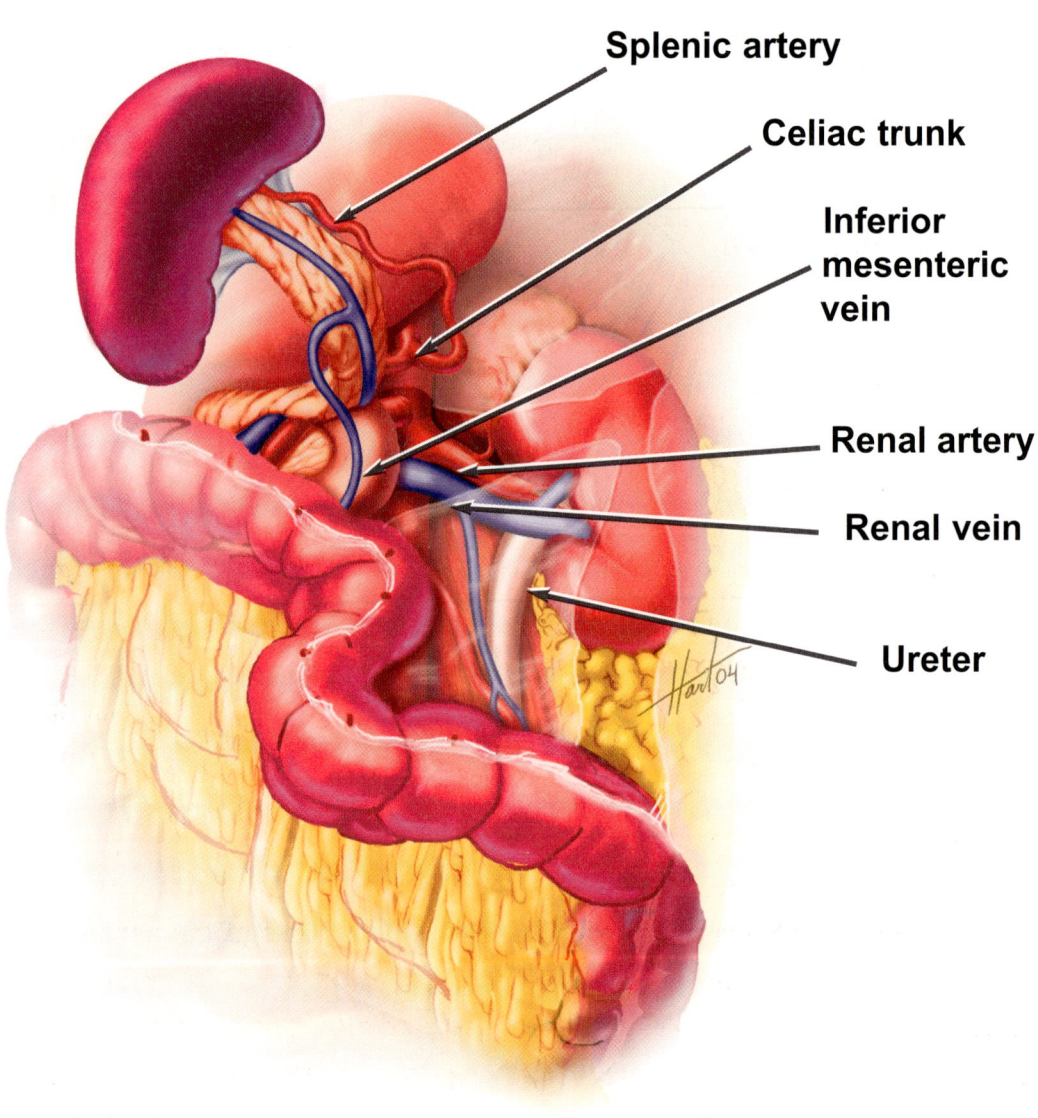

IVC Exposure

- Cattel Braasch maneuver or right side medial visceral rotation

- Kocher maneuver

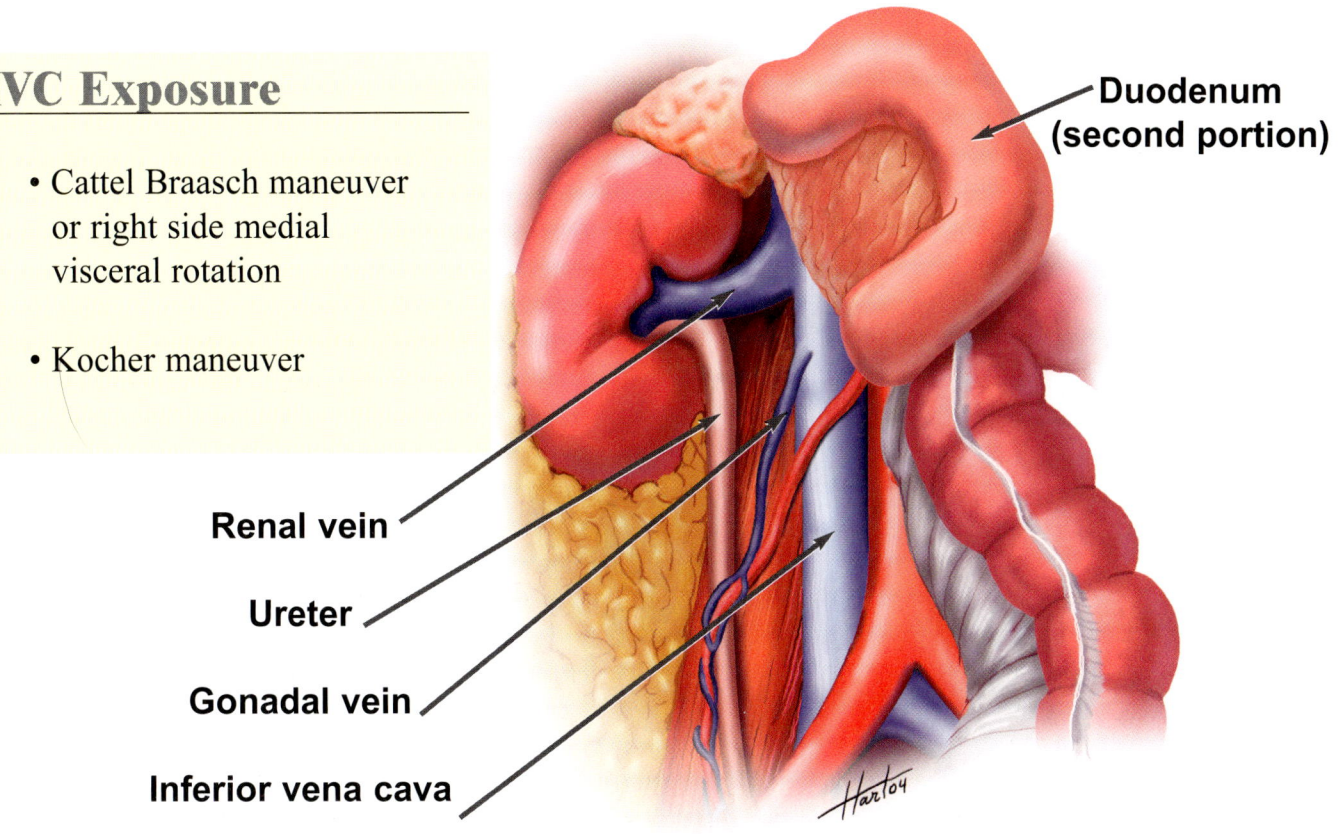

IVC Exposure

Exposure of the retroperitoneum on the right side of the abdomen can be gained by a right medial rotation maneuver, or the Cattel Braasch maneuver. This includes dissecting the cecum, the ascending colon, and the hepatic flexure at the white line of Toldt and reflecting the colon and the base of the mesentery medially and superiorly. The ascending colon and its mesentery are then placed in the left upper quadrant. This provides excellent exposure of the bifurcation of the aorta and the vena cava, the presacral artery, and the gonadal vessels. It also allows for excellent exposure of the ureter and the kidney.

Performing an extended Kocher maneuver can help gain access to and exposure of the vena cava, the posterior aspect of the head of the pancreas, and the duodenum. The duodenum and the head of the pancreas are bluntly dissected away from the vena cava and rotated medially. The dissection must be taken to the medial aspect of the IVC. The posterior aspect of the pancreas is inspected for evidence of bile, which is characteristic of an injury to the biliary tree or duodenum. This also provides excellent exposure to the right kidney and the renal pedicle vessels.

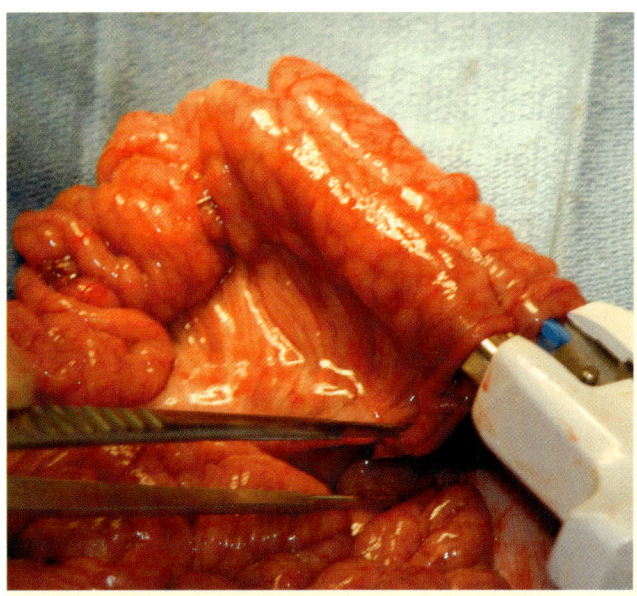

Stable Patient

- Re-exploration of bowel and areas of mesenteric hematoma
- Definitive bowel repair
- Finally repair of non-life threatening injuries, i.e. diaphragm, bladder

Colonic Injury

- Primary repair or anastomosis
- Colostomy
- Risk factors for complications:
    Hemodynamic instability
    Severe fecal contamination
    Transfusions
    Single agent antibiotic prophylaxis
    Delay in operation

Stable Patient

It is important to re-explore the bowel and look specifically at areas of mesenteric hematoma in the patient who is hemodynamically stable at the end of the exploratory laparotomy. Areas to inspect and evaluate include the entire superior abdomen, both diaphragms, and the inferior abdomen, as well as the pelvis to specifically exclude an injury to the bladder.

Colonic Injury

The management of colonic injuries has evolved over the past 30 years. Colonic management originally involved performing a diverting colostomy in any injury to the colon with fecal spillage. The diversion was classically carried out with a defunctionalizing diverting colostomy. Today, selective colostomy is performed, and a primary repair of injuries to the colon is often possible.

In order to safely manage the multiply injured patient, it is essential to fully evaluate the patient and the colonic injury. A primary repair of the colon may be considered for the hemodynamically stable patient who has a colonic injury with minimal fecal spillage or a small injury involving the antimesenteric border of the colon. A significant number of units of blood should not have been required for the resuscitation.

A diverting colostomy is a good, safe option for the patient who has multiple injuries; has required a number of units of blood for resuscitation; has acidosis, hypothermia, and coagulopathy; and has a wound of more than 50% of the lumen of the colon, a significant volume of fecal spillage, or a high-velocity gunshot wound.

Antibiotic therapy in penetrating injuries to the abdomen is an important issue. If colonic injury is a possibility, antibiotics covering gram-positive and gram-negative organisms and anaerobes for bacteroides need to be administered in the periresuscitative phase. Exploratory laparotomy can confirm or exclude an injury to the colon. There is no further need for antibiotics if there is no colonic injury. If there is injury, the degree of spillage will determine the duration and intensity of antibiotic coverage. At a minimum, perioperative antibiotic coverage should be included in the treatment regimen. A longer course of antibiotics is recommended when there is significant peritoneum soilage.

Unstable Patient

The unstable patient is described as the severely injured patient who has been hemodynamically unstable, acidotic, hypothermic, and coagulopathic. Frequently, this patient has had a significant volume of hemorrhage and has needed multiple blood transfusions to become euvolemic. A general ooze from injured organs and the incision provides clinical evidence of coagulopathy. Although the patient may currently have a normal blood pressure, the anesthesia team has had to aggressively transfuse crystalloid and colloid to maintain a normal blood pressure.

The unstable patient is not a candidate for definitive reconstruction. It is best to shorten the duration of the operative procedure and move to the intensive care unit for continued metabolic resuscitation. The unstable patient is a candidate for damage control procedures.

Unstable Patient

- Hemodynamic lability
- Acidotic
- Hypothermic
- Coagulopathic
- Not a candidate for reconstruction
- Damage control instead

Damage Control

- Allows for further stabilization in the ICU setting with the intent of returning to the operating room for more definitive management

- Goal to return as soon as patient is stabilized hemodynamically as well as metabolically

Damage Control

Damage control is defined as a procedure that allows for further stabilization in the intensive care unit with the intent of returning to the operating room for definitive management when the patient becomes metabolically stable. The patient should be normalotic, normothermic, not coagulopathic, and have no base deficit prior to returning to the operating room for a definitive surgical repair. This resuscitative process may take a number of hours.

When a stable state has been attained, it is important to make sure that the operating team is also physically able to return to the operating room and carry out the definitive procedures. It may be more effective to delay the return to the operating room for a number of hours until the operating room team, the blood bank, and the anesthesia team are fully ready to proceed with a major operative procedure.

Deciding on an optimal time to return to the operating room involves making some judgment calls. The time period may be only 2 to 6 hours, although it may be necessary to delay the return to the operating room for as long as 24 to 48 hours in order to attain a stable physiologic state.

Damage Control Techniques

For solid organ injury or nonsurgical bleeding:

- Packing

- Fibrin glue

- Avitene

- Thrombin

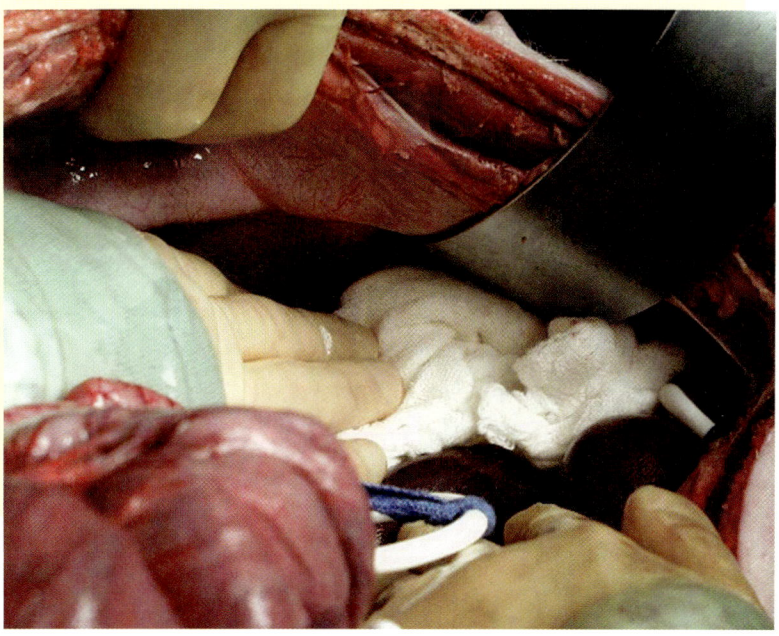

Damage Control Techniques

Damage control procedures in solid organ injuries involve the use of various local hemostatic agents. Any active bleeding from the surface of the solid organs such as the liver must be controlled with a ligature or surgical clip. Surface oozing should be tamponaded using digital compression.

Hemostatic agents are effective when there is minimal oozing from the cut surface. The hemostatic agent is directly applied to the oozing surface, and an abdominal pack is placed on the organ to exert primary pressure on the hemostatic agent and to tamponade the bleeding. In order for the hemostatic agent to be effective, it cannot be washed off the surface of the organ by excessive bleeding. Different agents, including fibrin glue, Avitene, thrombin, and Gelfoam, have been employed with varying degrees of success.

It is important to remember that local hemostatic agents will not control significant arterial or venous bleeding. This kind of bleeding needs to be controlled surgically.

Contamination must be quickly and effectively controlled in the severely injured patient who is a candidate for a damage control procedure and has injuries to the small and/or large bowel. Rapid control can be achieved by a number of methods, which control contamination but are not designed to definitively repair the

Damage Control Techniques

Bowel injuries:

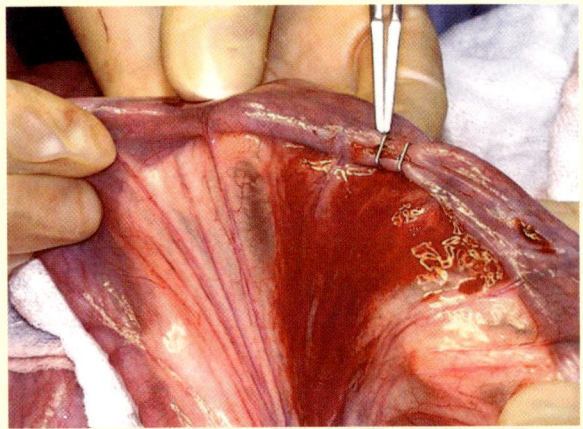

- Skin stapler

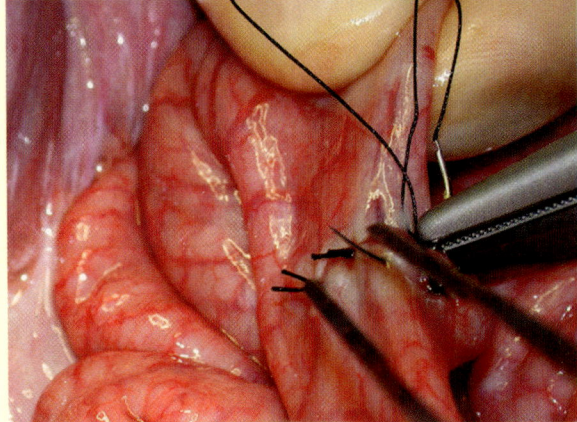

- Primary single layer closure

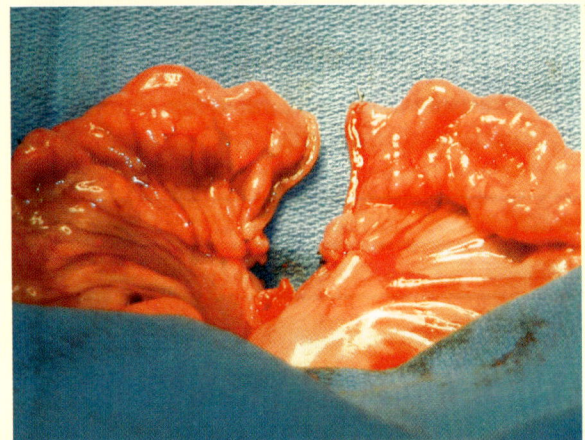

- Resection without anastomosis

injury. Small enterotomies in the small or large bowel can be controlled with the use of a staple. A few staples can easily and effectively stop any effluent from passing through the enterotomy. Similarly, a single-layered rapid closure with interrupted or continuous sutures can effectively control contamination. Another effective technique involves using a stapling device to resect an injured portion of the bowel. An attempt to complete the anastomosis is not necessary, as the main goal of the procedure is to minimize the patient's time in the operating room and then quickly move to the intensive care unit for definitive resuscitation.

Damage Control Techniques

Closure of the abdomen is a significant challenge in a severely injured trauma patient who has had multiple transfusions and has acidosis, coagulopathy, and abdominal packs in situ to tamponade ongoing bleeding. The ability to bring the fascia together in a primary abdominal closure should be carefully evaluated. If the fascia is under significant stress, as evidenced by difficulty in approximating the fascia in the midline or sutures beginning to tear on closing the abdomen, it is best to abandon the primary closure and utilize different techniques for temporary closure. A number of techniques have been used with considerable success.

Damage Control Techniques

For abdominal closure:
- towel clips
- Bogotá bag
- mesh
- occlusive dressing
- Ioban/Vi-Drape
- zipper or Velcro

Towel Clips

The towel clip closure is designed to quickly approximate the skin with the use of multiple towel clips placed in the midline. The advantage to this technique is that it is very easy to apply the towel clips and the entire closure can be effected in a short period of time. The disadvantages are that the towel clips are metal and radiopaque and therefore will exclude any attempt at diagnostic angiography and/or a therapeutic selective angiographic embolism of bleeding vessels. Similarly, the metal towel clips will render a CT scan or an MRI impossible to perform. Another problem with this method of closure is that the patient will have significant discomfort from the towel clips.

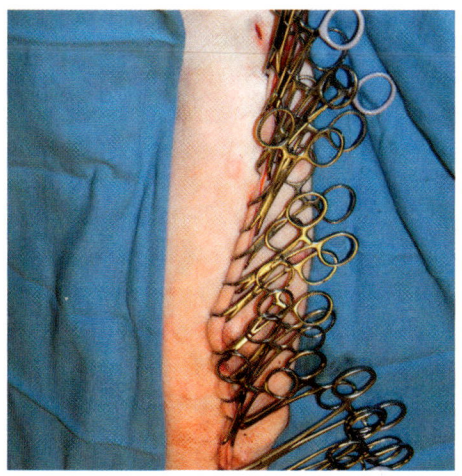
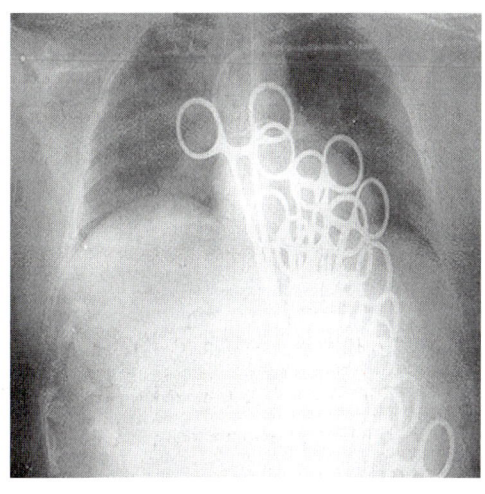

Bogotá Bag

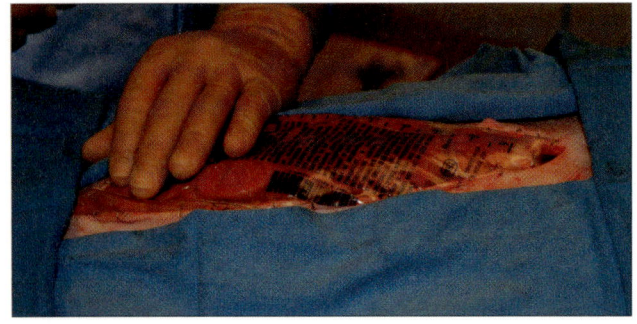

The Bogotá bag closure, which was developed in Bogotá, Colombia, is an effective, fast, simple, and inexpensive method of closing the abdomen. The procedure involves obtaining a 2-liter urology irrigation bag. The bag is opened widely and then placed over the open abdomen and fashioned to the laparotomy incision. Next, it is either sutured or stapled to the skin. This method is rapid, easy to perform, and gives a view of the abdominal viscera through the transparent bag, providing visual evidence of the viability of the bowel and allowing visual quantification of the amount of ongoing bleeding.

Mesh

Different types of mesh closures have been used. A number of these materials are porous, and although they are effective in containing eviscerated viscera and providing visualization of the bowel, the effluent of blood and serum can be difficult to contain. An Esmarch rubberized dressing can also be sutured

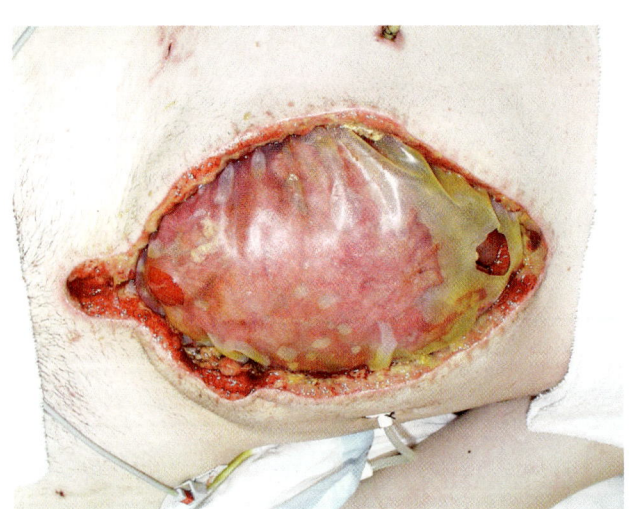

to the skin or fascia, creating an effective closure of the abdomen. However, this material is usually opaque so it is difficult, if not impossible, to visualize the bowel. A fenestrated plastic dressing, which is placed over the abdominal contents and guided into the lateral paracolic gutters on either side of the abdomen, effectively contains the viscera. A suction catheter such as a Jackson-Pratt drain is placed superiorly and inferiorly to collect effluent. A sterile operating room pack is placed over the drape, and an Ioban dressing is placed over the entire abdomen to effectively close the wound. The disadvantage of these methods is that care must be taken to be sure that the effluent is adequately collected and that the skin does not macerate under the dressing.

Damage Control

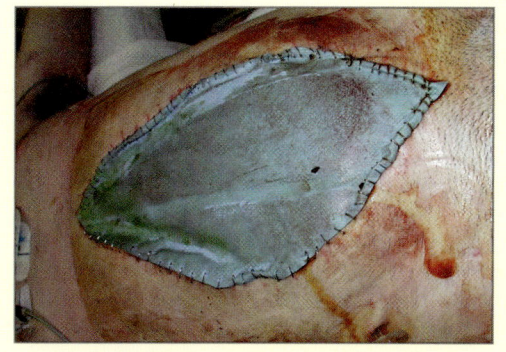

- Abdominal Closure Occlusive Dressings -Esmarch

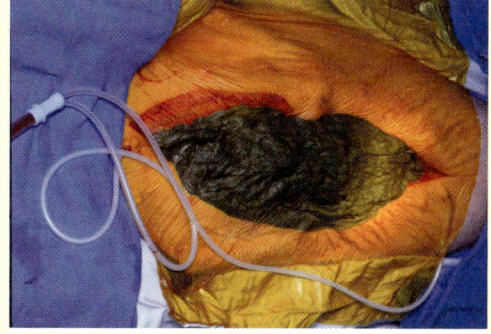

- Abdominal Closure Vacuum

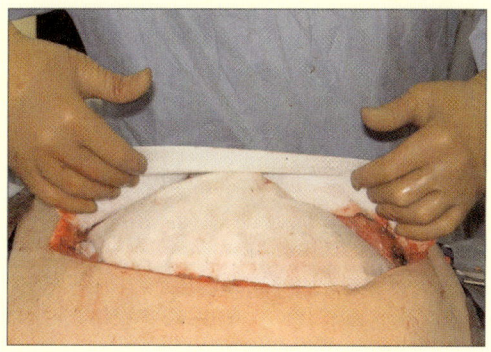

- Abdominal Closure Wittmann Patch (Velcro)

Velcro Dressings

The use of Velcro dressings has been a useful addition to abdominal closures. This technique employs a Velcro-type dressing sutured to the fascia and tailored to come together in the midline. The Velcro is then advanced every four to six hours, bringing the fascia closer together. It is very difficult to create a compartment syndrome with this method, since the Velcro will unfasten as the abdominal pressures increase. Excess Velcro can be trimmed off and readjusted as the third space losses allow for abdominal content to gradually become smaller. Another major advantage to this method is that the abdomen can be re-entered for a definitive procedure by simply unfastening the Velcro at the midline.

Abdominal Compartment Syndrome

It is important to identify the early signs of an impending abdominal compartment syndrome. At the end of a difficult exploratory laparotomy with significant blood loss and the potential for a substantial degree of third space losses, the index of suspicion of a compartment syndrome should be high.

It is important to observe the peak inspiratory pressure on the ventilator as the abdomen is being closed. If it rises by 15 to 20 mmHg during the abdominal closure, it is very likely that the abdominal viscera are compressing the diaphragms. Obviously, this compromises the ventilation of the patient and alerts the surgeon to the fact that continued fascia-to-fascia closure of the abdomen will result in intraabdominal hypertension, and extreme ventilatory embarrassment. Fascial closure will also result in increased pressure on the renal venous vasculature, causing oliguria.

If the pressure in the retroperitoneum increases to greater than the pressure in the IVC, there will be a decreased venous return with a resulting decrease in cardiac inflow. Ultimately, this will lead to a decrease in cardiac output and hypotension. It is critical to identify this impending situation, abandon the abdominal fascial closure, and switch to a procedure, which allows for creatively closing the abdomen without increasing intraabdominal pressure.

Abdominal Compartment Syndrome

- **Causes:** Bowel wall edema
  Intraabdominal packing
  Third spacing

- **Signs:** Hypotension
  Oliguria
  Ventilatory difficulty
  Bladder pressure > 25 mmHg

- **Treatment:** Release of pressure

ADVANCED TRAUMA OPERATIVE MANAGEMENT

Selected Readings

Chapter 1 - Trauma Laparotomy

Hirshberg A, Mattox KL. (eds) Surgical Clinics of North America: Damage Control Surgery. August 1997.

Johnson JW et al. Evolution in damage control with exsanguinating penetrating abdominal injury. J Trauma 2001;51:261-271.

Johnson JW et al. Hepatic angiography in patients undergoing damage control laparotomy. J Trauma 2002;52:1102-1106.

Simon RJ et al. Impact of increased use of laparoscopy on negative laparotomy rates after penetrating trauma. J Trauma 2002;53:297-302.

Nicholas et al. Changing patterns in the management of penetrating abdominal trauma: the more things change, the more they stay the same.
J Trauma 2003;55:1095-1110.

Feliciano DV et al. Trauma Damage Control. In: Moore EE, Feliciano DV, Mattox KL, eds. Trauma. 5th ed. 2004 McGraw-Hill:877-900.

Tips From the Masters

There are a number of safe methods to manage blunt and penetrating trauma in the operating suite. The following technical surgical tips have been successfully used by the authors to deal with difficult or challenging operating situations.

Chapter 1: Laparotomy

TABLE OF CONTENTS

Abdominal Closure in the Damage Control Procedure 28
Lenworth M. Jacobs, MD

Wittmann Patch: Staged Abdominal Repair (STAR):
For Penetrating Abdominal Trauma 30
Dietmar H. Wittmann, MD

Packing Techniques and Vac Pack Abdominal
Wall Closure After Damage Control 34
Michael F. Rotondo, MD

Towel Clip Abdominal Wall Closure 37
John P. Welch, MD

Stab Wound to the Cecum 39
Fred A. Luchette, MD

Sigmoid Colon Laceration 41
Brad Cushing, MD

Low Velocity Gunshot Wound to Descending Colon 43
Demetrios Demetriades, MD

Laceration to the Colon and Spleen 44
Paul E. Collicott, MD

Incontinuity Resection of Multiple (4) Contiguous Small Bowel
Lacerations Utilizing the Stapler 46
William F. Fallon, Jr., MD

Multiple Small Bowel Stab Wounds 48
Alasdair K.T. Conn, MD

Multiple Stab Wounds to Small Bowel 50
Blaine Enderson, MD

Distal Colorectal Irrigation 52
Lenworth M. Jacobs, MD

**Totally Diverting Loop Colostomy with
Non-Contaminating Distal Irrigation** 54
Kimball I. Maull, MD

Damage Control of the Abdomen with Penetrating Injury 56
C. William Schwab, MD

Measurement of Intraabdominal Pressure 58
Marc D. Palter, MD

The Browner Pelvic Stabilizer 60
Bruce D. Browner, MD

Coagulation Sandwich 62
Lenworth M. Jacobs, MD

Topical Hemostatic Agents in Trauma 64
Jameel Ali, MD

A FAST Examination for Thoracoabdominal Injuries 66
Grace S. Rozycki, MD

TECHNICAL OPERATIVE PROCEDURES:

HOW I DO IT

Abdominal Closure in the Damage Control Procedure

Lenworth M. Jacobs, MD, MPH, FACS

Scenario

A 24-year-old woman was involved in a motor vehicle crash. She sustained a Grade IV liver injury and a Grade V splenic injury. The liver injury was managed with packing and local control. A splenectomy was performed. At the end of the procedure, the abdominal viscera were protruding through the midline incision and the fascia could not be closed. Upon trying to close the fascia, the peak inspiratory pressure (PIP) on the respirator was observed and was found to increase by 15 mmHg. It was clear that an attempt to continue primary fascial closure would tear the fascia and induce abdominal hypertension and create an abdominal compartment syndrome. A creative closure of the abdomen was necessary.

- Closure
- Visceral herniation
- Fascia tearing on closure
- Diaphragm compression
- Rising peak inspiratory pressure on fascial closure

Procedure:

The advancing silo technique

A large sheet of Marlex mesh was sutured to the fascia with a #2 continuous Prolene suture. A second sheet was sutured to the fascia on the other side of the incision. The omentum was drawn down over the small bowel to cover the bowel. These two leaves were then used to contain the viscera. The two leaves were pulled up vertically. A #2 continuous suture was then used to sew the two leaves of the Marlex mesh together. The first stitch brought the apex of the fascia together at the xiphoid. This ensures that the small bowel will not herniate through a small defect at the apex of the closure. The two leaves were approximated along the length of the wound and a similar procedure was performed at the inferior end of the wound to prevent herniation. The repair formed a silo which contained the viscera. Since the mesh is transparent, the bowel can be observed for viability. Special attention needs to be paid to the neck of this hernia where the bowel protrudes out of the abdominal wall. The bowel and its vascular supply can be pinched and kinked at the fascia and cause ischemia of a loop of bowel. The problem is easily solved by manually moving the bowel and releasing the pressure on the vascular supply. The bowel is then observed to return to a pink, well-perfused state.

The wound is then re-examined in four to six hours. The bowel is then eased back into the abdomen and the silo is then pinched and cinched closed. Usually the suture line can be advanced by about an inch. A second layer of #2 Prolene is then placed. These two leaves were then used to contain the viscera. This procedure is performed in the intensive care unit. At six-hour intervals, the procedure is repeated. If there is more rapid mobilization of fluid, the procedure can be repeated at shorter intervals. The silo is advanced with multiple suture lines. This procedure gradually returns the bowel into the abdomen until the fascia can be closed primarily.

The peak inspiratory pressure on the respirator should be observed at the beginning and end of each advancement. This maneuver will ensure that the closure is not creating an abdominal compartment syndrome.

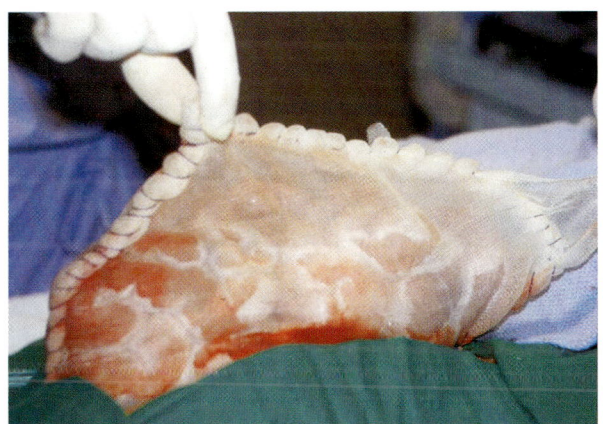
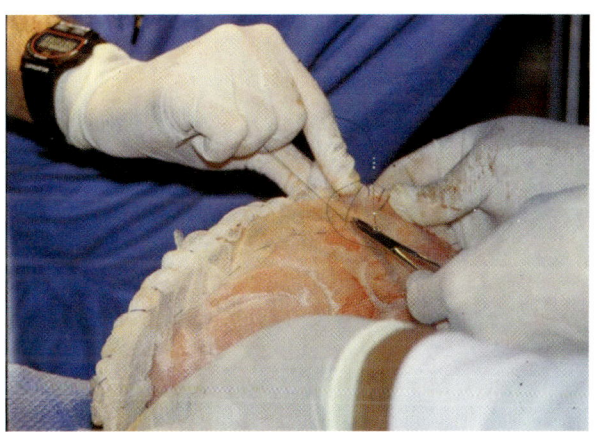
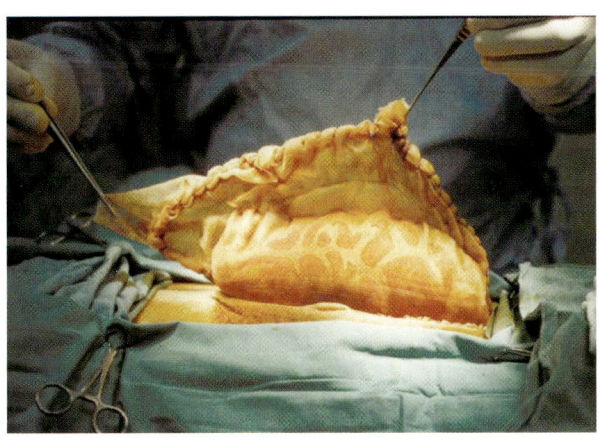
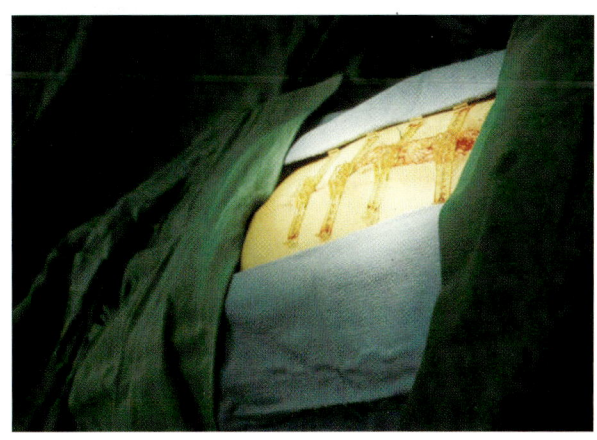

TECHNICAL OPERATIVE PROCEDURES:

HOW I DO IT

Wittmann Patch Staged Abdominal Repair (STAR) For Penetrating Abdominal Trauma

Dietmar H. Wittman, MD

Scenario

A 27-year-old man presented 45 minutes after a gunshot injury with a wound penetrating the abdominal wall 5 cm below the umbilicus. In spite of vigorous resuscitation with crystalloid during transport he remained hypotensive. He was immediately taken to the operating room. The abdomen is distended and dull to percussion suggesting abdominal hypertension from hemorrhage.

Operative management:
Staged Abdominal Repair (STAR)

A full-length midline incision from xiphoid to the symphysis provides sufficient access to the injuries. As the incision is opened further, edematous bowel protrudes. There are multiple ileal perforations. Blood comes from a source within the pelvis. Clotted blood is scooped out of the abdomen and the extent of the injury inspected. The projectile has also injured the internal iliac vein, the presacral venous plexus, and has perforated the sigmoid colon twice.

A clean pack is brought into the pre-sacral space and the internal iliac vein is freed, clamped and ligated. There is still considerable bleeding from the sacral venous plexus. The patient temperature is 35.8°C. New packs are inserted into the pre-sacral space which controls bleeding. A second dose of 2 grams of cefotaxime and 500 mg metronidazole is given intravenously.

The sigmoid perforations are débrided, connected and closed with single layer 4-0 PDS. To avoid time consuming repairs of the six irregular small bowel perforations, the entire 20 cm segment is resected and both ends are stapled deferring anastomosis to the next abdominal entry (STAR#2) when the patient has been rewarmed and his hemodynamics and coagulation have stabilized and peritoneal edema has decreased.

The abdomen is now irrigated with 8 liters of Ringer's lactate and then quickly closed temporarily using the artificial bur with hypobaric wound shield (HBS) to provide closure over the edematous intestines, to prevent complications of compartment syndrome, to avoid exogenous contamination, and to measure protein losses for meaningful replacement.

Artificial bur closure

The softer loop sheet is sutured to the right fascia using a running looped #1 Nylon suture.

The stitches are 2 cm apart and 2 cm into the fascia and 1 to 2 cm into the bur. The sheet with loops facing outwards is then pushed between the parietal and visceral peritoneum of the other side of the incision covering the abdominal contents.

The harder hook sheet is similarly sutured to the left fascia, and the hooks are gently pressed into the loops of the loop sheet. Because of the massive peritoneal hypertension in this case the hook sheet does not need trimming to fit the wound opening.

The space above the bur sheets is now packed with Kerlix wrapped around tubing that was used during the operation for suctioning. It stays connected to the intraoperative suction pump, which must continue suctioning until the wound is hermetically sealed and the tubing is connected to a transportable suction pump.

The wound including Kerlix and at least 15 cm of skin surrounding the wound is now covered with a self-adhesive sterile plastic drape. A mesentery is formed between the tubing and the skin to avoid any fluid leak around the tubing. It is important to keep suction running continuously (even during transport) to avoid fluid leaks between the skin and the drape that would open a path for exogenous contamination.

Also planned subsequent abdominal entries, STAR #2 through STAR #5 are scheduled immediately with the charge nurse in the operating room to make sure that all subsequent abdominal entries are happening at 24-hour intervals.

28 hours later

Hemodynamics have stabilized, coagulation is normal, and there is no evidence of further hemorrhage. 3580 mL of slightly hemorrhagic fluid has been collected via the hypobaric tubing, and the peritoneal fluid protein content is 30% of serum levels. These protein losses have been replaced by intravenous fresh frozen plasma. Antibiotics were continued every 12 hours because of the potentially contaminated pack within the pelvis. Antibiotic concentration in the peritoneal fluid was four to ten times above the MIC of intraperitoneal pathogens isolated. There was no fluid leak underneath the hypobaric wound shield.

STAR# 2

The wound shield and Kerlix are removed and the bur hook sheet pulled off the loop sheet and folded using a laparotomy pack to cover the hooks. The loop sheet is then pulled to open the abdomen. The peritoneal fluid is reddish clear, and the bowel is edematous. Before removing the presacral pack, the stapled end of the ileum is reconnected using a 4-0 running PDS suture to form a single layer anastomosis. (Alternatively stapling of the

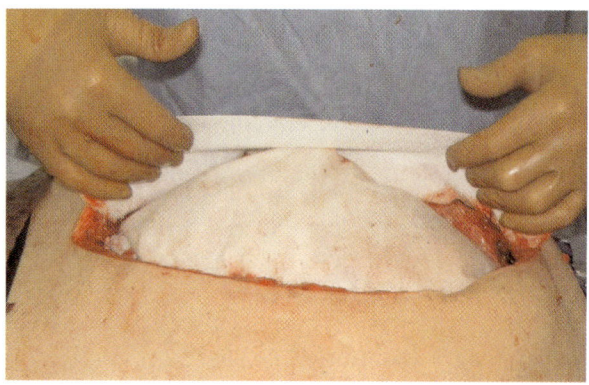

anastomosis has the advantage that the bowel edema is gently squeezed out while hand-sewn sutures may loosen as edema decreases). The presacral packs are now gently removed. There is only some minor oozing from the presacral space. Inspection of the sutured sigmoid reveals no leak and no necrotic tissue around the sutures.

All four quadrants of the abdomen are irrigated with Ringer's lactate. A new pack is brought into the pelvis, and the abdomen is closed by pulling the bur sheets together with some tension to reapproximate the fascia. A hypobaric shield is performed as described for the original procedure.

24 hours later

The patient has been stable with no fever and slight leucocytosis. The peritoneal fluid was yellowish clear with a protein content of 50% of serum protein. The patient continues to be on TPN. Diuresis has been introduced to reduce peritoneal edema and permit fascial reapproximation.

STAR # 3

The bur is opened as described above. There is still some bowel edema. Neither the small bowel anastomosis nor the sigmoid colon suture is leaking and the peritoneal fluid is clear and peritoneal inflammation is much improved. The pack is removed from the pelvis. There is no further hemorrhage. The peritoneal cavity is then washed with 6 liters of Ringer's lactate and closing the burr permits reapproximating the fascia up to a 7 cm gap.

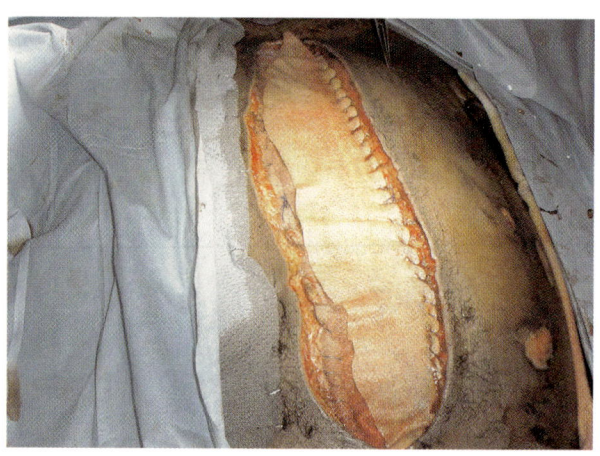

STAR # 4

After reopening the bur the abdomen looks ready for final closure. An abdominal x-ray is performed to identify any laparotomy sponges that may have been left. Meanwhile all suture lines appear to be healing well. There is no leak, no necrosis, and no new pathology. The bur sheets are pulled and the fascia edges are approximated. Both sheets are then removed and multiple fascial #1 PDS sutures are placed. The surgeon ties each single fascial suture. There were no complications postoperatively.

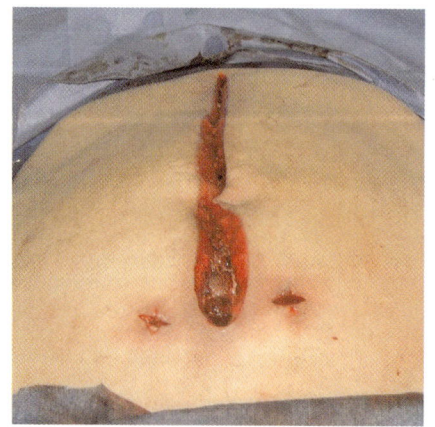

Critical Details: Lessons learned over 15 years with STAR

- Handle tissue and fascia gently, replace packs often

- Exert some tension to the fascia with the bur and the hooks on the sheets

- Perform deferred anastomoses early, avoid colostomies

- Stick to 24-hour intervals. Avoid transmural feeding tubes

- Final fascial closure at the end of STAR tolerates more tension than closure after a single laparotomy

- Obtain an abdominal x-ray at the last STAR to account for packs

- Prevent contamination of wound in the intensive care unit

- Give antibiotic one half hour prior to STAR entry

- Know antibiotic tissue concentration in peritoneal fluid

- Measure intraabdominal pressure

- Replace lost proteins with fresh frozen plasma

- Obtain initial informed consent for multiple abdominal entries

References

Wittmann DH: Newer methods of operative therapy for peritonitis: In Nyhus LM, Baker RJ, Fischer JE, (eds) Master of Surgery, Third edition Little Brown and Company, Publishers, Boston, pp. 146-152, 1996.

Wittmann DH. Chapter 160: Compartment Syndrome of the Abdominal Cavity. In RS Irwin, FB Cerra, JM Rippe (eds) Intensive Care Medicine, 5th Edition, Lippincott-Raven Publishers, pp. 164-1709, 2002.

Wittmann, DH. Chapter 37: Status of the open abdomen in patients with uncontrolled intraabdominal infection with sepsis. Deitch, Vincent & Windsor (eds). Sepsis and Multiple Organ Dysfunction. WB Saunders, London, New York, pp. 308-316, 2002.

TECHNICAL OPERATIVE PROCEDURES:

HOW I DO IT

Packing Techniques and Vac Pack Abdominal Wall Closure After Damage Control

Michael F. Rotondo, MD, FACS

Scenario

A 26-year-old thin male presents with a transabdominal gunshot wound just below the right costal margin in the midclavicular line with a palpable bullet located on the left just above the iliac crest in the mid-axillary line. He is initially confused, combative, and hypotensive.

Management: *Initial resuscitation and damage control laparotomy*

The need for operation is immediately recognized upon discovery of the right upper quadrant penetration and the palpable left flank bullet. After obtaining large bore peripheral intravenous access, at which time blood is obtained for type and crossmatch, and performance of an abbreviated neurologic exam, the patient undergoes rapid sequence induction and intubation for immediate airway control. Resuscitation is initiated with warm crystalloids and universal type O blood. The patient is fully exposed and examined for additional penetrations or palpable missiles. No other injuries are identified. A rectal examination is completed, which reveals gross blood. A Foley catheter is placed which reveals clear urine. A nasogastric tube is placed which reveals gross blood. A single directed abdominal film is obtained to determine the presence of additional missiles or fragmentation within the abdomen. No other missiles are identified with the exception of a large caliber bullet in the left flank soft tissues. The initial temperature is 35°C.

The patient's total resuscitation time is 12 minutes and he is taken to the operating room for exploratory laparotomy. At this point, two factors are critical to this patient's outcome. The first is that the operating room is totally prepared to receive this patient. The second is that the surgical team is well aware of the time course. In this particular scenario, the total time to the operating room is less than 15 minutes. This includes rapid sequence intubation, large bore intravenous access, placement of a nasogastric tube and Foley catheter, performance of digital rectal examination, and obtaining a single film to determine trajectory. It is clear from the information available that the patient has a torso injury confined to the abdomen likely to involve the liver or other major vascular structures, the stomach, small bowel and colon and unlikely to involve the genitourinary system. Because of the transabdominal trajectory and the persistent hypotension, this patient should immediately be identified as a candidate for damage control. In this regard, time is of the essence and attentiveness to the amount of time of resuscitation and operation is important in determining the outcome of this patient.

The patient is brought to the operating room and placed on the table in a supine position. The patient is prepped and draped from chin to knees and two suction devices are placed on the operative field, including a device for blood scavenging and autotransfusion. A midline incision is performed. The peritoneum is identified and a small opening is created and a cell saver suction device is inserted. 2.5 liters of gross blood are evacuated and the peritoneum is further opened throughout the extent of the incision. Four quadrant and central retroperitoneal packing then ensues. The Bookwalter retractor is set up for general exposure. As the blood pressure is normalized, the supraceliac aortic clamp may be removed one click at a time as tolerated.

At this point, the packs should be systematically removed and it is my practice to remove the packs that are least likely to be involved with hemorrhage first. This creates more room in the abdomen for exposure of the bleeding area. Systematic tracking of the trajectory of this missile should then take place starting at the right upper quadrant. A large stellate laceration to the dome of the right lobe of the liver is identified with an additional wound located just medial to the gallbladder and through the medial segment of the left lobe of the liver. This is easily controlled with perihepatic packing with minimal immobilization of the liver. Further exploration reveals a through-and-through injury to the stomach, which is primarily repaired in two layers. Four holes in the mid-jejunum are managed by primary stapled resection without anastomosis and a through-and-through injury to the sigmoid colon with significant tissue loss is likewise managed by simple stapled resection. Exit into the retroperitoneum on the left, anterior and lateral to the ureter and the psoas muscle is noted. Total operation time is 54 minutes.

- Apply plastic drape to surgical towel

- Cover the viscera with the plastic

- Place closed suction drains

- Apply a second adhesive plastic dressing to seal wound

- Apply low wall suction

Procedure: *Packing techniques and temporary abdominal wall closure after damage control*

The patient, however, is cold with a temperature of 34°C, coagulopathic with evidence of non-mechanical bleeding, and acidotic with a base deficit of −9. The liver is then re-examined for pack integrity. It is generally my practice to replace the perihepatic packing at this time and to be certain that care is taken to judiciously place the packs in order to control bleeding. Aggressive overpacking leading to hepatic necrosis is to be avoided. The number of packs placed around the liver is also noted and recorded.

Procedure: *Vac-Pack dressing*

If skin only closure is not possible, a Vac-Pac dressing is placed by first inserting a nonstick material in contact with the intestinal viscera. This is achieved by applying an adhesive plastic dressing to a surgical towel and then placing the surgical towel within the abdomen such that the abdominal viscera are below the level of the fascia in contact with the plastic non-stick surface of the towel. Two 10 Fr. Jackson-Pratt drains are then placed in the gutters created by the towel and subcutaneous tissues and brought out superiorly without a subcutaneous tunnel. A subcutaneous tunnel creates unnecessary tissue damage, which can lead to scarring later and subsequent difficulty with flap closure. Benzoin is then applied to the skin and additional towel or Kerlix dressings are placed above the level of the previously placed towel and Jackson-Pratt drains. A second adhesive plastic dressing is then placed to seal the wound and the Jackson-Pratt drains are placed to low wall suction. This achieves a vacuum closure.

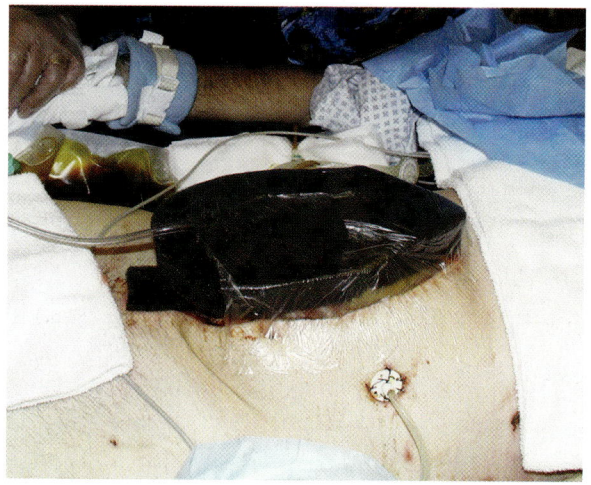

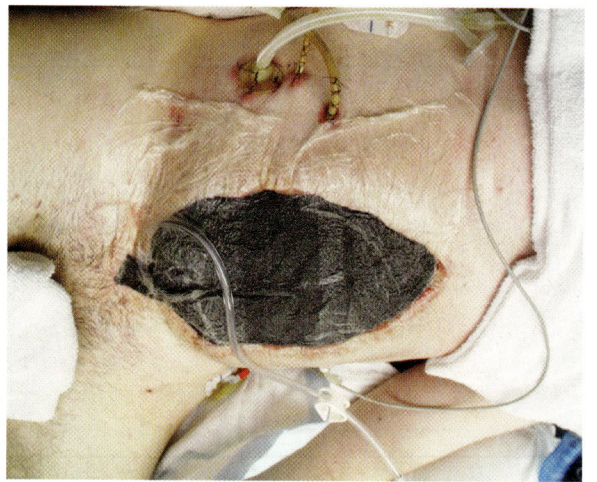

The patient is then transported back to the intensive care unit for additional resuscitation.

TECHNICAL OPERATIVE PROCEDURES:
HOW I DO IT

Towel Clip Abdominal Wall Closure

John P. Welch, MD, FACS

Scenario

A 35-year-old male presented following a head-on motor vehicle accident. He was alert but tachycardic with a blood pressure of 85 systolic. A chest x-ray showed several fractured ribs on the right, and his abdomen was distended. A FAST ultrasound examination showed free intraabdominal fluid. A peritoneal lavage was grossly positive. In the operating room a deep laceration of the right lobe of the liver was bleeding actively. Ongoing bleeding was difficult to control unless the liver wound was packed.

Management

Massive bleeding from injuries to organs such as the liver or to major vessels is frequently complicated by hypothermia and coagulopathy. These problems serve to worsen the bleeding and frequently the safest maneuver is to close the abdomen rapidly (once surgical or major vessel bleeding is controlled and areas of ooze are controlled by pressure) and to return the patient to the intensive care unit where warming, correction of the coagulopathy, improvement of hemodynamics and ventilatory support can occur.

Procedure

I have found that an expeditious abdominal wall closure in such a damage control situation is done easily with a large number of towel clips. I prefer short clips since they only cover a small area adjacent to the wound and are easily tucked under the wound dressing, consisting of sterile gauze or towels covered with an adhesive drape. Clips are placed in a parallel fashion about 1 cm to 2 cm apart and 1 cm to 2 cm from the edge of the incision. In most cases the patient remains on a ventilator, and abdominal wall pressures are well controlled. Approximation of the skin and some of the underlying subcutaneous fat is sufficient to prevent evisceration except if the bowel is massively dilated. Clips can be easily removed if an abdominal compartment syndrome develops. Fascial closure with or without mesh usually is done a few days later when the patient has stabilized and abdominal distention and edema have subsided. If fascial retraction occurs, abdominal wall closure might require use of mesh.

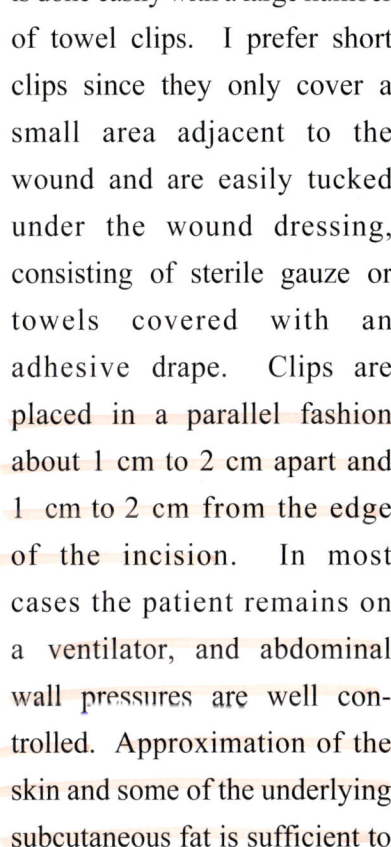

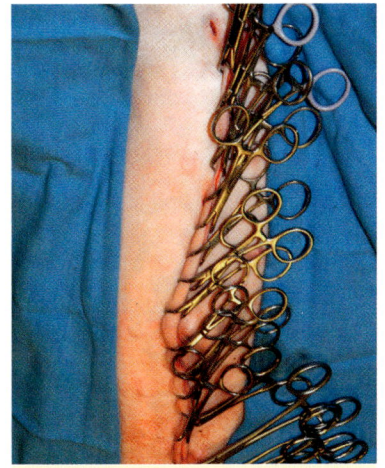

- Use **short** towel clips
- Place **1 to 2 cm apart**
- Place **1 to 2 cm from the edge of the incision**

A drawback of towel clip closure is interference with imaging procedures. If desired, a portion of the wound, skin and subcutaneous tissue, can be closed with a running heavy suture such as #1 PDS or Prolene to facilitate imaging, such as angiographic embolization. After several days, erythema and localized abscesses can develop at towel clip skin puncture sites. If the clips are left for more than a week, there is some risk of breakdown of skin and secondary wound infection. I have also seen herniation of small bowel into the subcutaneous fat in a patient whose return to the operating room for removal of the clips was delayed because of recurrent DT's. He eventually developed a small bowel obstruction.

In most cases of abdominal trauma, the abdominal wound can be closed moderately rapidly with primary fascial closure, whereas a distended abdomen can be closed with some form of mesh or silastic sutured to the fascia. I only employ the towel clip closure in situations when very expeditious abdominal wall closure is needed, usually in cases of damage control surgery following trauma or in hemodynamically unstable patients developing acute intraoperative complications such as an acute myocardial infarction.

References

Burch JM, Ortiz VB, Richardson RJ, Martin RR, Mattox KL, Jordan GL Jr.: Abbreviated laparotomy and planned reoperation for critically injured patients. Ann Surg 215(5): 476-84, 1992.

Feliciano DV, Burch JM: Towel clips, silos, and heroic forms of wound closure. In Maull KI, ed, Advances in Trauma and Critical Care, Vol. 6. Chicago: Mosby Year Book, 1991.

TECHNICAL OPERATIVE PROCEDURES:

HOW I DO IT

Stab Wound to the Cecum

Fred A. Luchette, MD, FACS, FCCM

Scenario

Prehospital personnel transported a 25-year-old male to the emergency department after sustaining a stab wound to the right lower quadrant with a steak knife. The physical examination is consistent with peritonitis. On exploration there is a 3 cm laceration to the anterior surface of the cecum with extensive fecal soilage. Further exploration identifies a right-sided Zone II hematoma of the mesentery with 600 cc of free blood in the abdomen.

Management

Broad-spectrum antibiotics that provide coverage for gram-positive organisms, gram-negative organisms and bacteroides are administered immediately. A generous midline incision is utilized to allow a complete exploration of the peritoneal cavity and to evaluate for associated injuries.

- Mobilize the right colon
- Limited ileocecectomy
- Primary anastomosis
- Two layer closure
- Leave the skin open

There is obvious need for further exploration to assess for a through-and-through laceration involving the retroperitoneal portion of the cecum. One should also recognize the potential for associated injuries to the right kidney and ureter, vena cava and iliac vessels. Initial management is directed at minimizing ongoing hemorrhage followed by minimizing further contamination. Hemorrhage is controlled by digital pressure until the ureter is identified. The cecal wound is temporarily closed with Babcock clamps or sutures.

Procedure

Retroperitoneal exploration and repair of injuries

To allow complete evaluation of the cecum and right retroperitoneum, the right colon is mobilized. Beginning at the base of the cecum, the white line of Toldt is incised cephalad to the level of the hepatic flexure. The hepatic flexure is mobilized by blunt and sharp dissection to the midline with exposure of the duodenum and if necessary the pancreatic head. The ascending colon and the mesentery are mobilized to the midline. Any bleeding from the mesentery is controlled with sutures. The right kidney and right ureter are now explored from the renal pelvis to the level of the iliac vessels to indentify any injuries. Finally, the external iliac artery and vein are inspected for a laceration.

If the cecal wound is through-and-through, a limited ileocecectomy is performed especially if the mesenteric hematoma is a vascular injury that will compromise the bowel. The mesenteric vessels should be explored. If the laceration is in proximity to the mesenteric side of the colon or there is any suggestion or concern that the bowel will be devascularized, one should proceed with a resection and primary anastomosis. Otherwise, if there is maintenance of the collaterals on the mesenteric side of the colon, the injured mesenteric vessels should be suture ligated. The anastomosis is completed using either a one-layer or two-layer suture technique. A stapled anastomosis is an acceptable alterative. An alternative management to resection is to perform two separate closures of each laceration particularly if there is no significant vascular injury. The initial layer is completed in a through and through fashion with a running 3-0 absorbable suture. A reinforcing layer of 3-0 silk Lembert sutures are placed. The fascia should be reapproximated with a mono-filament suture and the skin left open and allowed to heal by either delayed primary closure or secondary intention.

Chapter One - Trauma Laparotomy

TECHNICAL OPERATIVE PROCEDURES:

HOW I DO IT

Sigmoid Colon Laceration

Brad Cushing, MD, FACS

Scenario

A 25-year-old healthy male sustained a .45 caliber pistol wound that entered at his umbilicus and exited in the left posterior flank. He was normotensive and non-tachycardic. It was clear from the exam and trajectory that the bullet had traversed the peritoneal cavity. The rectal exam was non-bloody. The injury had occurred approximately 30 minutes ago. He was taken directly to the operating room. No consideration was given to the performance of a single shot intravenous pyelogram, although it is useful.

Management

He was placed supine on the operating table, a dose of a second generation cephalosporin was administered and after induction of general anesthesia, a Foley catheter was inserted. The urine was non-bloody.

A midline incision was made with the umbilical swerve to the right to leave more room for a left-sided ostomy should it be needed. The fascia was divided for the full length of the incision before entering the peritoneum so that intraperitoneal blood would not obscure the view and render the cautery unusable. The peritoneum was then entered and free blood aspirated clear. There was a large amount of stool contamination in the peritoneum. The small bowel was eviscerated to the right. The retroperitoneum was inspected and no bleeding or injury noted. A destructive lesion of the sigmoid colon was noted involving 70% of the circumference. The edges were devascularized and there was a small contiguous rent in the mesentery. Kocher clamps were applied to the open edges of the colon to prevent further spillage of stool. The remainder of the abdominal contents were inspected and no injuries noted. The patient remained hemodynamically stable.

Based on the data presented in the practice guidelines for penetrating colon

- 70% of circumference involved

- Large amount of fecal contamination

- Damaged colon is resected

- Stapled primary anastomosis

- Abdomen irrigated with saline

- 24-hour broad-spectrum antibiotics

injuries presented by the Eastern Association for the Surgery of Trauma, the decision was made to resect and primarily repair the colonic injury. In the absence of data to support the superiority of hand-sewn or stapled anastomoses and given the easy mobility of the colon at this level, I decided to use a GIA stapled anastomosis. A GIA stapler was fired across the colon, one staple line approximately one inch proximal and a second staple line one inch distal to the injury. Both staple lines were placed in clearly vascularized, undamaged areas of the colon. The damaged colon was thereby resected. Small bleeding points in the mesentery were ligated. Non-crushing bowel clamps were placed approximately four inches back from the ends of the bowel after stool was manually squeezed from the area that was to be anastomosed. The colon segments were placed side-by-side and small openings were made in the existing staple lines to allow insertion of the GIA stapler anvils. The stapler was inserted into each colon segment. It was then fired along the antimesenteric side of the bowel. The small amount of remaining stool was aspirated and the suture line inspected to assure circumferential closure and hemostasis. Another staple was fired to close the last opening. This method of GIA staple use consumes more staple cartridges than other methods routinely used in elective cases but stool spillage and manipulation is minimized. The bowel clamps were removed. The mesentery was inspected for a rent that would allow an internal hernia and none was seen.

The bullet tract as it exited the colon through the back was irrigated and a single bullet fragment removed, thus reducing the likelihood of later abscess formation. The entire abdomen was then irrigated with warm normal saline without antibiotics or other bacteriostatic solution. The abdominal fascia was closed with a continuous slow absorbing suture and the skin was left open with the intention of delayed primary closure on post-op day four.

Postoperative care included antibiotics for 24 hours (see EAST practice guidelines). A nasogastric tube was not placed. Rapid diet advancement, following the colon surgery postoperative pathway for elective surgery was utilized. The patient was discharged on postoperative day four after delayed primary closure of the wound and before flatus or a bowel movement. He was called by the surgery staff on postoperative day six and was doing well. He was seen in clinic on postoperative day twelve and noted to be doing well without signs of infection.

TECHNICAL OPERATIVE PROCEDURES:
HOW I DO IT

Low Velocity Gunshot Wound to Descending Colon

Demetrios Demetriades, MD, FACS

Scenario

A 24-year-old male was shot with a low velocity bullet to the left lower quadrant. He presented to the trauma center 20 minutes after being shot. He required two units of blood to become normotensive. There was a 2 cm defect in the mesenteric border of the colon with feces throughout the abdomen. There are no other injuries.

Management

The patient needs to go to the operating room for an exploratory laparotomy. I would give perioperative antibiotics. Ampicillin and sulbactam provide broad spectrum coverage. The first dose is given before the patient is taken to the operating room. The abdomen is entered through a midline incision. A full exploratory laparotomy is performed. The colonic injury is identified and any further spillage is immediately controlled. The colonic injury is débrided back to viable tissue. I then repair the colon in one or two layers using absorbable 3-0 Vicryl. The omentum is then placed over the repair if this is feasible. The peritoneum is then irrigated with warm saline. The abdomen is then closed. The skin is left open for secondary closure to prevent a wound infection.

There is excellent class I evidence that for non-destructive colon injuries primary repair is the best treatment option, irrespective of any so called risk factors.

- Perioperative antibiotics

- Resection and primary anastomosis

- Omentum over the repair

- Irrigate abdomen with saline

- Leave the skin open

TECHNICAL OPERATIVE PROCEDURES:

HOW I DO IT

Laceration to the Colon and Spleen

Paul E. Collicott, MD, FACS

Scenario

A 24-year-old male presented to the emergency room, the apparent victim of an aggravated assault during which he sustained a stab wound to the left upper quadrant. The entrance wound measures approximately 2 cm in length and is located just beneath the left costal margin in the anterior axillary line. The patient remained hemodynamically normal in the emergency department with crystalloid resuscitation and was brought to the operating room after being administered prophylactic antibiotics and tetanus toxoid.

- Minimal fecal spillage
- Splenic hilar laceration
- Hemoperitoneum
- Primary double layer colonic repair
- Splenectomy
- Closed suction drainage

Operative Findings

There is a 2 cm laceration of the splenic flexure of the colon on the antimesenteric surface as well as 700 cc of free blood in the peritoneal cavity with extensive clots about the hilum of the spleen.

Procedure: *Laceration to the colon and spleen*

After satisfactory induction of general endotracheal anesthesia, the abdomen is sterilely prepped and draped and a midline incision made. Upon entering the peritoneal cavity, the above operative findings are noted. Blood is evacuated and the left upper quadrant is packed. Abdominal exploration is carried out revealing no further evidence of active bleeding in the remaining quadrants. The packs are gently removed from the left upper quadrant and there is noted to be a 2 cm laceration of the antimesenteric surface of the splenic flexure with minimal fecal spillage.

The laceration is approximated with Babcock clamps and the splenic flexure is mobilized. During the mobilization of the splenic flexure, there is noted to be a significant amount of clot at the hilum of spleen. Since there is no other injury noted to the colon, it is felt that the laceration of the splenic flexure was tangential with the knife creasing the colon and penetrating the hilum of the spleen. Therefore, it was felt necessary to explore this area further to inspect the tail of the pancreas.

The spleen is mobilized to the midline by dividing its various attachments. During the course of this mobilization, active bleeding ensues from the hilum of the spleen and it is elected to proceed with a splenectomy. The hilar vessels are serially clamped and ligated utilizing absorbable sutures and the spleen is successfully removed. Upon inspection of the body and the tail of the pancreas, no hematomas or further injuries are noted. The diaphragm is intact. The area is then irrigated with copious amounts of saline.

Attention is then directed to the previously identified splenic flexure injury. Due to minimal fecal contamination, primary double-layered suture repair is carried out. This area is then further irrigated with copious amounts of saline and a closed suction drain is placed in the splenic fossa and brought out through a separate stab wound posteriorly. Accurate positioning of the previously placed nasogastric tube is then confirmed and the wound is closed in layers. The patient tolerated the procedure well and received two additional liters of crystalloid during the procedure.

TECHNICAL OPERATIVE PROCEDURES:

HOW I DO IT

Incontinuity Resection of Multiple (4) Contiguous Small Bowel Lacerations Utilizing the Stapler

Stapled Small Bowel Resection

William F. Fallon, Jr., MD, MBA, FACS

Scenario

A young male patient was the victim of multiple gunshot wounds to the torso during a robbery. He was initially hypotensive but responded to crystalloid resuscitation. An urgent laparotomy was planned due to the nature of his torso injury.

Management

Upon arrival, a rapid primary survey is performed to determine the status of the patient's airway, breathing and hemodynamics. A thorough search for all entrance and exit wounds is essential to avoid missed injury. Intravenous access is obtained and fluid resuscitation begun. Arterial blood gas determination is performed and a specimen sent for type and cross match. Imaging studies include a chest radiograph and KUB. Bladder catheter and nasogastric tube are inserted. A first generation cephalosporin antibiotic is initiated and tetanus status determined. The patient is taken to the operating room for an exploratory laparotomy.

Procedure: *Stapled small bowel resection*

My standard trauma laparotomy prep is nipples to knees. The abdomen is draped using an iodoform impregnated adherent plastic sheet with wide pockets on all four sides. The abdomen is entered through a long midline incision and packed in all four quadrants with large pads. Once the patient's hemodynamic status is confirmed to be stable with anesthesia, the packs are removed. A thorough examination commences and includes running the bowel. In this case, four discrete mid-jejunal enterotomies are identified and controlled using Babcock clamps. These through-and-through lacerations can be used to restore intestinal integrity using the linear cutting stapling device in the manner of creating side-to-side functional end-to-end anastomoses. The injured loops are secured with sutures to assist in stabilizing the two limbs for insertion of the stapler. The enterotomies function as the openings in the bowel wall. The antimesenteric borders are approximated and secured in place with sutures. The operative field is protected with clean laparotomy pads to control contamination. A linear stapling device is inserted into each of the openings. The length of the instrument selected will determine the size of the anastomoses. The stapler is engaged, fired, and removed. The staple line is inspected for bleeding. The now common opening is then grasped with Allis clamps and a transecting stapler placed across the opening, using the clamps to assure complete closure. The stapler is fired and the excess amputated with curved Mayo scissors as this material crosses two staple lines together and is difficult to amputate with a blade. There is no mesenteric defect to deal with using this technique. The intestine is re-inspected once more at the completion of the procedure to ensure that there is no bleeding from the staple line on the bowel or the mesentery.

Surgical judgment regarding the proximity of the lacerations will determine the type of repair selected. Alternatively, the most proximal and distal injury sites can be used to perform the anastomosis. In this scenario, a mesenteric window is created and a longer transecting stapler is employed after the anastomosis has been fashioned with the linear stapler. This stapler excludes the opening created by the linear stapler as before. Once the segment of small bowel has been amputated from its mesentery, the mesenteric window can be closed with interrupted absorbable suture. The middle two lacerations are incorporated in the resected specimen.

- The laceration can be used to restore intestinal integrity

- Intestinal loops are used to stabilize the limbs for stapler insertion

- The mesentery is stapled leaving no defect

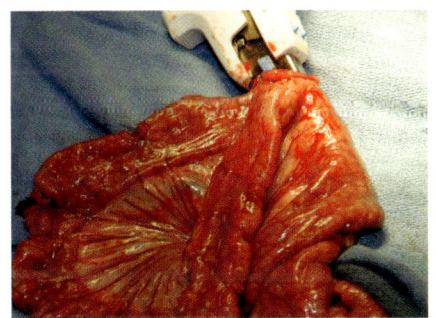
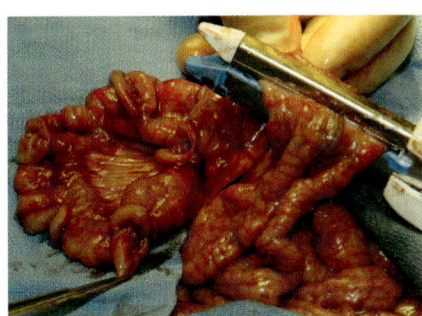
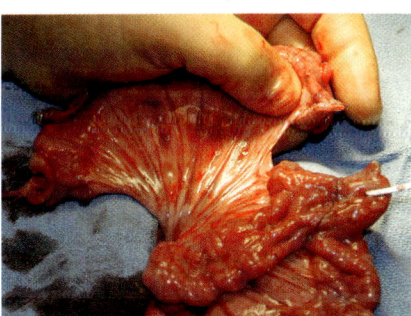
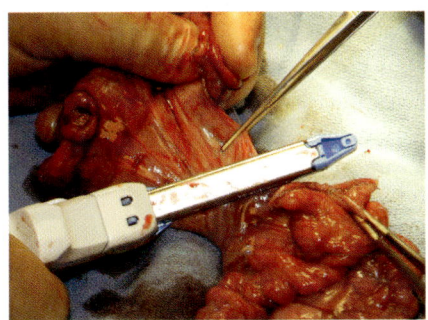
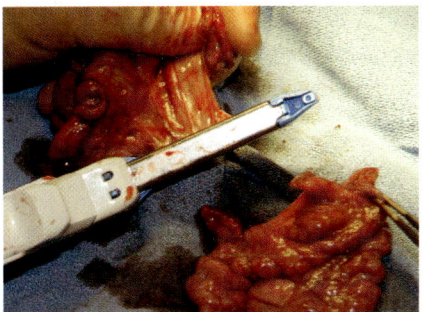
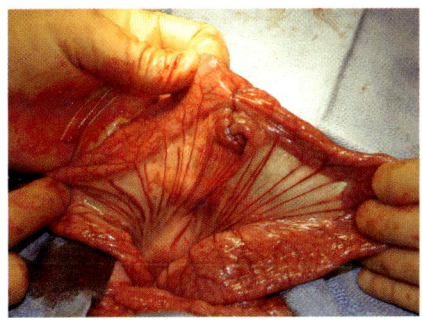

TECHNICAL OPERATIVE PROCEDURES:

HOW I DO IT

Multiple Small Bowel Stab Wounds

Alasdair K.T. Conn, MD, FACS

Scenario

A patient arrives with six stab wounds to the proximal ileum with significant succus entericus coming from each of the wounds. The wounds are within three feet of each other and two of them involve the mesenteric border. There are no other wounds.

Management

Preoperative antibiotics should have been given to this patient, either in the emergency department or at the time of induction of anesthesia. A generous midline incision to allow a complete exploratory laparotomy is a quick, satisfactory initiation to the operation.

As I explore the small bowel, I apply a non-crushing clamp to the proximal small bowel to decrease further contamination; and as I explore the small bowel looking for further injuries, I apply a non-crushing clamp to the distal bowel - again, to control contamination. As the wounds are identified, I usually also try an Allis or a Babcock clamp to approximate the wound edges, both for identification and for easy relocation of the injuries. I also try to envision the tract of the knife and mentally try to count the number of injuries to the bowel. Stab wounds to the bowel with an entrance to the bowel but no exit can occur, but are unusual.

- Non-crushing bowel clamps control contamination

- Small bowel in continuity resection of multiple wounds

- Stapled anastomosis

- Interrupted sutures close the mesentery to prevent internal herniation

In this case, two lacerations involve the mesenteric border and as there are six stab wounds within three feet, I would quickly consider a small bowel resection rather than primary closure. Although there is a tendency to perform resections and anastomoses using the traditional inner layer of chromic catgut and outer layer of interrupted silk sutures, I think that in the trauma patient time must be of the essence. "Show me an operation that takes more than two hours or requires more than two units of blood, and I will demonstrate a surgical complication" is a quotation from Warren, one of the fathers of American surgery. Having once decided to perform the resection, I would now try to do it as expeditiously as possible. Isolating the bowel proximal and distal to the injury and using a GI stapler, the damaged bowel is now isolated. The mesentery can now be quickly controlled using isolated silk ties, so one is now soon ready for reanastomosis.

The quickest way is again to use the stapler. I usually place two holding sutures of 3-0 silk to keep the bowel together; use the scalpel to make two stab wounds into the proximal and distal segments and introduce the stapler into each limb. After firing and making sure that the anastomosis is patent, one can then close these small stab wounds with an additional application of a stapler - although I personally prefer interrupted sutures. I do not think a second layer is necessary. Interrupted sutures can then be used to close the mesentery and prevent an internal herniation.

I have found the small bowel to be extraordinarily forgiving, and providing one does not close it under tension or with any ischemia, small bowel leaks are uncommon. Thorough irrigation with warm saline and then closure of the abdomen without drain should complete the operation. In good hands, this should be completed in less than one hour. In healthy individuals, I always use a running suture to close the fascia, and this speeds up the closure.

TECHNICAL OPERATIVE PROCEDURES:

HOW I DO IT

Multiple Stab Wounds to Small Bowel

Blaine L. Enderson, MD, MBA, FACS, FCCM

Scenario

A 30-year-old man was stabbed in the abdomen and sustained six 1 cm stab wounds within three feet of each other in the proximal small bowel, combined with a hematoma in the mesentery.

Management

Indications for exploration of patients with stab wounds to the abdomen are often less clearcut than those with gunshot wounds, however, patients with hypotension, peritoneal signs, and evisceration must be explored. Prior to the incision, broad-spectrum antibiotics, such as a third generation cephalosporin must be given. This occurs more reliably if a protocol is established to give the antibiotics in the emergency department prior to moving to the operating room. The operating room should be prewarmed to help prevent hypothermia. The abdomen is explored through a generous midline incision to allow complete exploration.

Upon entering the abdomen, the priorities are: 1) control of hemorrhage; 2) control of contamination; 3) identification of all injuries; and 4) repair of all injuries. To control hemorrhage, all quadrants should be rapidly packed with laparotomy pads, and are then carefully removed to clear shed blood and examined systematically for active bleeding. The abdomen is examined to evaluate the path of the stab wound and to identify injuries to any organs. The bowel is evaluated from the ligament of Treitz to the ileocecal valve, controlling any injuries with Babcock clamps to prevent further contamination, until all injuries are identified. The colon must also be examined carefully.

> • If multiple wounds are involved in a short segment of bowel, it is quicker and safer to resect that portion of the bowel

Procedure:

Small bowel sutured repair

Attention is then turned to the mesenteric hematoma. If large, expanding, or obviously still bleeding, the mesentery should be opened to identify and ligate the bleeding vessels. If small it may be observed, although if it is near the bowel, it must be explored enough to ensure that there is not a hidden bowel injury. If exploration does not allow satisfactory control of the bleeding or obviously devascularizes a segment of bowel, the bowel and mesentery can be resected and a primary anastomosis performed.

Once the mesenteric hematoma is controlled, attention is returned to the bowel injuries. Stab wounds rarely require much débridement and usually can be closed primarily. With six holes over three feet of small bowel, I would try to preserve as much bowel as I could by primary repair. I close small bowel holes transversely with a single-layer running closure, with 3-0 silk sutures. The bites should be full thickness with a minimal amount of mucosa.

If multiple wounds involve a short segment of bowel, it is often quicker and safer to resect that portion of bowel with repair of only one or two of the holes. I use a linear cutting stapler to divide the bowel and to do the anastomosis. This can be done in the standard fashion, by transecting the bowel proximally and distally to the area of injury. After dividing the mesentery between clamps and ligating the vessels, the two ends of the bowel are anastomosed by inserting the linear cutter at the antimesenteric portion of each, firing it to create the functional end-to-end anastomosis and then using the stapler to close the defect in the bowel.

Procedure: *Damage control stapled resection*

An alternative method that I use in a damage control situation or when the segment is small is to pass one portion of the linear cutter in the proximal-most injury of the segment being resected and the distal-most injury, and stapling the two portions together. A second load of the stapler is then used to close the resulting defect and to transect some or all of the mesentery with removal and anastomosis of the injured segment in only two loads of the stapler, rather than four as above.

Upon completion of the anastomosis, the bowel is run again to ensure no missed injuries. The abdomen is irrigated with five to ten liters of warm saline to help with any residual contamination, and the abdomen is closed. Perioperative antibiotics should not be continued for more than 24 hours.

TECHNICAL OPERATIVE PROCEDURES:

HOW I DO IT

Distal Colorectal Irrigation

Lenworth M. Jacobs, MD, MPH, FACS

Scenario

A 37-year-old man presents with a penetrating injury from a gunshot wound to the rectosigmoid colon at the peritoneal floor with fecal spillage below the peritoneum in the presacral space.

Management

Immediate preoperative antibiotics to cover gram positive and gram negative organisms as well as bacteroides should be given. A generous midline incision allows for a complete exploratory laparotomy to identify any other injuries.

The injury to the rectosigmoid is identified by opening the pelvic peritoneum and delivering the distal sigmoid and proximal rectum into the wound. The full extent of the injury is identified and evaluated. The wound is débrided back to viable tissue and then a two-layer closure is performed using a continuous 3-0 absorbable suture for the mucosa followed by 3-0 interrupted silk sutures to the serosa. The pelvis is then irrigated with at least two liters of warm saline to remove any solid or liquid fecal material. The liberal use of saline irrigation reduces the bacterial colony count. A closed suction drain is placed in the most dependent part of the pelvis close to the wound.

If there is significant fecal spillage in the retroperitoneal space, a small transverse incision is made posterior to the anus and anterior to the coccyx and a finger introduced into the most dependent area of the presacral space. A presacral Penrose drain is then placed in this space and brought out through the incision in the perineum.

Procedure: *Distal colorectal irrigation*

There is a high likelihood that this wound will leak. For this reason, a diverting colostomy with irrigation of the distal section of the colorectum is indicated.

The proximal sigmoid colon is drawn up into the wound. The colon is then divided. The distal end of the colon is identified and a large Foley catheter with a 30 mL balloon is introduced into the colon. The balloon is then inflated to secure the catheter in the colon.

The lower part of the operating table is lowered to allow full access to the anus. The anus is dilated and clear anesthesia tubing is introduced into the anus and advanced for two to three inches. The corrugation of the tube allows it to be held in place by the anal sphincter. Saline is then injected through the Foley catheter with a 50 mL syringe. The contents of the colon can be observed through the clear anesthesia tubing. The irrigation is continued until clear saline is observed through the anesthesia tubing at the anus. The effluent is directed into a 2-liter bottle by the anesthesia tubing. This procedure elegantly contains all the fecal content and prevents fecal contamination of the operating room.

At the end of the irrigation, the distal end of the colon is brought up as a mucous fistula at the inferior aspect of the incision. The abdomen is then closed in layers. If there was severe fecal contamination and a significant risk of a wound infection, the skin should be left open. The proximal end of the colon is brought up through the abdominal wall and matured.

The mucous fistula can be used to perform a contrast study weeks or months later prior to considering closing the colostomy to verify that the rectosigmoid injury is completely healed.

- Rectosigmoid injury with infra-peritoneal presacral fecal spillage

- High likelihood of leakage and pelvic abscess

- Diverting colostomy

- Colonic irrigation

- Pelvic irrigation

- Contrast study prior to colostomy closure

Jacobs LM, Plaisier B: "An Efficient System for Controlled Distal Colorectal Irrigation", J of ACS, 178:305-306, 1994.

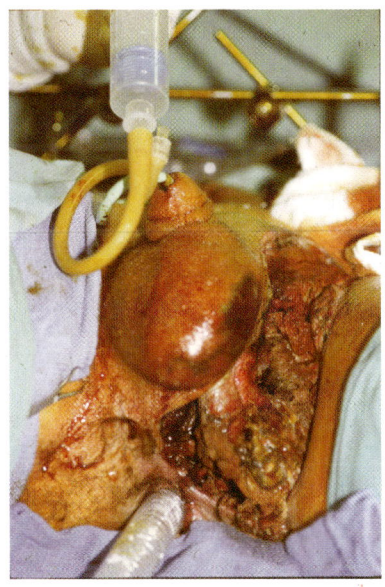
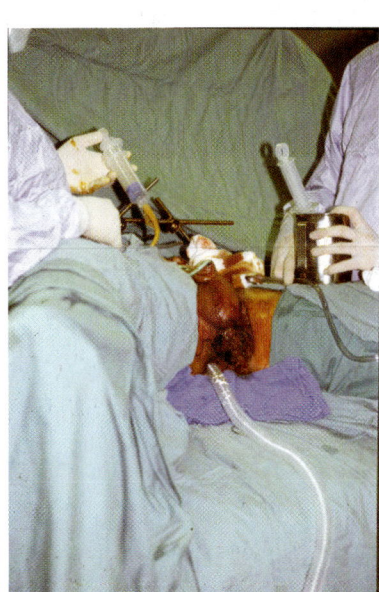
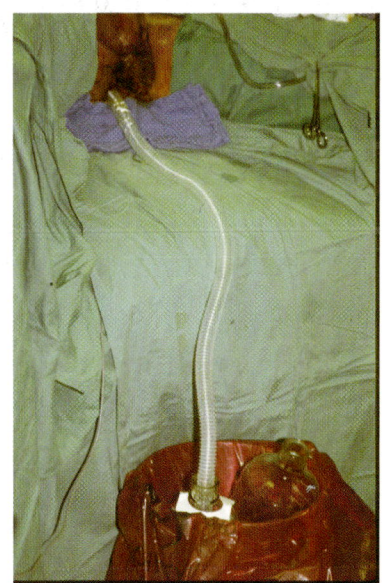

24 year-old male with an open pelvic fracture and perineal laceration.

TECHNICAL OPERATIVE PROCEDURES:

HOW I DO IT

Totally Diverting Loop Colostomy With Non-Contaminating Distal Irrigation

Kimball I. Maull MD, FACS

Scenario

A 26-year-old motorcyclist is struck by an oncoming vehicle as he attempts to make a left turn. He braces himself by extending his right leg and sustains a vertical shear pelvic fracture with a deep perineal laceration.

Management

Resuscitation is continued in the emergency unit and the perineal laceration is packed to control bleeding. On examination, the laceration is seen to enter the pelvic retroperitoneal space alongside the rectum for a distance of 10 cm to 12 cm. The anal sphincter appears intact. Fecal diversion is indicated.

- Loop sigmoid colostomy
- Flexible bridge
- Stapled colonic diversion
- Foley catheter through purse string
- Distal irrigation
- Active colostomy proximal to staple line

Procedure: *Totally diverting loop colostomy with non-contaminating distal irrigation*

The patient is placed in the modified lithotomy position on a fracture table and is draped to allow access to the perineum. An oblique left lower quadrant incision is made and a loop of sigmoid colon is brought through. A small defect is made in the sigmoid mesentery and a flexible plastic bridge is passed and sutured to the skin. Using absorbable 3-0 sutures, the exteriorized segment is fastened to the peritoneum and external fascia. A standard non-cutting stapler is passed through the mesenteric defect and the colon is stapled, thereby interrupting flow of bowel contents into the distal segment.

A purse string suture is placed in the distal loop, a stab incision is made and a 18 Fr. irrigating catheter is passed into the distal lumen. Traction is held on the purse string suture to prevent reflux of luminal contents. The assistant between the patient's legs dilates the anus and carefully inserts a retractor, providing egress for rectal contents. Washouts are begun via the irrigating catheter and continued until clear. The irrigating catheter is removed and the purse string suture is tied securely. The colostomy can be opened immediately or delayed, allowing the stomal site to seal. To complete the colostomy, the colonic lumen is entered proximal to the staple line, resulting in a totally diverting loop colostomy.

Reference

Sachatello CR, Maull KI: Rapid Totally Diverting Loop Sigmoid Colostomy with Noncontaminating Rectal Irrigation. Am J Surg 134:300, 1977.

- The incision for stoma site may be placed higher on the abdominal wall if an external fixation device is to be used

- When closing the colostomy, it is essential to confirm the presence of the staple line in the resected stomal segment

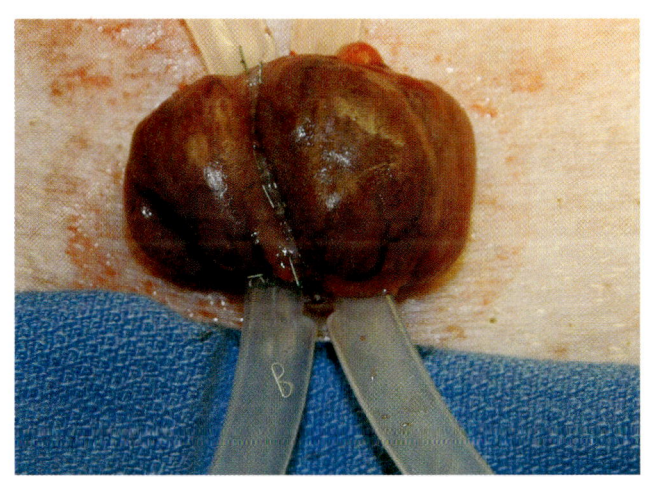
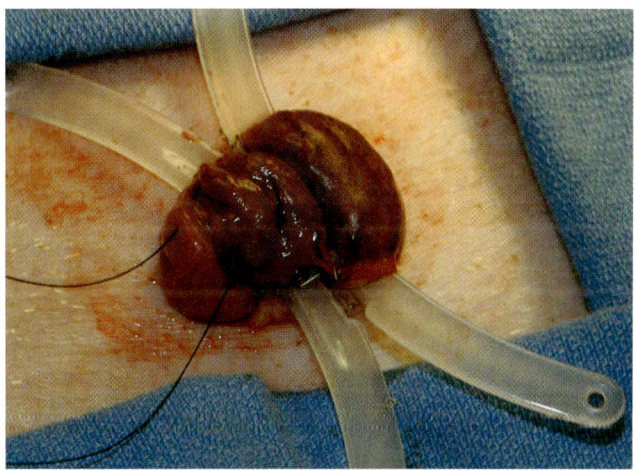
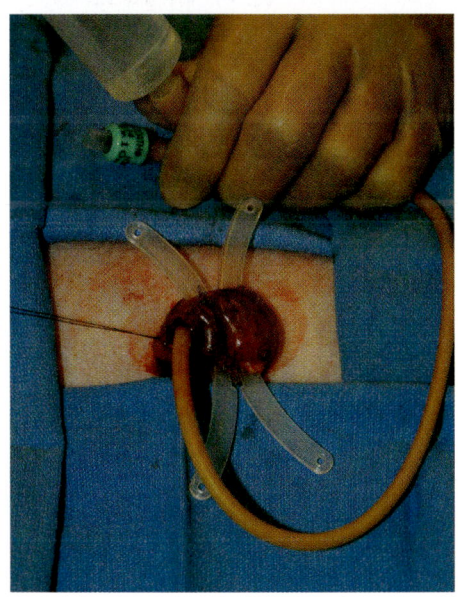
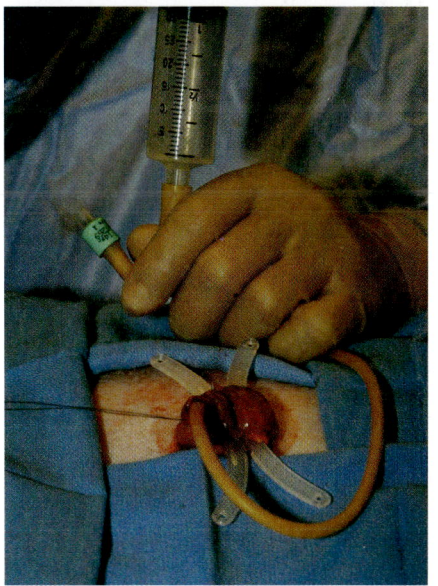

TECHNICAL OPERATIVE PROCEDURES:

HOW I DO IT

Damage Control of the Abdomen with Penetrating Injury

C. William Schwab, MD, FACS

The experience with damage control of the abdomen with penetrating injury in the early 1990's afforded us an opportunity to make just about every judgment about closing the abdomen. In those days, we sought to close the abdomen at damage control laparotomy, or at the end of the first operation in the abdomen. What we failed to recognize is that reperfusion injury of the bowel and viscera is a dynamic process and goes on for 8 to 24 hours after the initial exsanguinating event. We attempted to close the abdomen initially by forcing the fascia together or using plastic to create synthetic silos.

- Leave the abdomen open in damage control surgery

- Look horizontally across the patient's abdomen. If any bowel is visible leave the abdomen open

- Bladder pressures are continuously displayed

- Integrate all data on the patient into the decision to leave the abdomen open

This technique resulted in loss of fascia and at times terrible infection with foreign bodies, and overall more open abdomens. Upon recognizing the problem of the dynamic abdomen leading to increased abdominal pressure and abdominal compartment syndrome, we chose to leave all abdomens open if we performed a damage control laparotomy. One of the best measures that I have used to prove this principle to trainees is to have them back away from the operating room table and look horizontally across the patient, particularly the abdomen. If any bowel is visible above the fascia, we make the point that in the next few hours that bowel and visceral edema will protrude those organs another two to six inches above and out of the abdomen. Most times the viscera and the bowel are already well above the skin level with the abdominal opening made by the incision, representing a wide fish mouth, diverting skin and subcutaneous fat. Therefore, we have made it our practice to leave all damage control laparotomies open initially followed by use of some form of vac-pack dressing.

In the intensive care unit, we routinely measure vital signs, peak and plateau inspiratory pressures, bladder pressure and urinary output. Bladder pressure is constantly displayed on an electronic monitor as routinely measured via a

Foley catheter. Although bladder pressure is one of the key determinants for detection of abdominal compartment syndrome, it is not the only one. My most important clinical trick is to watch the overall picture of the patient and integrate all the numbers listed above. Clinically, I have found people with relatively low bladder pressures that have all of the physiologic manifestations of abdominal compartment syndrome. Lastly, a patient with an abnormal bladder may exhibit a false high or low bladder pressure. This is something commonly seen when there is primary injury to the bladder, with repair of the bladder, and with placement of suprapubic tubes. In those cases bladder pressure should be considered inaccurate and other parameters and the overall clinical picture closely watched.

TECHNICAL OPERATIVE PROCEDURES:

HOW I DO IT

Measurement of Intraabdominal Pressure

Marc D. Palter, MD

Scenario

A young male involved in a motor vehicle crash presents with severe hypotension. He is taken to the operating room where multiple intraabdominal injuries are found and addressed. At the time of closure he is hypothermic and diffusely oozing from a coagulopathy, but is easily closed. He requires ongoing resuscitation with large volumes of crystalloid and blood products in the intensive care unit. He is initially rewarmed and becomes hemodynamically stable. However, several hours later he becomes difficult to ventilate with minimal urine output.

Management

Any patient with major visceral or vascular injuries who received massive resuscitation should be considered at risk for development of the abdominal compartment syndrome. These patients will often have continued capillary ooze because of a multifactorial clotting deficiency and progressive retroperitoneal and visceral edema. It may have been difficult to obtain tension-free closure of the abdomen in these patients at the conclusion of their operative procedure. Patients who have undergone damage control laparotomies are especially at high risk if their abdomens are closed primarily. Furthermore, certain nonoperated patients resuscitated from profound shock are also at high risk for developing this syndrome.

Elevated intraabdominal pressure has serious physiologic consequences. The patients typically have a tensely distended abdomen. The intraabdominal hypertension initially affects pulmonary function by compromising ventilation and causing a significant rise in peak airway pressure. The patient develops severe, acute hypercarbia and respiratory acidosis. Increased levels of ventilatory support may be only temporarily effective in compensating for the deteriorating pulmonary function.

Pressure on the inferior vena cava will lead to decreased venous return and a fall in cardiac output. Cardiac function will be further compromised from the increased afterload caused by the intraabdominal

- The Foley catheter is an excellent way to measure intraabdominal pressure

- An arterial transducer is used to measure pressure

- The anterior surface of the pubis is the zero point

hypertension. Inotropic agents and further volume resuscitation will often have only transitory improvement in hemodynamics.

Renal dysfunction is manifest by initial oliguria which is followed by anuria. Elevated intraabdominal pressure causes decreased renal artery flow leading to a falling glomerular filtration rate. Placement of ureteral stents in an attempt to bypass obstruction of the ureters secondary to direct compression is not useful.

There is no definitive critical value for elevated intraabdominal pressure. Significant organ dysfunction has been observed with intra-abdominal pressures ranging from 15 to 40 mmHg. The decision to surgically decompress the abdomen should be based on the clinical presentation of ventilatory difficulty and oliguria rather than any absolute number. The measurement of intraabdominal pressure helps to confirm the diagnosis and helps to establish the effectiveness of any decompressive procedure in relieving intra-abdominal hypertension. One of the various techniques for temporary abdominal wall closure should be utilized.

Procedure: *Measurement of intraabdominal pressure*

The gold standard method for measuring intraabdominal pressure uses the patient's indwelling Foley catheter. The tubing of the drainage bag is clamped a few centimeters distal to the aspiration port of the catheter. One hundred mL of sterile saline is injected into the bladder via the aspiration port. The tubing is unclamped just enough to allow for the fluid to flow just past the point of the clamp and then reclamped. Since these are typically intensive care unit patients, an arterial pressure transducer setup can be used to measure the pressure. An 18 to 19 gauge needle is connected to the end of the pressure transducer tubing and inserted into the aspiration port. The anterior surface of the pubis can be used as the zero point.

Reference

Palter, MD, Cortes, V: Secondary Triage of the Trauma Patient. In: *Critical Care Medicine*, Civetta JM, Taylor RW, Kirby RR eds., Lippincott-Raven, Philadelphia, 1997:1053.

TECHNICAL OPERATIVE PROCEDURES:

HOW I DO IT

The Browner Pelvic Stabilizer

Bruce D. Browner, MD, FACS

Scenario

A 32-year-old male was involved in a motor vehicle crash and was transported to the trauma center in shock with a blood pressure of <90 systolic. The field personnel have noted a tender compressible pelvis. There were no MAST trousers available for compression and splinting, so the patient was transported on a long backboard.

Management

In the emergency center, the presence of an externally rotated or vertically displaced, externally rotated pelvic ring disruption must be confirmed by an AP screening x-ray, to cause the patient to be a candidate for mechanical reduction and stabilization of the pelvic ring disruption by the application of the pelvic stabilizer. Other fracture patterns including undisplaced, lateral compression, acetabular, and pelvic wing fractures are not appropriate for mechanical compression.

Ninety percent of patients with hemorrhage associated with pelvic ring disruption have torn veins as the primary source of bleeding. Early reduction of the intrapelvic volume via mechanical compression will tamponade the venous bleeding by compression of the pelvic hematoma. Stabilization of the mobile hemipelvis will reduce pain and promote hemostasis.

> Reduction of intrapelvic volume via mechanical compression will tamponade venous bleeding

Following application of the pelvic stabilizer, hemodynamic parameters should improve if torn veins are the primary source of bleeding. If the patient remains hemodynamically unstable requiring massive transfusion, this may be an indication that the source of pelvic bleeding is an injured artery. In these instances, the patient should receive emergent selective pelvic angiography and embolization.

Procedure:
Browner external pelvic clamp

For maximum benefit, the pelvic stabilizer should be applied within the first hour of admission to the emergency center. In the majority of cases, an anterior site just above the acetabulum can be selected for application of the stabilizer pins. This site is located by imagining a line, which extends

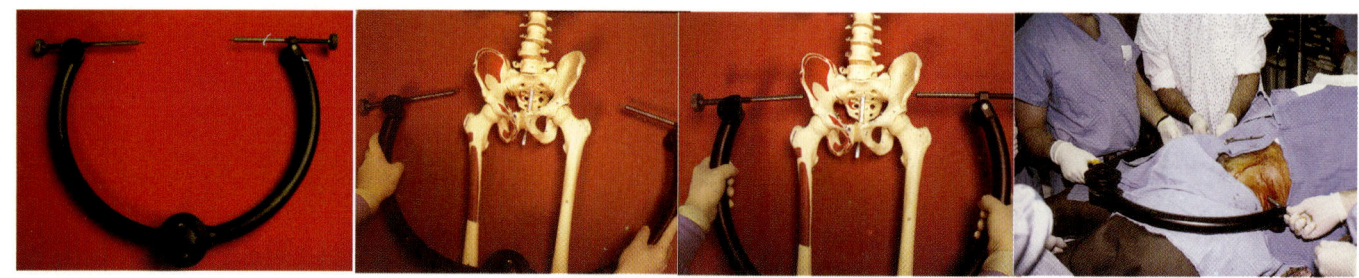

for a point three fingerbreadths posterior to the anterior superior spine of the pelvis to the tip of the greater trochanter. The site for pin insertion is at the center of this line. This point is just above the acetabulum in a dense area of bone, which will resist pin penetration. In certain instances such as associated anterior column acetabular fractures or anterior skin wounds, a posterior site for pin insertion should be selected which lays over the sacro-iliac joints. The sciatic notch and superior pelvic rim should be avoided.

The device can be applied without C-arm control. Local anesthetic is used after identification and preparation of the intended pin sites. The skin and deeper tissues are infiltrated with 2% Xylocaine. Two centimeter incisions are made and extended down to the bone by blunt dissection with a Kelly clamp.

When vertical displacement is part of the pelvic injury pattern, manual longitudinal traction is utilized to reduce the vertical component. External rotation of the pelvis is reduced by application of the stabilizer. The ratchet gear in the center of the stabilizer is disengaged to allow the device to be opened. Sterile pins are then inserted in the pin holders. The clamp is then brought together so that the pins enter the incisions and the spiked pin tips come up against the outer cortex of the pelvis on both sides. As the device is closed down, the ratchet gear will allow only compression. Using the knobs at the ends of the tubular arms the alignment of the pins should be adjusted so that they come to lie along a single axis. This will decrease the likelihood of pin disengagement. Final compression is achieved by tightening the knobs on the pin holders on either side. Compression is continued until a firm end point of reduction is achieved. Radiographic confirmation can then be obtained to assess the reduction.

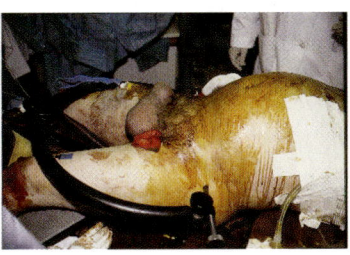

The device can be rotated from the thighs to the chest to allow access to the abdomen or the perineum

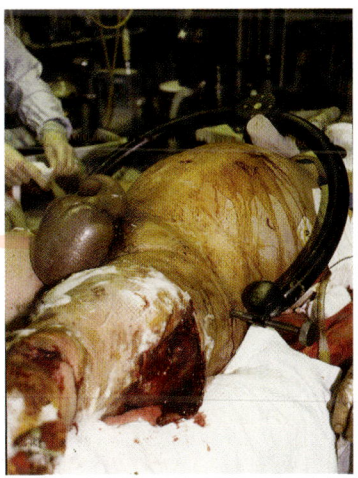

The device can be rotated from the thighs to a position across the chest to allow access to the perineum or to place the hips in the lithotomy position. The device is intended to provide temporary pelvic stabilization. It may be necessary to keep it in place for several weeks until the patient's condition permits definitive internal and/or external fixation of the pelvic ring injury.

Reference

Buckle RM, Browner BD, Morandi M: Emergency Reduction for Pelvic Ring Disruptions and Control of Associated Hemorrhage Using the Pelvic Stabilizer. Techniques in Orthopaedics Vol. 9, No. 4, 1994.

TECHNICAL OPERATIVE PROCEDURES:
HOW I DO IT

Coagulation Sandwich

Lenworth M. Jacobs, MD, MPH, FACS

Scenario
A 34-year-old man was involved in a motor vehicle crash where he sustained blunt trauma to the right side of his chest and abdomen. He was hypotensive and had a tender, distended abdomen.

Management
The patient was rapidly resuscitated with two large 14 gauge intravenous lines. He was transfused with crystalloid and type specific blood. A chest x-ray showed no hemopneumothorax and a FAST examination showed free blood in the abdomen and a significant liver injury to the right lobe. The patient became hypotensive to 60 systolic and his abdomen continued to distend. He was taken directly to the operating suite. An exploratory laparotomy was performed using a midline incision. All four quadrants of the abdomen were packed with laparotomy packs. A stellate tear of the right lobe of the liver was found to be oozing.

Procedure:
Hemostatic coagulation sandwich

Abdominal laparotomy packs are placed above and below the right lobe of the liver. A hand is placed on either pack and primary manual pressure is applied for five minutes by the clock. This procedure controlled the bleeding. On removal of the packs some oozing from the lacerated parenchyma of the right lobe of the liver is noted.

This type of bleeding is an indication for a local hemostatic agent. The Hemostatic Coagulation Sandwich is a useful adjunct in this situation. A two-inch by four-inch Gelfoam patch is placed on a surgical towel. A bottle of Avitene powder (microcrystalline collagen) is emptied onto the Gelfoam sheet.

The handle of a scalpel is used to spread the Avitene over the surface of the Gelfoam. A vial of thrombin is then emptied onto the Avitene. The surface should be

- The bleeding surface should be dried with a pack

- Place the sandwich face down on the wound

- Mold into the crevices

- Primary pressure for five minutes

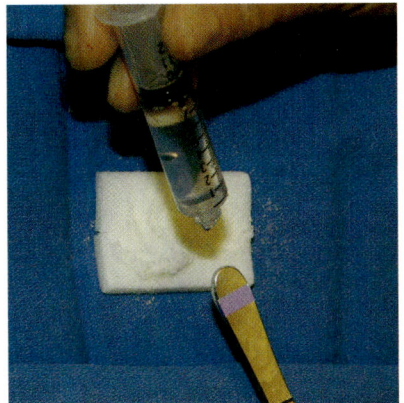 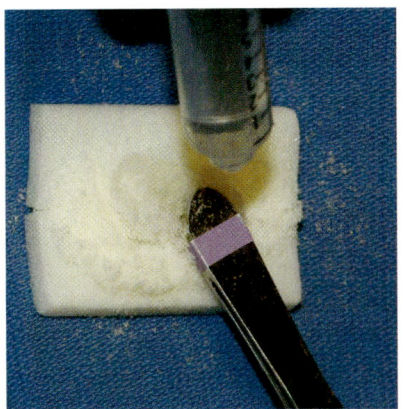 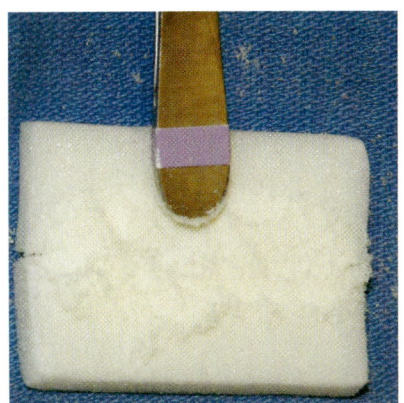

dried with a laparotomy pack immediately before the Gelfoam/Avitene/thrombin pack is pressed and molded to the parenchyma of the liver. This sandwich is now placed face down onto the oozing surface. The thrombin moistened Avitene allows the coagulating mixture to be applied directly to the surface and the firm consistency of the Gelfoam traps the coagulant on the parenchyma and promotes maximal coagulation.

An abdominal laparotomy pack is then placed on the back of the Gelfoam and continuous primary digital pressure is applied for five minutes by the clock. At the end of this period of time, the laparotomy pack is gently peeled off of the Gelfoam leaving the coagulation sandwich densely adhered to the liver parenchyma. The surface is inspected to be sure that oozing has stopped. If there are small areas which need further coagulation, another sandwich is applied. The sandwich is then left in place and the abdomen is closed.

TECHNICAL OPERATIVE PROCEDURES:

HOW I DO IT

Topical Hemostatic Agents in Trauma

Jameel Ali, MD, FACS

Before considering topical hemostatic agents one must ensure that the bleeding is not from major vascular disruption or a diffuse systemic process. Major vascular disruption requires direct surgical control. In diffuse bleeding such as occurs in the coagulopathic patient from massive transfusions, acidosis and hypothermia, the mainstay of hemorrhage control is packing and the institution of damage control techniques. After stabilization in the intensive care unit where normothermia is achieved as well as the control of coagulopathy by the use of fresh frozen plasma, and platelets, and specific factors including recombinant factor VIIA, the patient is then returned to the operating room for more definitive management.

Topical hemostatic agents are most useful in controlling local bleeding from raw peritoneal surfaces, on the surface of solid organs such as the liver, spleen, kidney or pancreas.

Management

Achieving as dry a field as possible is important by suction, adequate exposure, electrocoagulation and the application of packing and gentle pressure for 10 to 15 minutes. The packing is then slowly removed and if there is no further bleeding then no further action is required. If there is still localized bleeding after removal of appropriately placed packs the use of topical hemostatic agents is indicated.

The use of techniques such as high frequency coagulation and argon beam coagulation are very effective topical hemostatic agents. In most instances, however, I use Surgicel, Gelfoam, Avitene (microfibrillar collagen) or fibrin glue, alone or in combination.

Procedure: *Smooth surface*

If the bleeding arises from a raw surface without crevices or cavities I cover the surface with a sheet of Surgicel large enough to cover the entire area and then apply a

- Achieving a dry field is important

- Packing and gently apply pressure for 10 to 15 minutes

- Generous portions of Gelfoam wrapped in Surgicel are effective in crevices

- Fibrin glue is very effective for raw surfaces

dry abdominal pack for 10 to 15 minutes. The pack is then gently removed and if the bleeding has stopped then there is no further action required.

Irregular Wounds

When the bleeding arises from a crevice or a cavity, I will use generous portions of Gelfoam wrapped in Surgicel to pack the wound tightly and apply pressure with an abdominal pack for 10 to 15 minutes. It is important to remove the abdominal pack very gently so that in the process of withdrawing the pack the Surgicel or Gelfoam does not become dislodged.

I have also found Avitene to be very effective in controlling hemorrhage from crevices and cavities but this material is much more difficult to handle without spillage. To decrease spillage from the crevice or cavity, I usually cover the material with a layer of Surgicel and then also apply gentle pressure with abdominal packs for 10-15 minutes after which the sponges are again removed. The use of the Surgicel also prevents adherence of Avitene to the sponge and prevents its dislodgement when the sponge is removed.

I have found fibrin glue to be very effective for localized bleeding from a large raw surface such as the resected edge of the liver, raw surface of a partial splenectomy, partial nephrectomy or pancreatectomy. The main disadvantages are the time for preparation, cost and the reported risk of severe hypersensitivity reactions. When I use this agent, I use generous amounts to cover the entire bleeding surface and avoid immediately applying sponges over the surface until the agent becomes adherent and solidified over the bleeding surface.

TECHNICAL OPERATIVE PROCEDURES:

HOW I DO IT

A FAST Examination for Thoracoabdominal Injuries

Grace S. Rozycki, MD, RDMS, FACS

Scenario

A 19-year-old construction worker fell 30 feet. He presents to the emergency department hemodynamically normal but with a respiratory rate of 18 and pain in his left thoracoabdominal area.

Management

Assessment of the patient's airway, breathing, and circulation are intact. While 2 liters of lactated Ringer's solution is infused, appropriate blood work including a blood sample for type and cross match are sent to the laboratory. The secondary survey is initiated and the surgeon performs the FAST examination.

Procedure: *Focused abdominal sonogram in trauma (FAST)*

Using the machine's annotation keys, the patient's name and identification number are recorded. Most machines have function keys that automate the recording of these data. Furthermore, the internal clock automatically labels each image with the date and time to one-hundredth of a second.

Developed for the evaluation of injured patients, the FAST is a rapid diagnostic test for assessing patients with potential truncal injuries. It surveys for blood in the pericardial sac and three dependent abdominal regions including Morison's pouch, the splenorenal recess, and the pelvis. The examination is performed during the American College of Surgeons Advanced Trauma Life Support secondary survey while the patient is in the supine position.

With the thoraco-abdominal area exposed, water-soluble ultrasound transmission gel is applied on the abdomen in four specific areas. A focused, limited examination for the detection of blood in dependent regions is conducted in sequence as follows: (1) pericardial area, (2) right upper abdominal quadrant, (3) left upper abdominal quadrant, and (4) Pouch of Douglas (Figure 1).

The transducer is oriented for sagittal sections and placed in the subxiphoid region. The pericardial region is visualized first so that the blood within the heart can be used as a standard to set the gain.

> • Excellent method of detecting blood in the pericardial sac and the three dependent areas of the abdomen

The subxiphoid approach through the longitudinal axis is used to identify the heart and examine for blood in the pericardial region. The normal examination of the heart is demonstrated in Figure 2A. The abnormal examination, with the arrow indicating hemopericardium, is demonstrated in Figure 2B.

The transducer is then placed in the right mid-axillary line region between the eleventh and twelfth ribs to identify the liver, kidney, and diaphragm and to examine for blood in Morison's pouch. The normal sagittal section demonstrating liver, diaphragm, and kidney is noted in Figure 3A and the abnormal section with fluid in Morison's pouch is shown in Figure 3B.

Next, the transducer is positioned on the left posterior axillary line between the tenth and eleventh ribs to visualize the spleen and kidney and to seek blood in the space between these organs and posterior to the spleen. The normal spleen and kidney are noted in Figure 4A and the abnormal examination, with fluid in the spleno-renal recess, is shown in Figure 4B.

The transducer is then oriented for transverse sections and placed midline approximately 4 cm superior to the symphysis pubis. The normal examination demonstrates the full bladder as an anechoic structure in Figure 5A and the abnormal examination demonstrates the bladder with surrounding hematomas as noted in Figure 5B. Required hard copies of the ultrasound images should be printed, saved and reviewed.

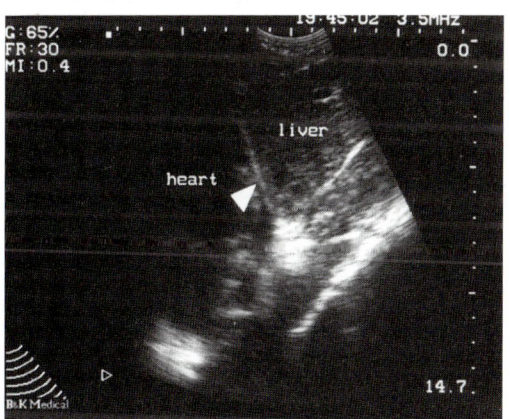

2A

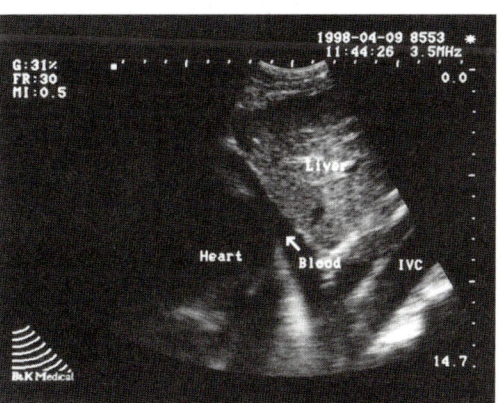

2B

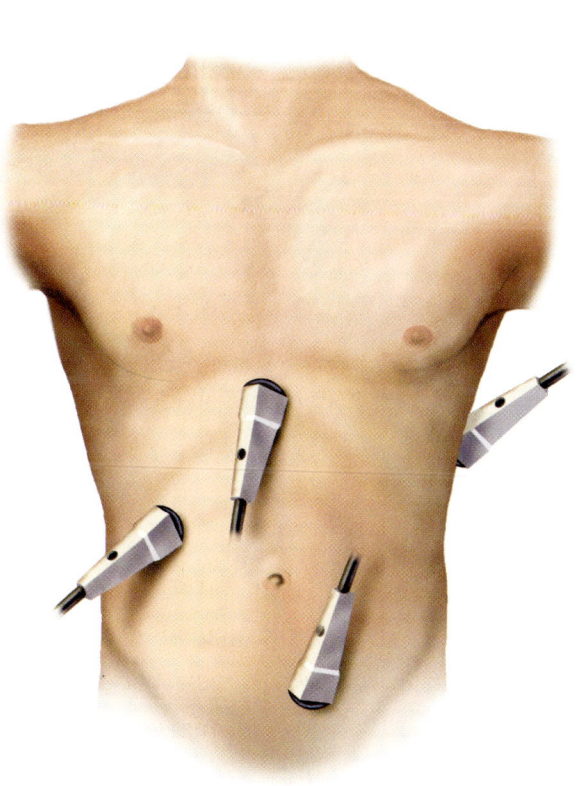

Figure 1

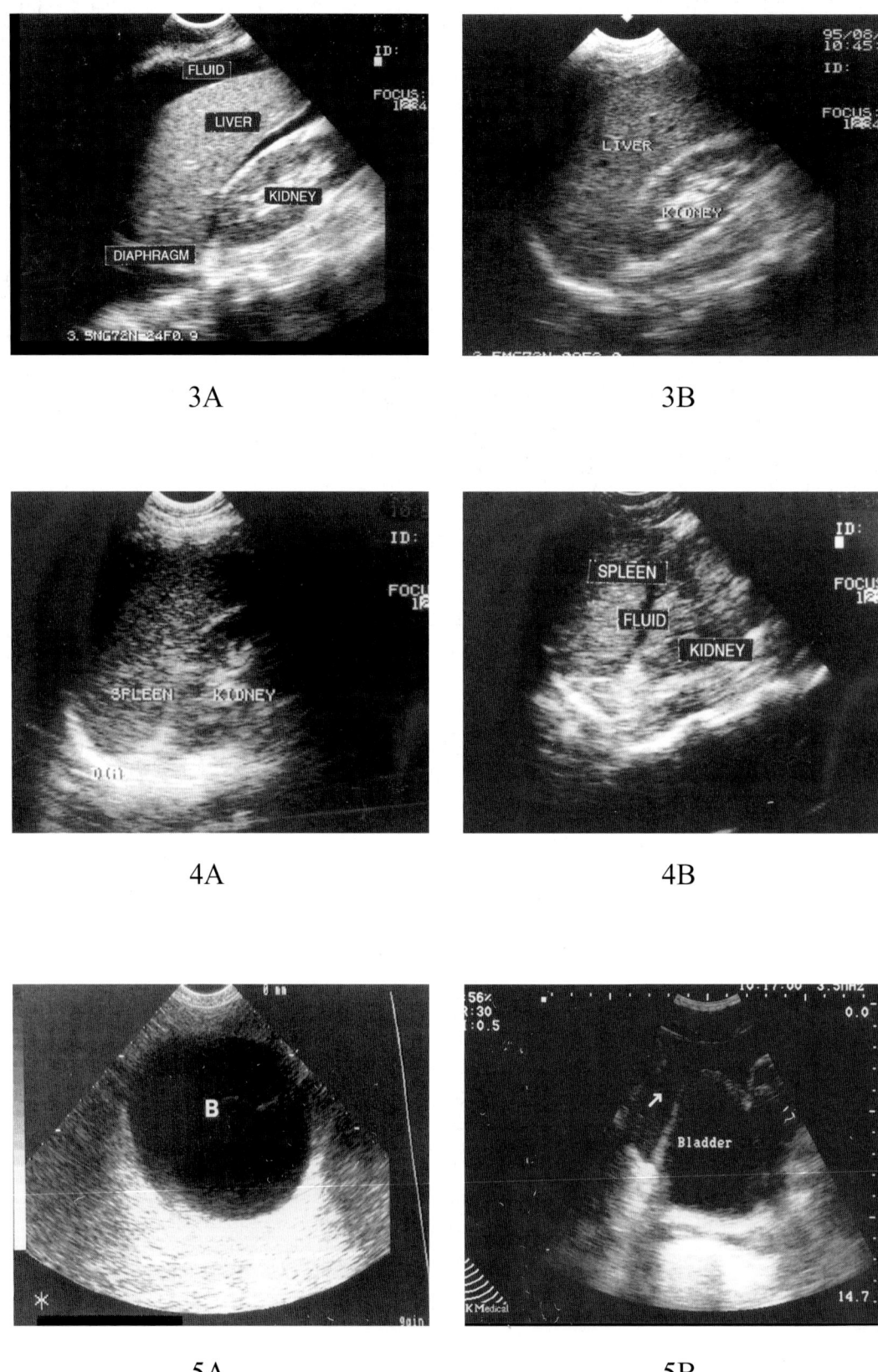

3A

3B

4A

4B

5A

5B

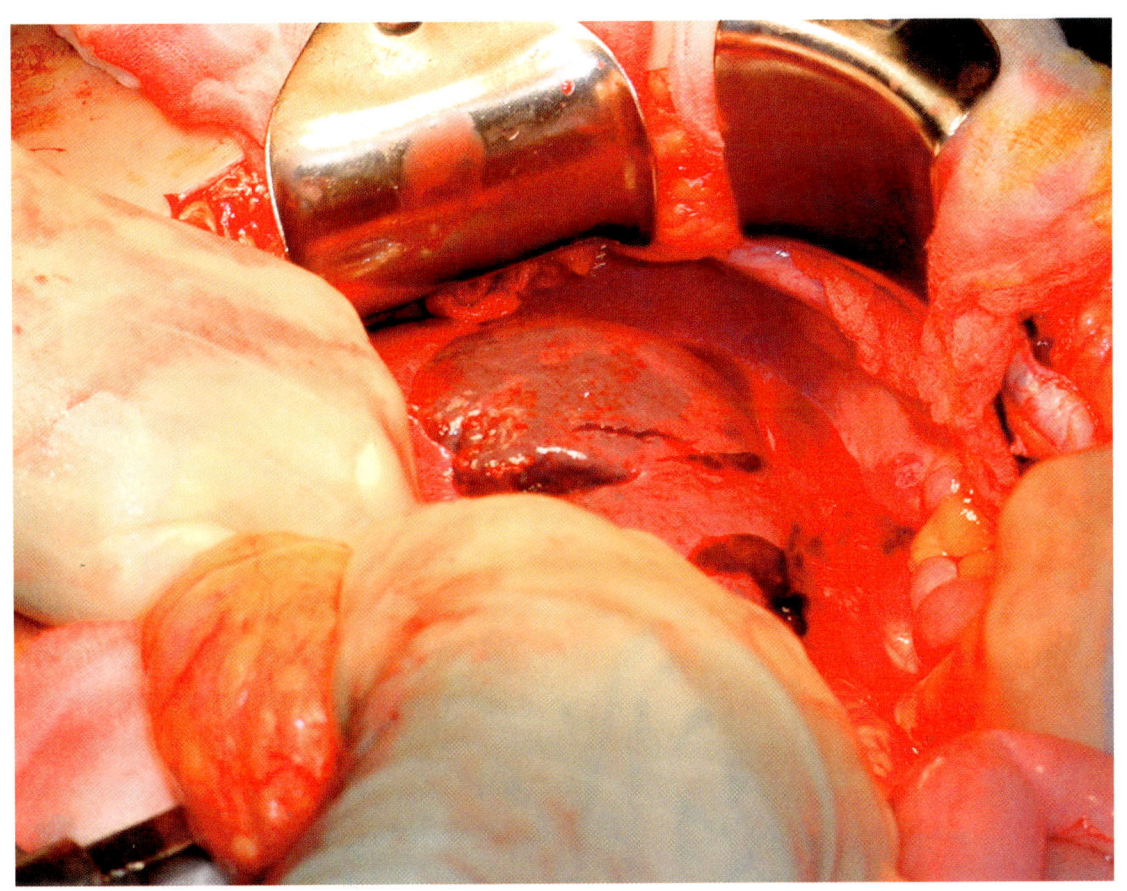

The Spleen & Diaphragm

Nonoperative Management

Improved understanding of the spleen's immunogenic properties prompted attempts at nonoperative and conservative management of splenic injuries in the pediatric population. Increased rates of splenic salvage in this group have led to the use of a similar approach in the adult population.

Splenic salvage is successful in 85% to 95% of hemodynamically stable patients with nonoperatively managed splenic injuries. However, it is successful in only 40% of patients who undergo immediate surgical intervention.

Nonoperative Management

- Increased salvage rate:
  85 to 95% with observation
  40% with immediate operation

- Balance:
  risk of bleeding (and transfusion)
  vs.
  morbidity of increased splenectomy rate

The surgeon must weigh the risks versus the benefits of splenic salvage and nonoperative therapy. The most significant risk is the potential for failure of conservative management, as indicated by recurrent or continued bleeding, and hemodynamic instability of the injured patient. In addition, it is well understood that transfusions are not without risk. Transfused patients are exposed to the risk of transmitted disease processes, immunologic compromise, and increased morbidity. However, the benefits of conservative therapy and splenic salvage include lowered morbidity rates resulting from the nonoperative approach, maintenance of the immunogenic capacities of the spleen, and prevention of the increased risk for overwhelming postsplenectomy sepsis (OPSS), a syndrome seen in a small percentage of splenectomized patients.

Indications for Operative Management: Pre-op Diagnosis

Spleen

Appropriate patient selection determines the success of nonoperative management of splenic injury. Inappropriate candidates for nonoperative therapy include trauma patients who are hemodynamically unstable as a result of splenic injury and patients with moderate or severe traumatic brain injury, in whom any episode of hypotension might result in secondary brain injury. Due to ongoing blood loss from the injured spleen, candidates for nonoperative therapy will occasionally require blood transfusions to maintain an adequate hematocrit.

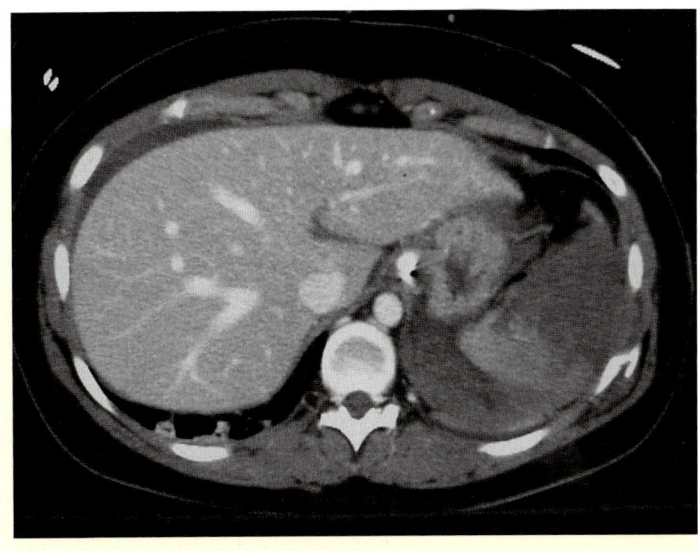

Pre-op Diagnosis

- Hemodynamic instability
- Moderate or severe traumatic brain injury
- Transfusion threshold met
- CT with high grade injury or contrast extravasation
  - possible angiography

Failure of nonoperative management is indicated when the maximum number of units of blood has been transfused to a patient. Although an exact number of maximum units has not been universally agreed upon, the maximum allowable number of transfusions must be established when the decision to manage a patient conservatively has been made. The patient should be moved to the operating room when this number has been exceeded.

In the past, patients with high-grade injury or contrast extravasation on a CT scan have gone directly to the operating room. Today, angiographic embolization for splenic salvage might be attempted if angiography is available and the patient is hemodynamically stable. However, in the presence of high-grade injury and contrast blush when angiography is not available, patients should be taken to the operating room for intraoperative attempts at splenic salvage, regardless of their hemodynamic stability.

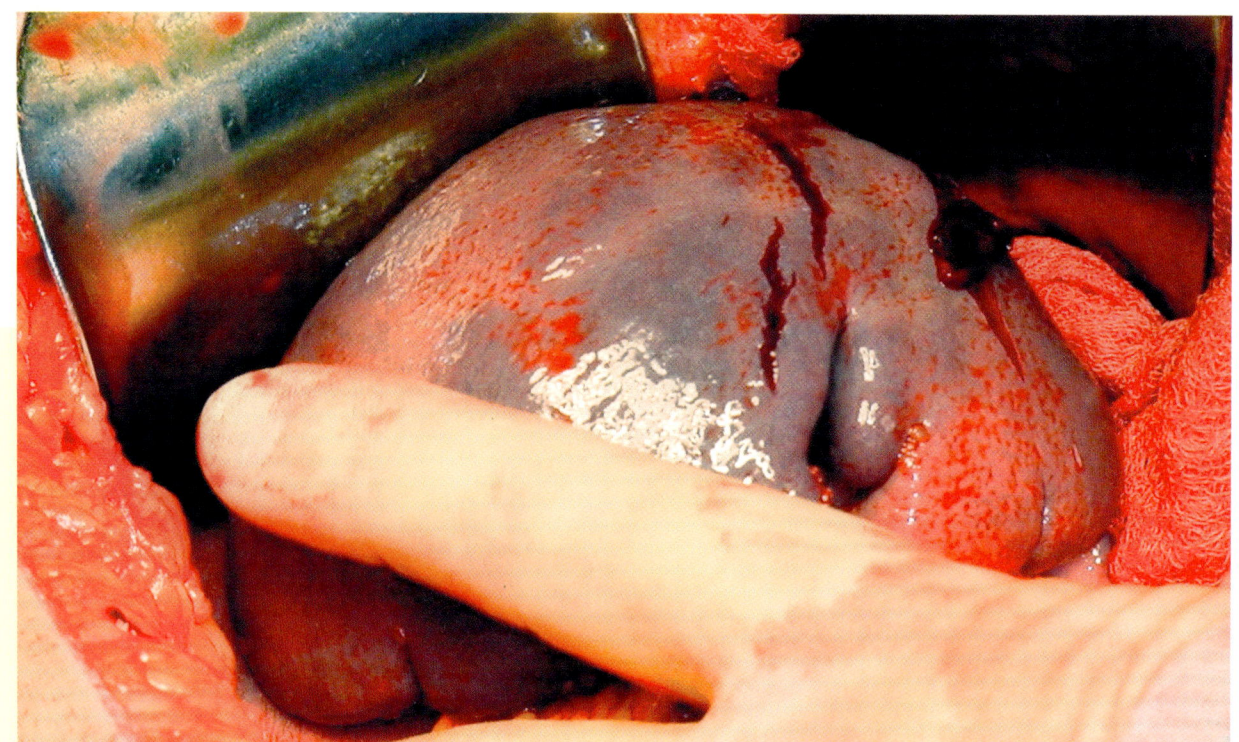

Intra-op Diagnosis

- Moderate or severe traumatic brain injury

- Actively bleeding or devascularized spleen

- Coexisting injury at high risk for hemorrhage

- Coagulopathy

Indications for Operative Management: Intra-op Diagnosis

Operative management for splenic injury is also an option when injury is diagnosed at the time of a celiotomy being performed for other injuries. Splenectomy should be seriously considered for patients who have a moderate-to-severe brain injury and active bleeding from the spleen, have a devascularized spleen and co-existing injuries that put them at high risk for hemorrhage, or are in a coagulopathic state at the time of surgery. The likelihood of splenic salvage is low in these patients. The time needed to try to control splenic bleeding is not justified, and a splenectomy should be performed instead.

Injury Grading

The Organ Injury Scale of the American Association for the Surgery of Trauma (AAST-OIS) is the most commonly used system for grading splenic injury. The AAST-OIS, which is also used for other organ systems, provides a consistent means of comparison for clinical description and decision making with respect to the management of the injured spleen. It is also the most useful tool for comparing splenic injuries in research. The scale assigns a grade, from I to V, to splenic injury based on CT findings. It is important to remember that the grade of injury can change to either a higher or a lesser grade if the patient is taken to the operating room and the spleen is directly visualized.

Injury Grading

American Association for the Surgery of Trauma - Organ Injury Scale (AAST-OIS)

- Most commonly used system

- Means of consistent comparison for clinical description / decision making and research

- Grade I to Grade V

- Based on CT or intraoperative findings

Low Grade

Grade I splenic injuries are injuries with subcapsular hematomas that occupy less than 10% of the surface area of the spleen, or lacerations and capsular tears that involve less than 1 cm of the parenchyma. Nonoperative therapy should always be attempted in a hemodynamically stable patient with no evidence of active bleeding.

Grade II splenic injuries are characterized by a subcapsular hematoma occupying between 10% and 50% of the surface area of the spleen, an intraparenchymal hematoma smaller than 5 cm, or a 1 cm to 3 cm splenic laceration showing no vessel involvement. As with Grade I injuries, patients with Grade II splenic injuries are managed with nonoperative therapy if they are hemodynamically stable with no evidence of active bleeding.

Low Grade

Grade I:
Subcapsular hematoma < 10% surface area
Laceration/Capsular tear < 1 cm deep

Therapy: non-operative if stable and not bleeding

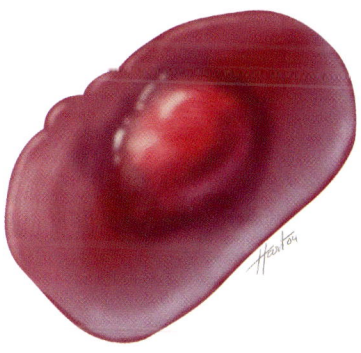

Grade II :
Subcapsular hematoma 10 to 50% surface area
Intra-parenchymal hematoma < 5 cm
Laceration 1-3 cm without vessel involvement

Therapy: nonoperative if stable and not bleeding

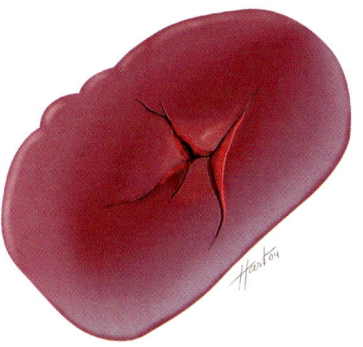

Moderate Grade

Grade III :
Subcapsular hematoma > 50% surface area or expanding.
Intraparenchymal hematoma.
> 5 cm Ruptured hematoma.
Laceration > 3 cm or with trabecular vessel involvement.

Therapy:
Observation
Surgery
Angiography

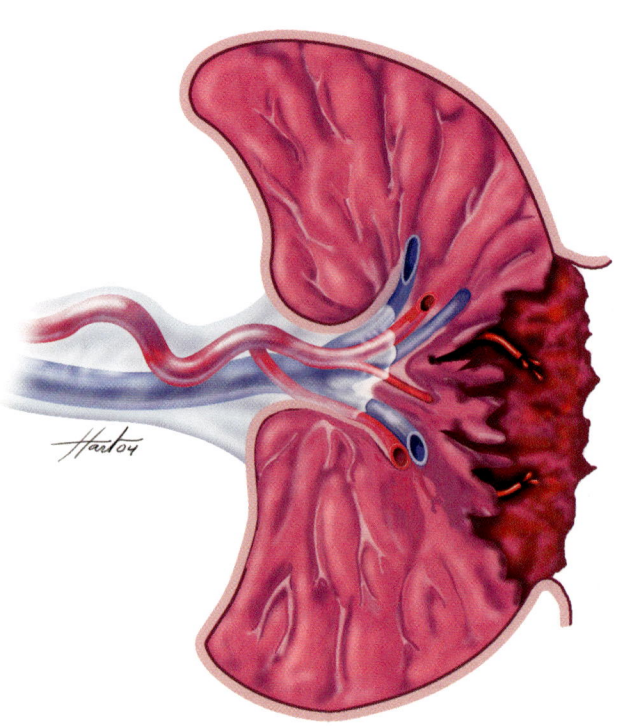

Moderate Grade

Grade III splenic injuries are more serious and more likely to have ongoing blood loss than Grade I and Grade II splenic injuries. Grade III splenic injuries are characterized by subcapsular hematomas that occupy more than 50% of the surface area of the spleen or are expanding, have an intraparenchymal hematoma larger than 5 cm, have a ruptured hematoma, or have lacerations larger than 3 cm into the parenchyma with trabecular vessel involvement. These injuries are frequently found to have a contrast blush on abdominal CT scan.

Unlike the patient with a Grade I or Grade II injury, a patient with a Grade III injury should be admitted to a monitored bed, preferably in the intensive care unit, although a step-down unit bed is acceptable. Constant hemodynamic monitoring and frequent monitoring of hemoglobin and hematocrit levels are essential. If the patient requires transfusions, it is important to determine the transfusion threshold above which the patient will be taken to the operating room when the decision for nonoperative therapy has been made. This threshold must not be exceeded.

Patients with contrast blush on the initial CT scan should be considered for angiography and embolization of the involved vessel. This may improve the chances for successful nonoperative management. Splenic salvage should be attempted intraoperatively if angiography is not available.

High Grade

Grade IV and Grade V injuries to the spleen involve splenic lacerations. A Grade IV splenic laceration is characterized by the laceration of segmental or hilar vessels that results in the devascularization of more than 25% of the splenic parenchyma.

Although splenic conservation may be possible for some patients with Grade IV injuries, it will almost always require angiographic study with embolization of the involved vessels. When angiographic embolization is not immediately available, the patient should be managed intraoperatively with a partial splenectomy and splenorrhaphy, or a total splenectomy if attempts at splenic salvage are unsuccessful or contraindicated.

High Grade

Grade IV :
  Laceration of segmental or
  hilar vessels causing major
  devascularization > 25% of spleen

Therapy:
  Partial splenectomy
  Total splenectomy

Grade V:
  Shattered spleen
  Injury of hilar vessels with
  completely devascularized spleen

Therapy:
  Splenectomy

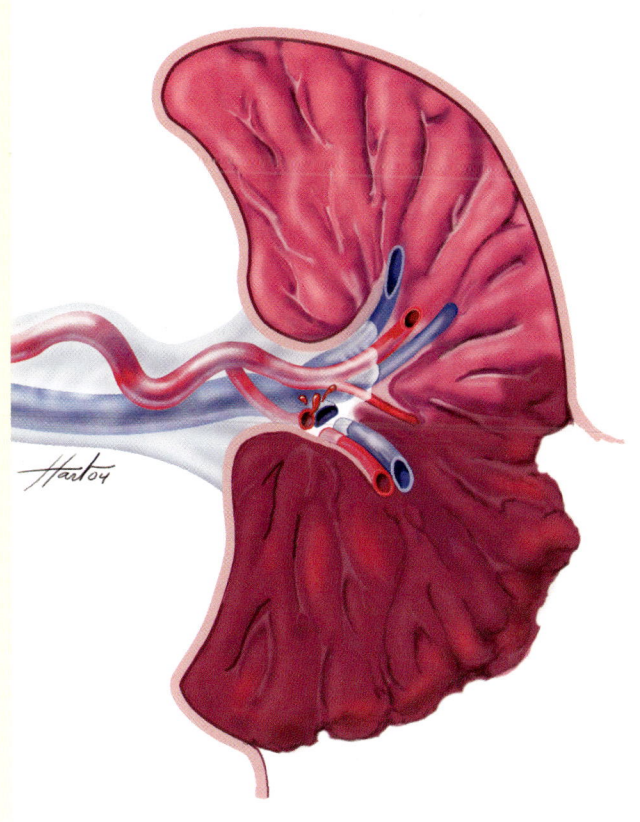

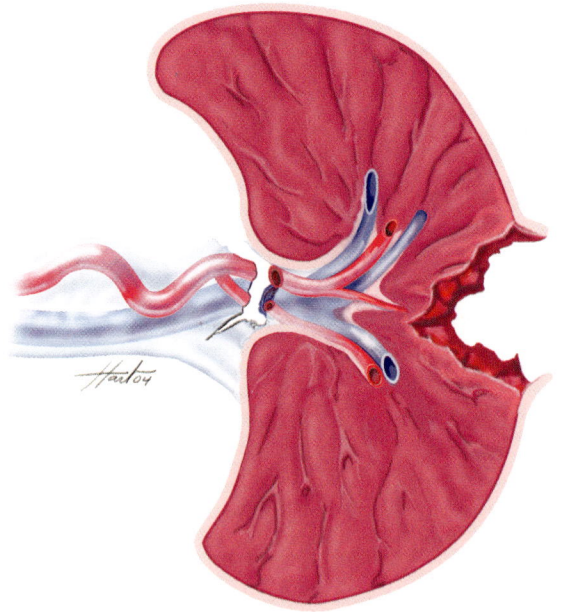

Grade V injuries of the spleen are characterized by a completely shattered spleen or a complete devascularization of the organ resulting from injuries of the hilar vessels. Nonoperative management is not indicated for Grade V injuries, and a splenectomy is required.

Technique First Step: Mobilization

As with all surgical procedures, the successful outcome of splenic surgery depends on exposure in the operating room. The goal of splenic surgery is to mobilize the spleen and bring it from a posteriolateral position to a midline position. In trauma, this is best accomplished through a midline incision extending from xiphoid to pubis. Using very gentle traction, the spleen is mobilized medially and the retroperitoneal attachments of the spleen (lienophrenic and lienorenal ligaments) are carefully divided. In the urgent setting, this can be done bluntly, but it is preferable to perform this sharply, using Metzenbaum scissors under controlled circumstances.

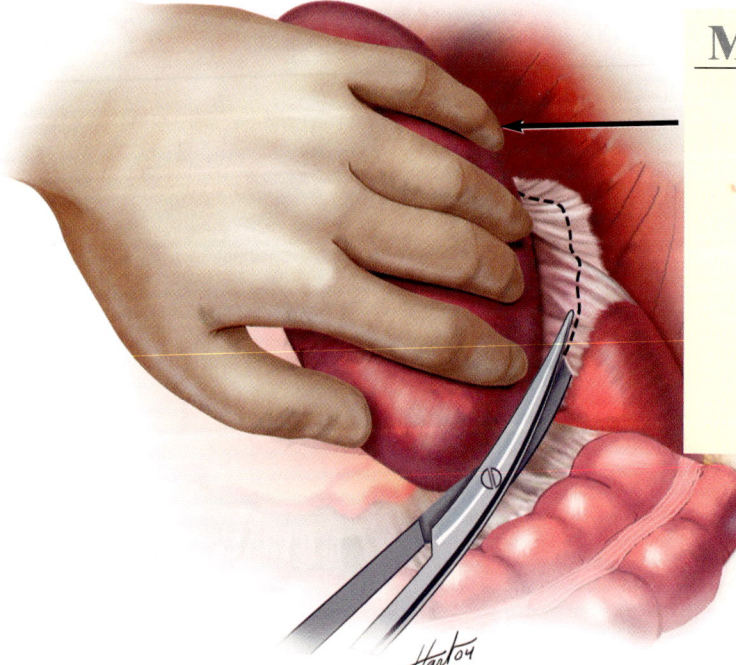

Mobilization

- Retract the spleen and divide phrenicolienal and lienorenal ligaments (attachments to retroperitoneum)

- Can be done bluntly in urgent setting

Once the retroperitoneal splenic attachments have been taken down, the surgeon can mobilize the spleen into a more anterior position by sweeping a hand posterior and medial to the spleen in front of Gerota's fascia. This maneuver will enable the operator to deliver the spleen from its posteriolateral position within the abdominal cavity to a much more medial position. At this point, the spleen can be mobilized so that it sits anteriorly within the abdominal wound. The short gastric vessels and the lienogastric ligament can also be divided if necessary.

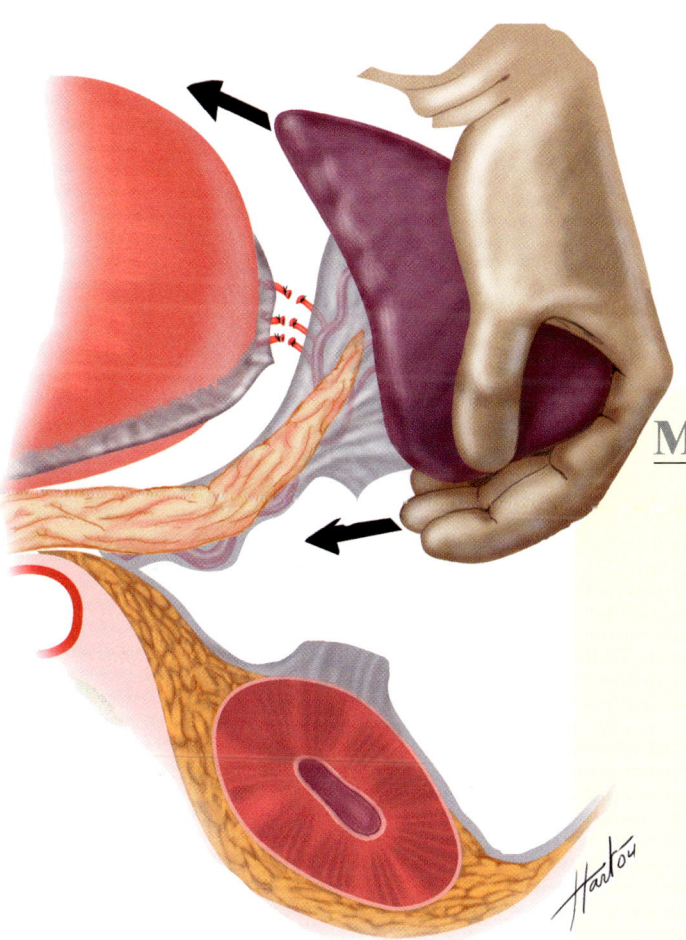

Mobilization

- Sweep bluntly behind the spleen, in front of the kidney

- Divide gastrolienal ligament/short gastrics if necessary

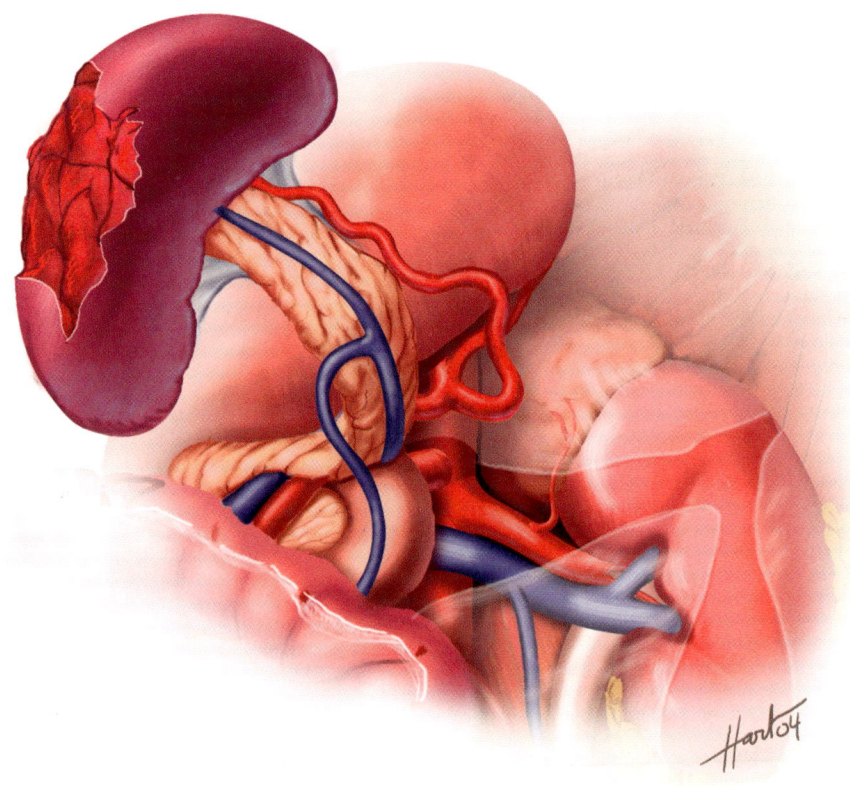

The spleen is out of the retroperitoneum and accessible

The spleen can be carefully inspected once it has been completely mobilized out of the retroperitoneum and is easily accessible as an anterior abdominal structure. A decision regarding whether to repair and save the spleen, or resect the spleen can be made more easily and safely this way. Caution should be taken during the process of mobilization and inspection to discern the position of the tail of the pancreas. This will help to avoid pancreatic injury.

Splenorrhaphy: Indications

Although splenorrhaphy is not always possible, it should be the goal when operating on a damaged spleen. As with nonoperative therapy, hemodynamic stability is a mandatory requirement if splenic conservation is being considered. In addition, there should be no indication of serious head injury or other potentially life-threatening injury or sources of bleeding. Splenic salvage is generally considered for patients who have failed nonoperative therapy and have Grade I, II, or III injuries to the spleen.

Indications

- Hemodynamically stable

- No serious head injury

- No other potentially life threatening injury

- Bleeding Grade I to Grade III injuries

Splenorrhaphy: Pledgeted Repair

Splenic parenchyma is extremely friable and must be handled with extreme care and gentleness. All devitalized splenic tissue must be resected.

Hemostasis can be achieved through a variety of means, including topical agents such as Avitene or Surgicel, fibrin glue, electrocautery, and an argon beam coagulator. Suture ligation of larger bleeders should be performed before applying topical agents.

Once hemostasis has been achieved, the splenic capsule can be approximated using absorbable sutures and pledgets. Pledgets allow the appropriate amount of tension to be applied to the sutures while preventing splenic capsular tears.

Blackened tissue indicates hemostasis, which can be achieved by the use of topical agents and electrocautery. Applying pledgeted sutures ensures no further bleeding from the open end of the spleen.

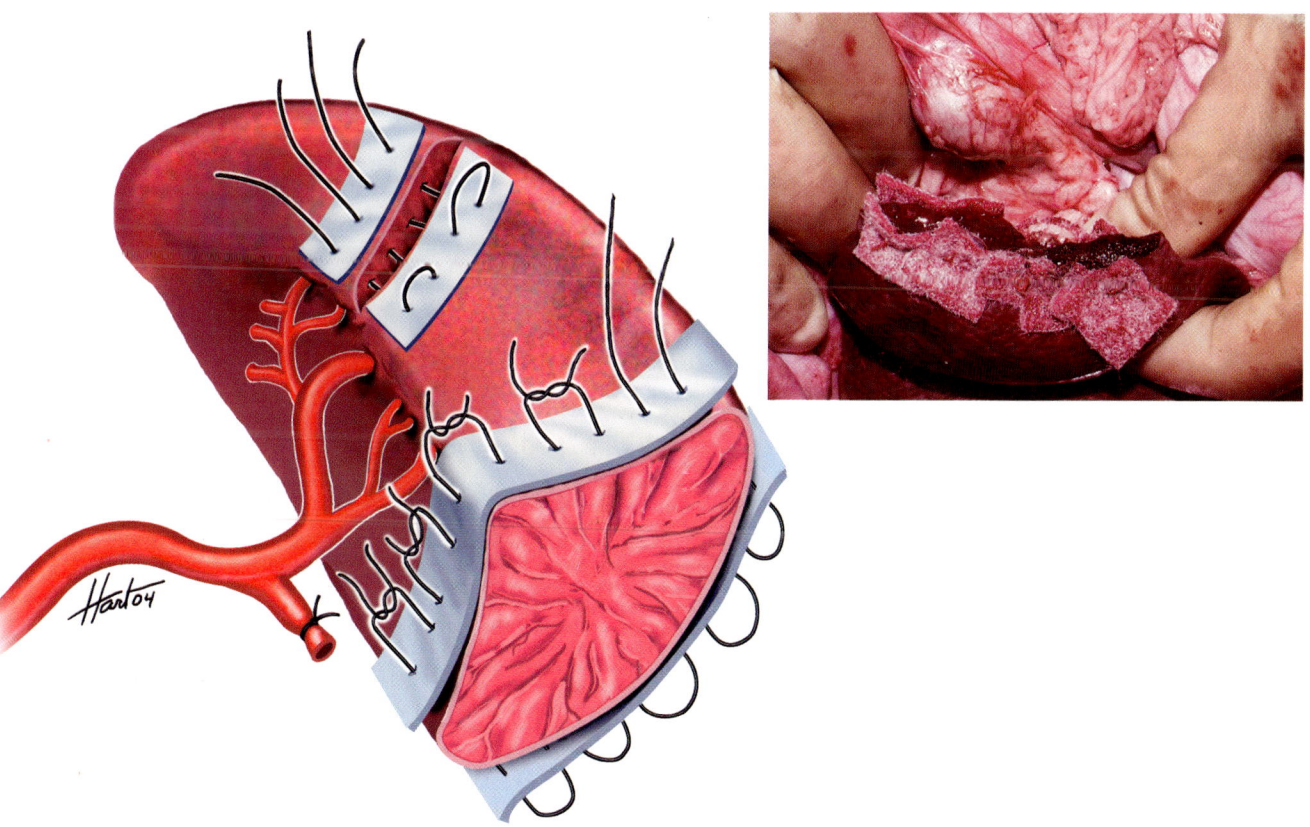

Splenorrhaphy: Mesh Wrap

Some surgeons advocate the use of an absorbable mesh wrap. This procedure is sometimes referred to as "bagging the spleen." The splenic remnant is surrounded by an absorbable mesh, with care being taken to keyhole the mesh around the splenic hilum. The spleen is then encircled by the mesh, which is sewn together. Additional sutures can increase the tension exerted by the mesh around the spleen. The goal is to appropriately and adequately tamponade any bleeding from the injured spleen.

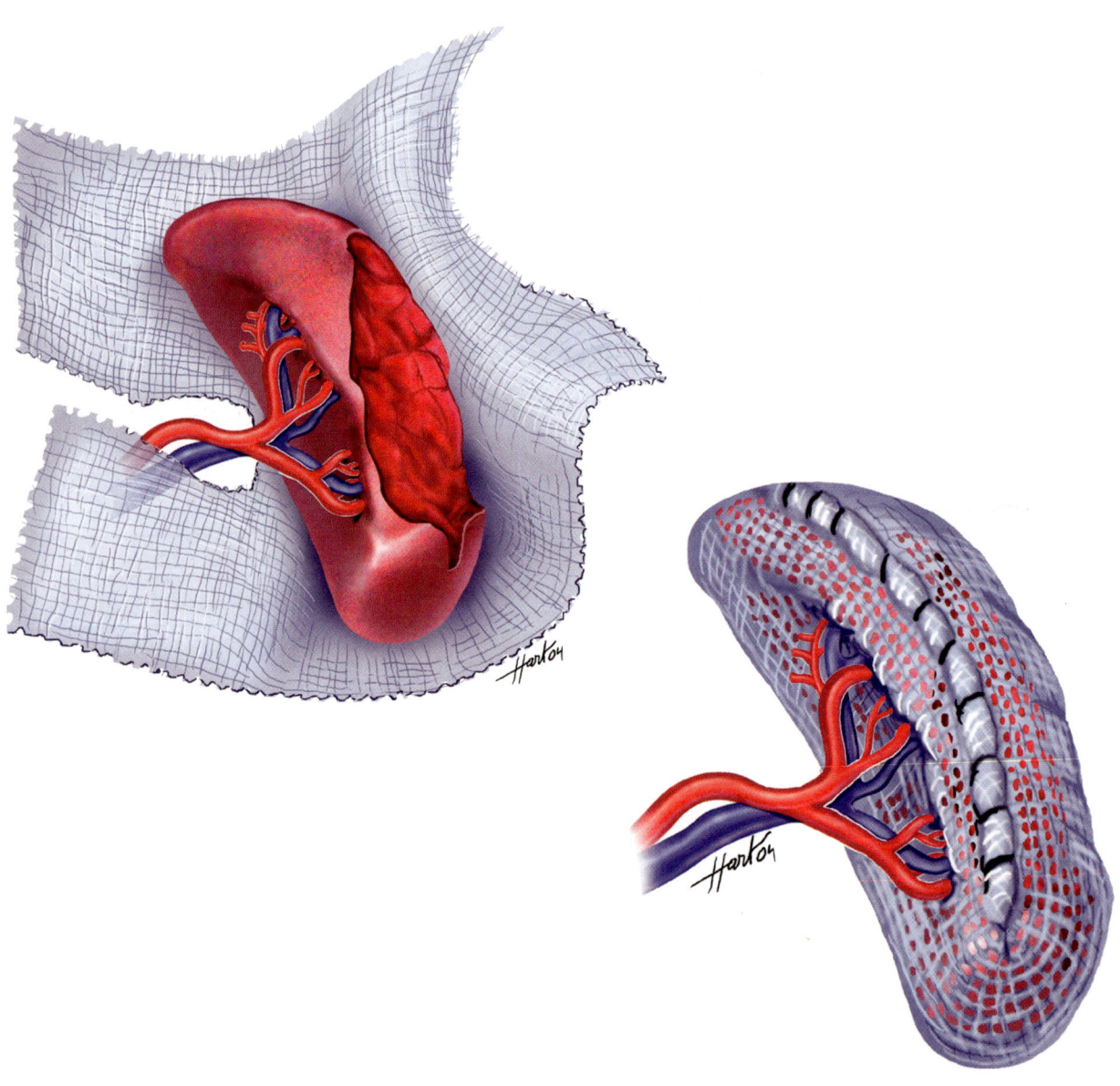

Splenorrhaphy: Omental Patch

Using an omental patch is another reliable technique that can be performed during a splenorrhaphy. Once hemostasis has been achieved within the injured portion of the spleen, a tongue of omentum can be laid into the defect and sewn into position using absorbable sutures, with or without pledgets, on either side of the defect.

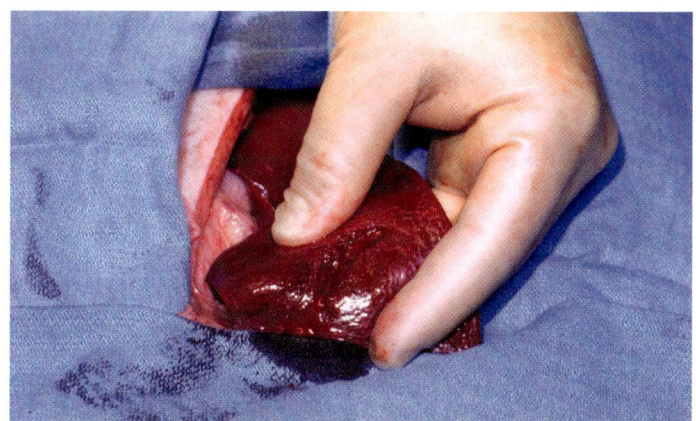

Omental Patch

Overlay laceration with a tongue of omentum held in place with absorbable sutures

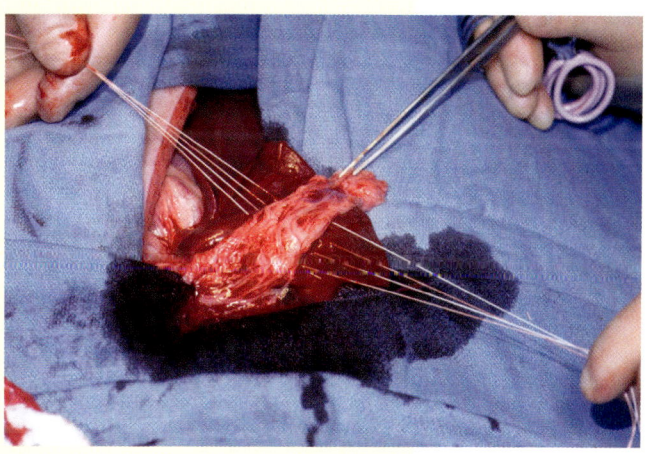

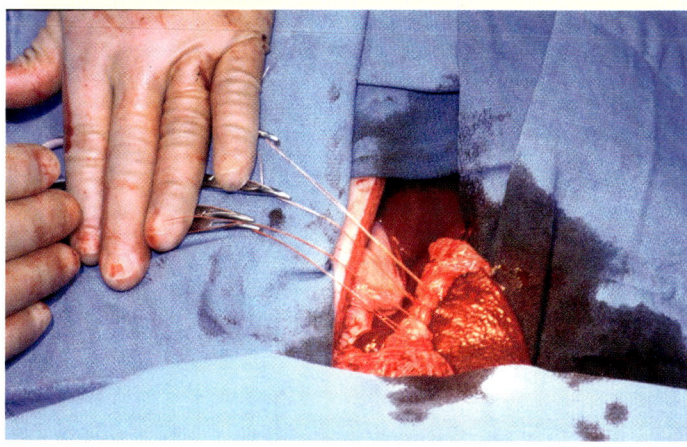

Splenorrhaphy: Partial Splenectomy

In some cases, a partial splenectomy is required before attempting splenorrhaphy. Partial splenectomy is indicated when a spleen exhibits significant damage to a pole with preservation of the majority of splenic tissue. It is also indicated when splenic damage is caused by vascular disruption to a portion of the spleen, but the vasculature has been preserved in the rest of the spleen. In these cases, the operator should perform an anatomic resection of the devitalized tissue after the appropriate vascular ligation. Once the damaged splenic tissue has been resected, a splenorrhaphy can be performed using techniques previously described. As mentioned earlier, great care must always be taken to identify and protect the tail of the pancreas, which normally abuts the splenic hilum.

Partial Splenectomy

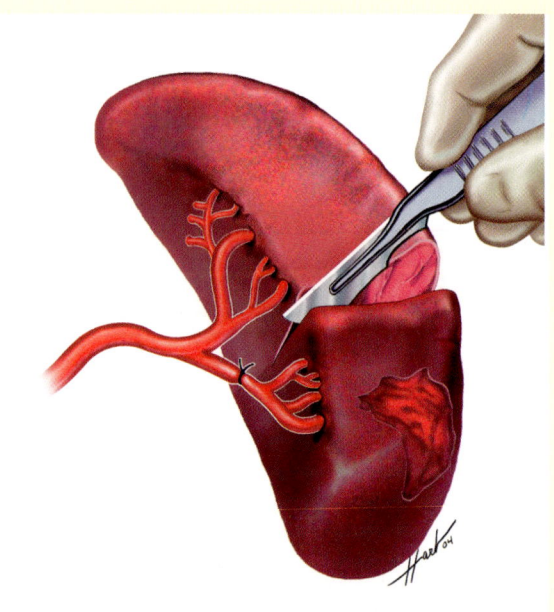

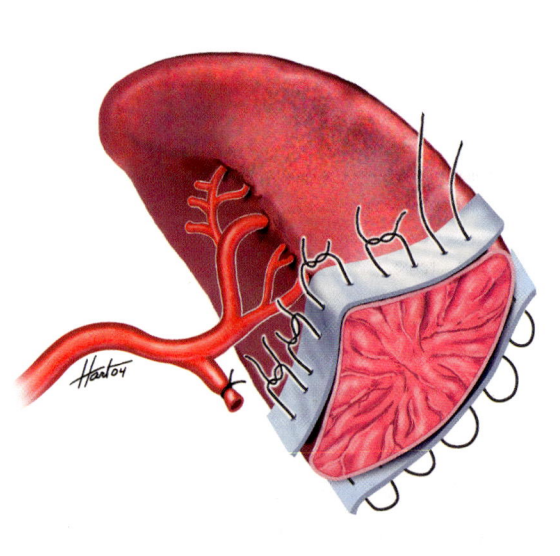

- Partial, anatomic resection after vascular ligation

- Pledgeted closure of raw surface

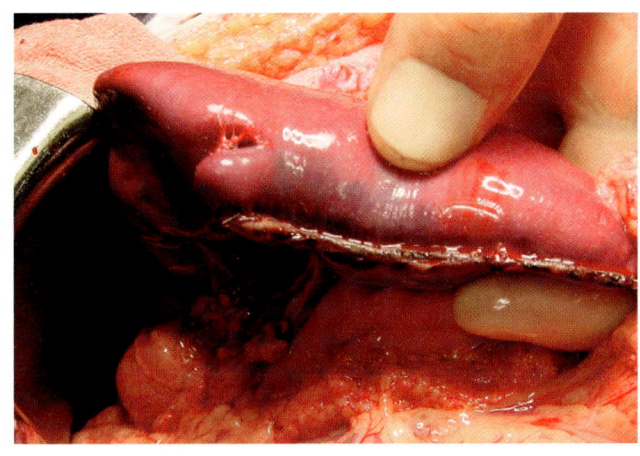

GIA stapled partial splenectomy

Splenorrhaphy: Partial Splenectomy Stapled

The size and shape of the normal human spleen is not ideal for stapling. However, in rare instances when the spleen is flatter than usual, a partial splenectomy and splenorrhaphy can be performed using either a GIA or TA stapler. The spleen must be adequately mobilized and inspected carefully, and the use of the stapler must be evaluated. Careful attention must be given to the spleen as the stapler is applied. More conventional splenorrhaphy techniques should be used if there is any evidence of a capsular disruption with application of a stapler. The stapled partial splenectomy can be a very effective and time efficient procedure.

Splenectomy: Indications

- Grade IV to Grade V injury

- Uncontrollable bleeding

- Unstable/ acidotic/ coagulopathic

- Comorbidity

- Other injury with potential for hemorrhage

- Serious TBI (to avoid secondary brain injury)

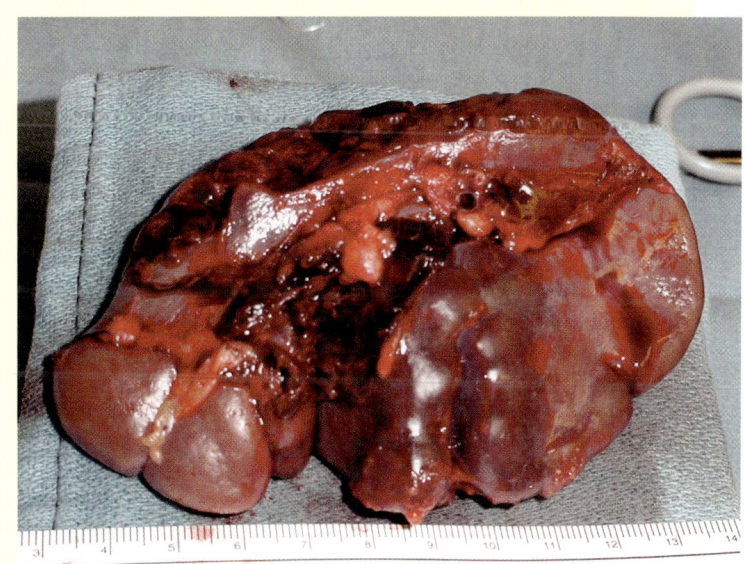

Splenectomy: Indications

Indications for splenectomy include either the failure of nonoperative conservative management of the injured spleen, or contraindications to nonoperative management. Although splenectomy is generally indicated for Grade IV and Grade V injuries, it is occasionally indicated for lesser degrees of injury. Any patient with a Grade I, II, or III injury who has failed nonoperative management is a candidate for splenorrhaphy. However, the patient may require splenectomy if all attempts at salvaging the spleen have failed.

Additional indications for splenectomy include uncontrollable bleeding from the spleen or other concurrent injuries, and significant splenic injury in the hemodynamically unstable patient who is acidotic, cold, and coagulopathic. Splenectomy should also be seriously considered for any patient with splenic injury and concomitant severe traumatic brain injury. Any episode of hypotension puts these patients at risk for secondary brain injury.

The same operative considerations for patients undergoing mobilization of the spleen for splenorrhaphy should be applied to patients undergoing splenectomy for trauma. The retroperitoneal splenic attachments should be either bluntly or sharply divided, and the spleen should be swept medially and up into the abdominal wound. This will facilitate exposure and identification of

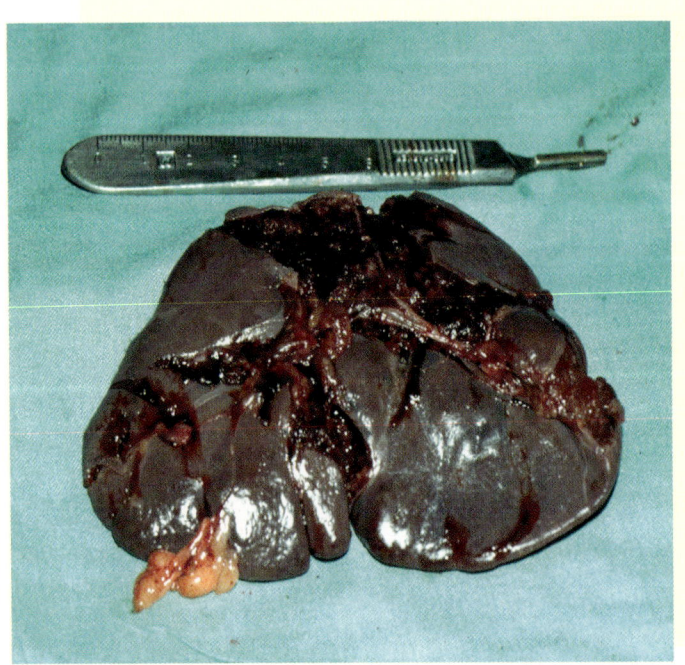

Indications

- Ligate and divide hilar vessels:
  - traditional ties
  - vascular Endo-GIA stapler

- Avoid the tail of the pancreas:
  - consider a drain if sufficiently concerned

critical structures, making it easier than working in the posterior aspect of the abdomen. Key structures to identify include the hilar vessels of the spleen, the tail of the pancreas, and the short gastric vessels.

Injury to the tail of the pancreas will result in comorbidity that is avoidable, and failure to identify and appropriately ligate the short gastric vessels can result in postoperative bleeding and hypotension. Although a mass suture ligature of all hilar vessels can be performed during damage control in an emergency situation, it is widely accepted that each vessel must be individually isolated and ligated, either with a suture ligature or a free tie. Vascular control can be accomplished with traditional ties or the vascular Endo-GIA stapler.

It cannot be stressed enough that the tail of the pancreas must be identified and carefully protected. If there is any question regarding the integrity of the tail of the pancreas once splenectomy has been completed, placement of closed-suction drainage should be performed.

Complications

As with any surgical procedure, splenectomy carries the potential for morbidity and mortality. The most common complications associated with splenectomy are OPSS, subphrenic abscesses, and pancreatic fistulas.

> **Complications**
>
> - Overwhelming post-splenectomy sepsis
> - Subphrenic abscess
> - Pancreatic fistula

Overwhelming postsplenectomy sepsis (OPSS), which is now well recognized, is very rare in the nonsplenectomized population because of the immunologic activity of the spleen. Specifically, the spleen participates in the immune response to encapsulated organisms such as pneumococci, meningococci, streptococci, and Haemophilus influenzae (H.flu). The incidence of OPSS in the normal (i.e., nonsplenectomized) population is well below 1%. Although seen in less than 1% of the nonsplenectomized population, the incidence of OPSS rises dramatically in the splenectomized population, especially in the pediatric age group. Concern for the possibility of OPSS should never prevent a clinically indicated splenectomy. However, knowledge of this syndrome should encourage splenorrhaphy and splenic preservation whenever possible.

Overwhelming Postsplenectomy Sepsis (OPSS)

- Encapsulated organisms:
  Pneumococcus
  Meningococcus
  H. Flu

- < 1% incidence

- More important in pediatric age range

- Immunization timing controversial

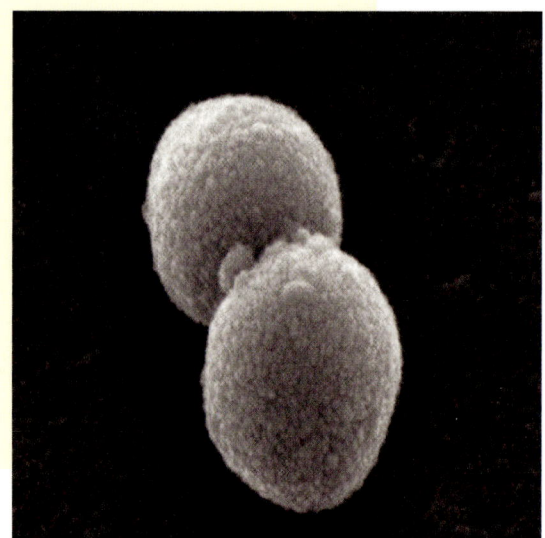

Streptococcus pneumoniae

When splenectomy is unavoidable, all patients should be immunized against encapsulated organisms with Pneumovax vaccine and H. flu vaccine. The timing of this immunization remains controversial. It has been suggested that immunization should be deferred for seven to ten days because of the up-regulation of the immune system after trauma and surgery. Others argue that this up-regulation is not a significant factor and encourage immunization as early as the immediate postoperative period while the patient is still in the postanesthesia care unit (PACU). The appropriate timing of booster immunizations also remains unknown. Level 1, randomized, prospective, controlled studies need to address these questions in order to find appropriate answers.

Sub-diaphragmatic Abscess

Although sub-diaphragmatic abscesses after splenic surgery are more common than OPSS, they are still very rare. Factors that contribute to the formation of subdiaphragmatic abscesses, which are more frequently seen after splenectomy than splenorrhaphy, include synchronous bowel injury (especially colonic injury) with peritoneal contamination, and pancreatic injury with a subsequent pancreatic fistula. In addition, the use of left upper quadrant drains after splenectomy has been shown to contribute to an increased incidence of subdiaphragmatic abscesses in the post splenectomy patient.

> **Sub-diaphragmatic Abscess**
> - More common with splenectomy than splenorrhaphy
> - Increased with synchronous bowel injury
> - Pancreatic fistula

Pancreatic Fistula

The pancreas is a relatively unforgiving organ, and morbidity due to injury is severe and sometimes difficult to manage. Damage to the tail of the pancreas during splenic surgery can result in many postoperative complications, including pancreaticocutaneous fistulas, pancreatic phlegmon, and peripancreatic abscesses. Damage to the pancreatic tail usually occurs during mobilization of the spleen and isolation of the hilar vessels. If injury to the tail is suspected or confirmed, and closed-suction drains have been properly positioned, the pancreatic fistula can be well controlled and managed conservatively.

> **Pancreatic Fistula**
> - Manage conservatively
> - Octreotide
> - Selective drainage

The use of octreotide remains controversial. Its benefits have been alternately supported and refuted in the surgical literature. Supporters of its use report a decreased volume in pancreatic exocrine secretions, and a faster resolution of pancreaticocutaneous fistulas. Other studies have failed to replicate these observations, and investigators have questioned the justification of the cost of using octreotide based on their results. Some of the most important factors in the success of nonoperative management of a pancreaticocutaneous fistula include distal feeding of an elemental diet, and wide closed-suction drainage of the injured pancreatic tail and the resulting pancreaticocutaneous fistula.

Diaphragmatic Injury

- High index of suspicion

- Penetrating based on location

- Blunt based on mechanism
  - any high energy injury

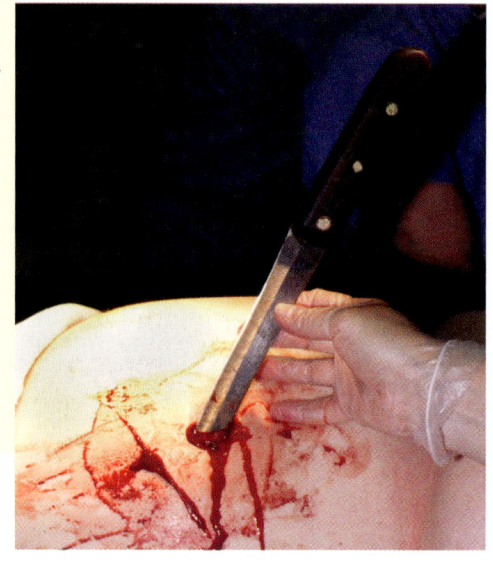

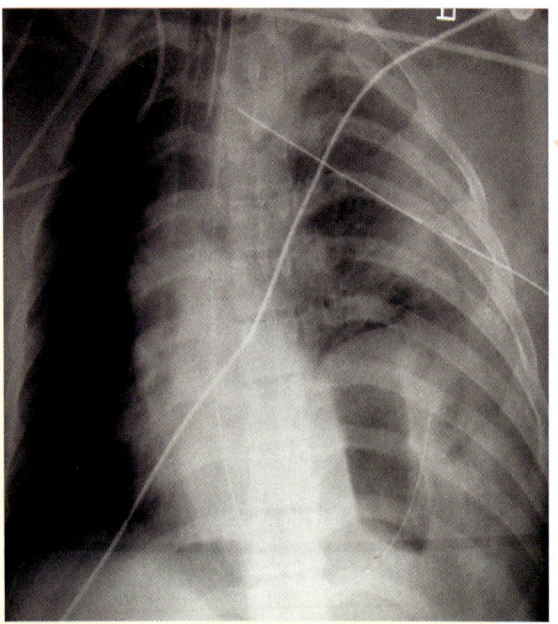

Diagnosis

- Physical exam:
  - decreased breath sounds
  - bowel sounds over lower thorax

- Radiographic:
  - CXR
  - CT scan
  - exploration:
    - laparotomy
    - laparoscopy or thoracoscopy

Diaphragmatic injuries can be very difficult to diagnose because they are frequently silent on initial presentation. It is important to maintain a high index of suspicion for diaphragmatic injury, especially in patients who have sustained penetrating trauma to the chest or abdomen. Although suspicions may be raised by the location of a wound in penetrating trauma, the trajectory of a knife or bullet may not be as expected, and diaphragmatic injury could have occurred even with a wound located away from the area of the diaphragm.

Diaphragmatic injury due to penetrating trauma is often much smaller in size than injury caused by blunt mechanisms. In fact, diaphragmatic injuries from blunt trauma result from high-energy injuries, and tend to be large rents that are usually obvious early on, usually occurring on the left side.

Diagnosis

A thorough and in-depth physical examination is probably the surgeon's best tool for diagnosing diaphragmatic injury. However, injuries from penetrating trauma are frequently small and may be missed entirely on a physical examination. In addition, neither hemidiaphragm is at greater risk than the other when the mechanism of injury is penetrating trauma. The subdiaphragmatic location of the liver will tend to protect the right hemidiaphragm from injury in blunt mechanisms, with the liver absorbing most of the energy. Therefore, the majority of cases involve injury to the left hemidiaphragm.

Blunt trauma tends to cause more disruption than penetration of the diaphragm. Physical examination is more reliable in these cases. Key findings on physical examination include decreased breath sounds on the side of diaphragmatic injury, and the presence of bowel sounds over the lower thorax on the side of injury. Radiographic indications on chest x-ray include an elevated or obscured hemidiaphragm on the side of injury accompanied by the presence of the nasogastric tube, or bowel loops in the chest. Findings on a CT scan can confirm the presence of diaphragmatic injury and the fact that the bowel has traversed the confines of the diaphragm on the affected side.

When a diaphragmatic injury cannot be ruled out by conservative, or noninvasive, work-up, laparoscopy, fluoroscopy, and a formal celiotomy or thoracoscopy may be required to establish or rule out the presence of diaphragmatic injury.

AAST-OIS for the Diaphragm

Grade I: Contusion

Grade II: Laceration up to 2 cm

Grade III: Laceration 2 cm to 10 cm

Grade IV: Laceration > 10 cm, < 25 cm^2 tissue loss

Grade V: > 25 cm^2 tissue loss

AAST-OIS for the Diaphragm

The AAST-OIS is also used to grade diaphragmatic injuries. A Grade I diaphragmatic injury is characterized by a contusion to the diaphragm without disruption of the normal anatomy. A Grade II injury is defined by a diaphragmatic laceration smaller than or equal to 2 cm in length. A Grade III injury is characterized by a laceration between 2 cm and 10 cm, and a Grade IV diaphragmatic injury is characterized by either a diaphragmatic laceration longer than 20 cm or diaphragmatic tissue loss less than 25 cm². A Grade V diaphragmatic injury is categorized by diaphragmatic tissue loss of more than 25 cm².

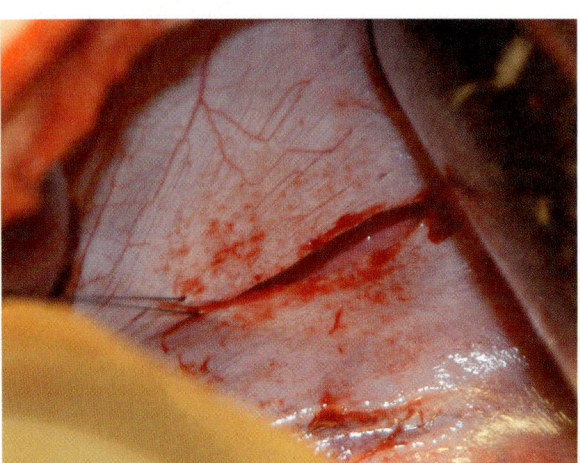

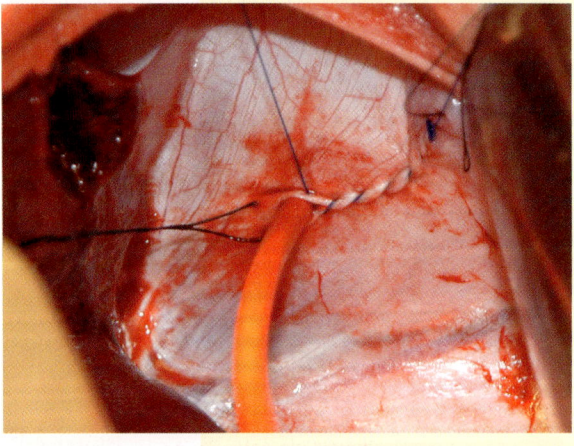

Treatment

- Laparoscopy
- Thoracoscopy
- Laparotomy
- Nonabsorbable suture
- Air tight closure
- Thoracostomy tubes

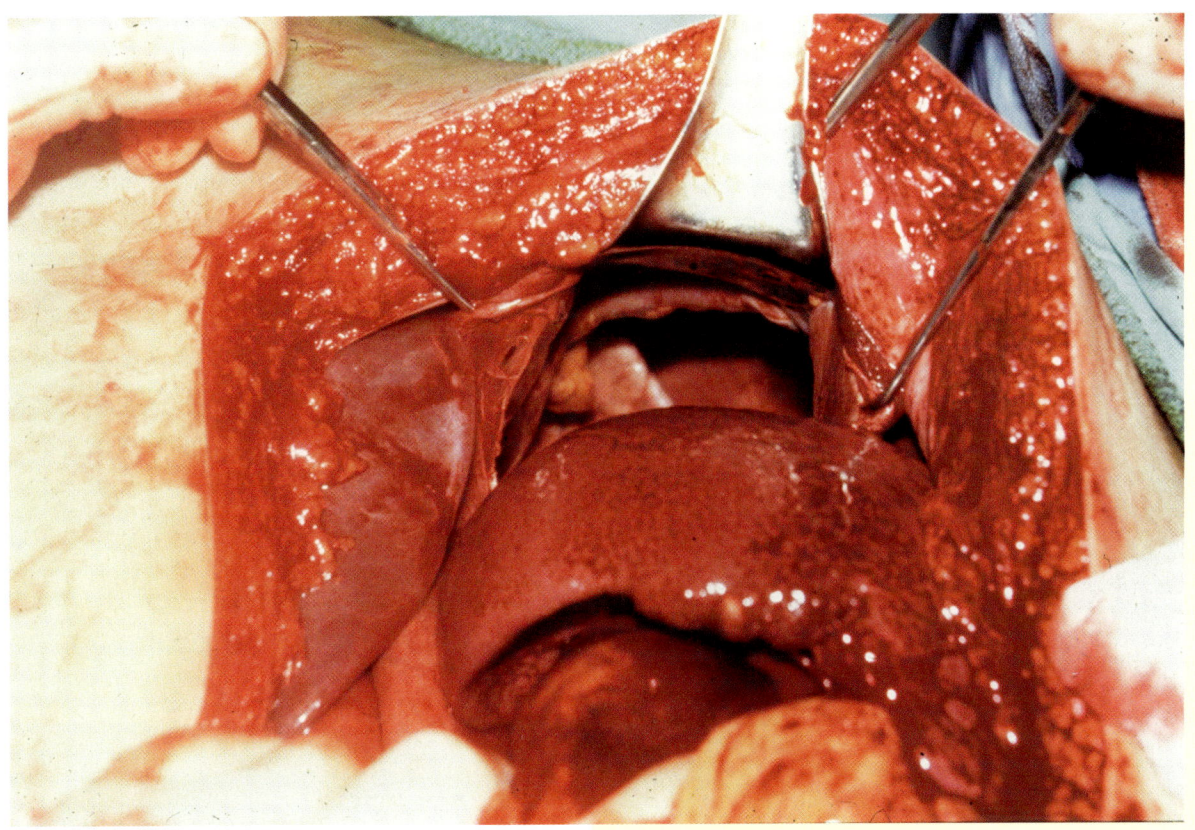

Diaphragmatic Injury: Treatment

Diaphragmatic injury must be repaired once it has been diagnosed. This can be done with either a formal laparotomy (especially when the patient is being explored for other injuries) or by using laparoscopic or thoracoscopic techniques.

Treatment

- Reattachment to chest wall
- Replacement with prosthetic patch

A nonabsorbable suture should be used for the repair, and interrupted or running sutures can be used at the surgeon's discretion. The closure, however, must be airtight. It is generally suggested that a thoracostomy tube be placed after the repair because there is usually parenchymal lung damage caused by the injury itself. When there has been concomitant bowel injury with soilage of the abdominal cavity, it is important to lavage the hemithorax with sterile saline to remove as much particulate matter as possible and minimize the risk for developing a postoperative empyema.

Late Complications

- Visceral herniation
  - colon
  - stomach
  - liver
  - small bowel

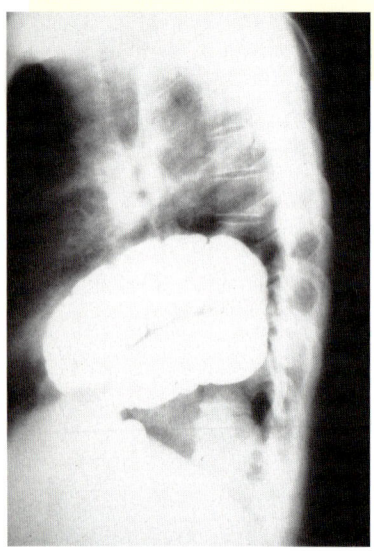

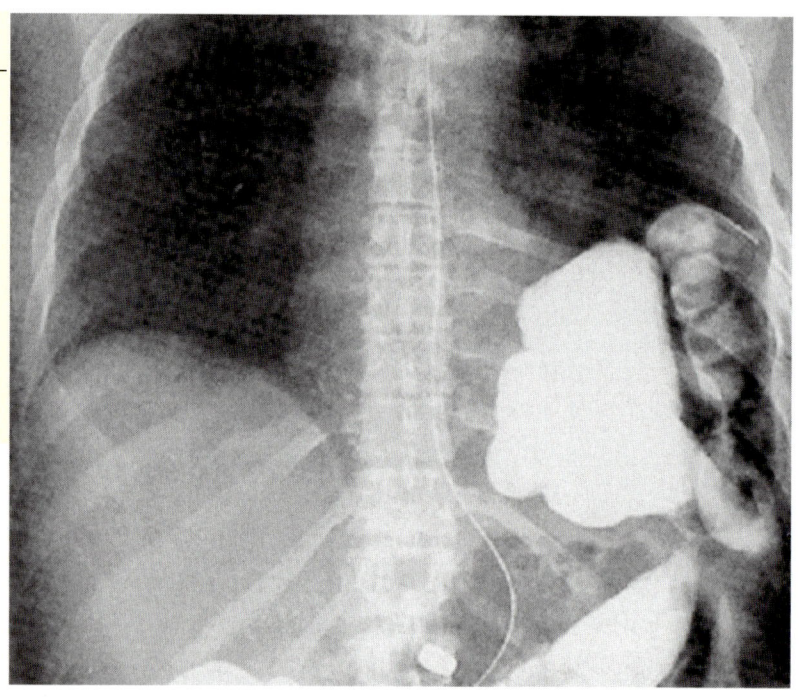

Treatment of Complex Injuries

High-grade diaphragmatic injuries can be very difficult to repair. These complex injuries may require inventive methods of diaphragmatic repair and/or replacement. Whenever possible, large diaphragmatic rents should be closed primarily, and diaphragmatic avulsions from the chest wall should be reattached using suitable surgical techniques. Nonabsorbable sutures, such as those for simple closures, should be used. The chest wall should be thoroughly irrigated, and a chest tube should be placed at the end of the repair.

A prosthetic patch may be needed to replace the diaphragm on rare occasions when tissue loss greater than 25 cm^2 precludes the surgeon's ability to reapproximate the diaphragm either to itself or to the chest wall. The patch cannot be porous, and it must be permanent. Good materials for this type of closure include Gore-Tex and silastic patches.

Late Complications

The diagnosis and repair of a diaphragmatic injury can be difficult, but the complications of an undiagnosed and unrepaired diaphragmatic injury can be catastrophic. In the best-case scenario, the consequence of visceral herniation of the colon, stomach, small bowel, or liver is respiratory compromise. In the worst-case scenario, these complications can cause vascular compromise to the herniated organ with necrosis, tissue death, and sepsis, and ultimately the death of the patient.

ADVANCED TRAUMA OPERATIVE MANAGEMENT

Selected Readings

Chapter 2 - Spleen & Diaphragm

Murray JA et al. Penetrating left thoracoabdominal trauma: the incidence and presentation of diaphragm injuries. J Trauma 1997;43:624-626.

Shackford SR. Spleen. In: Thal ER, Weigelt JA, Carrico CJ. Operative Trauma Management: An Atlas. 2nd Edition. McGraw-Hill. 2002;288-301.

Leppäniemi A et al. Occult diaphragmatic injuries caused by stab wounds. J Trauma 2003;55:646-650.

Asensio JA et al. Injury to the diaphragm. In: Moore EE, Feliciano DV, Mattox KL, eds. Trauma. 5th ed. 2004 McGraw-Hill;613-635.

Tips From the Masters

There are a number of safe methods to manage blunt and penetrating trauma in the operating suite. The following technical surgical tips have been successfully used by the authors to deal with difficult or challenging operating situations.

Chapter 2: The Spleen & Diaphragm

TABLE OF CONTENTS

Exposure and Management of a Grade V Shattered Spleen 95
Lenworth M. Jacobs, MD

Blunt Diaphragmatic and Splenic Injury 97
Brad Cushing, MD

Burst Wound of Dome of Diaphragm 99
David G. Burris, MD

Repair of Left Diaphragmatic Laceration 101
Glen Tinkoff, MD

Laparoscopic Repair of Diaphragmatic Injury 103
Rocco Orlando, III, MD

Stab Wound to Lower Pole of Spleen 105
Alasdair K.T. Conn, MD

TECHNICAL OPERATIVE PROCEDURES:

HOW I DO IT

Exposure and Management of a Grade V Shattered Spleen

Lenworth M. Jacobs, MD, MPH, FACS

Scenario

A 46-year-old man was involved in a motor vehicle crash with blunt trauma to the abdomen. He was initially hypotensive and presented with a contusion and tenderness in the left upper quadrant

Management

The patient is rapidly resuscitated with two 14 gauge intravenous lines through which 2 liters of crystalloid are rapidly infused. A chest x-ray shows normal lung parenchyma with no hemopneumothorax. The focused assessment with sonography in trauma (FAST) examination identified free fluid in the left upper quadrant. Blood is sent for type and crossmatching and a Foley catheter was placed which shows no hematuria.

The patient's blood pressure promptly returns to normal. A spiral CT scan was rapidly performed and showed a Grade V injury with a blush present in the splenic parenchyma. The patient is taken to the operating room for an exploratory laparotomy.

- The left hand is used to control the hilum

- The right hand performs the posterior splenic dissection

- Splenic artery is doubly ligated and suture ligatured

- Inspect the tail of the pancreas

Procedure: *Exposure of the spleen*

The abdomen is widely prepped and draped. A large midline incision is made from the base of the sternum to the pubis. The catheter that is attached to an autotransfusion collecting device is introduced into the peritoneal cavity and free blood aspirated. The peritoneum is then widely opened and clot scooped out and placed in a bowl on the table. All four quadrants are then rapidly packed. Attention is then turned to the left upper quadrant. The abdominal wall is retracted away from the contents of the left upper quadrant and the right hand introduced to palpate the spleen. The severe injury to the spleen is digitally confirmed. The surgeon's left hand is then used to digitally control the splenic hilar vessels. This effectively arrests all flow to the spleen and controls further hemorrhage. The fingers of the surgeon's right hand are then used to create a plane anterior to Gerota's fascia and posterior to the convex surface of the spleen. Dissection is used to open the plane in the retroperitoneum and it is carried medially until the posterior surface of the pancreas is palpated. The digital dissection is carried superiorly and inferiorly. Superiorly, the lienophrenic ligament or attachment is identified. This ligament needs to be sharply dissected with a scissors. The dissecting hand is then swept inferiorly and the lienocolic ligament is identified and divided sharply. Once these attachments are released, the entire spleen and the tail and body of the pancreas are mobilized using blunt dissection along the plane of the posterior aspect of the pancreas. The spleen and its vasculature along with the tail of the pancreas are then gently brought up into the wound. Once the entire spleen is on the anterior abdominal wall, the concave and convex surfaces are carefully inspected and a judgment is made as to the feasibility and appropriateness of a repair. In a Grade V laceration there is significant enough damage in multiple areas of the spleen that a repair is not indicated. Attention is then turned to the splenic hilar vessels. The splenic artery is doubly ligated and a 3-0 silk suture ligature is used to secure the splenic artery. The splenic vein is doubly ligated. Attention is turned to the short gastric vessels. It is essential to ligate the short gastric vessels as close to the spleen as possible. Care must be taken to not devascularize the greater curve of the stomach. Control of the vessels proximal to the greater curve of the stomach, which can include the gastroepiploic vessels, may lead to ischemia of the greater curve of the stomach with resulting necrosis and a gastric fistula. Once the splenectomy has been completed, the anterior and posterior surface of the tail of the pancreas must be inspected. If there is no damage to the tail of the pancreas, there is no need for closed suction drainage. The left upper quadrant is then irrigated with a liter of saline. The splenic artery is then inspected and the vasculature of the pancreas is then inspected again to be sure there is not a vessel which has been in spasm and is now bleeding. A laparotomy pack is then placed in the left upper quadrant and the exploratory laparotomy completed. At the end of the procedure, the pack is then inspected to see if there is further bleeding and/or clot evident. If there is, the bleeding vessel has to be identified and suture ligated. The pack is then removed and the abdomen closed.

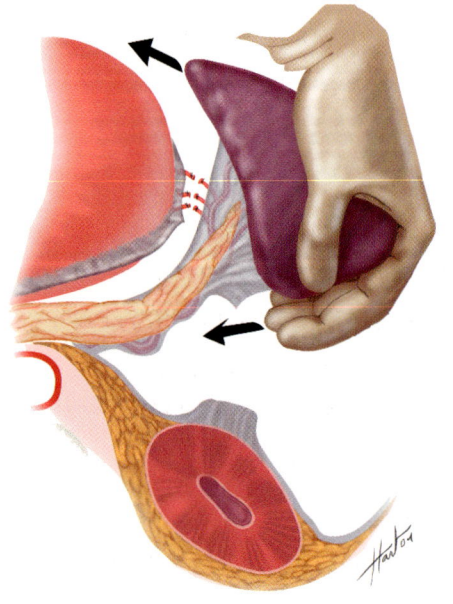

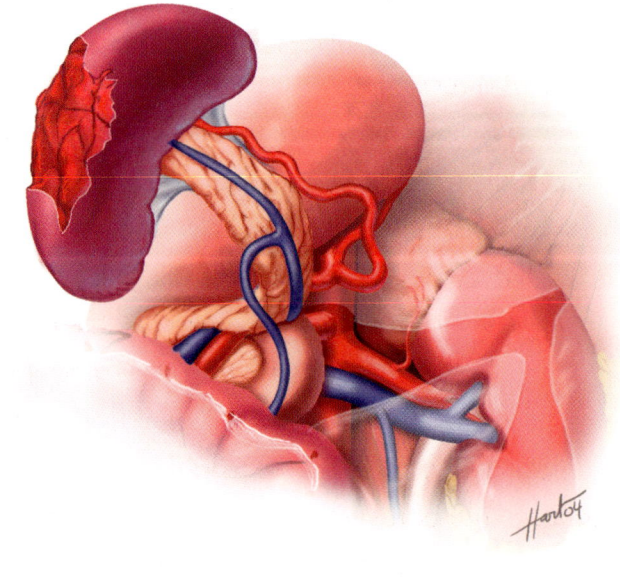

TECHNICAL OPERATIVE PROCEDURES:

HOW I DO IT

Blunt Diaphragmatic and Splenic Injury

Brad Cushing, MD, FACS

Scenario

The patient is an elderly woman driver who was involved in a same-side lateral crash. She is hypotensive in the resuscitation suite. Her chest x-ray shows a disrupted left hemidiaphragm and rib fractures without pneumothorax. Her FAST exam shows a large amount of blood in the peritoneum.

Management

She is taken directly to the operating room where she is intubated, large bore lines are established and blood transfusion is initiated. As this is accomplished, the cell saver with two attached sump suction systems are prepared. Her abdomen and left chest are prepped and draped. A midline abdominal incision is made from alongside the xiphoid, i.e. as high as possible, to below the umbilicus. The fascia is opened completely before the peritoneum is opened so that blood does not obscure the field. On entry to the peritoneum, a suction catheter is directed to the pelvis and another to the left upper quadrant. Hand exploration of the left upper quadrant reveals an 8 cm stellate laceration of the dome of the diaphragm and an actively bleeding macerated spleen with lacerations extending into the hilum. A laparotomy pad is placed over the spleen. The liver is intact on brief palpation. Laparotomy pads are not placed in all quadrants as this maneuver wastes blood, obscures vision, and reduces the mobility that will be needed to obtain good exposure.

- The hemorrhage from the spleen is controlled first

- Full mobilization and inspection

- All blood and clots removed from the chest

- Non-absorbable sutures to close diaphragm

Procedure

Pressure is held on the spleen while exposure is obtained. An Omni or Bookwalter retractor is placed. The extra time spent doing this is well rewarded by improved exposure and liberation of assistants. If a second assistant is available or the staff surgeon is letting the senior resident hold the primary instruments, they are positioned on the patient's right below the primary surgeon. The transverse colon and its mesentery serve as an excellent towel to exclude the contents of the lower abdomen from the field. It is elevated, moved to the left and swept along the left lateral abdominal wall. The assistant places the right hand on the mesentery and retracts it towards the pelvis beautifully exposing the lower pole of the spleen and the left upper quadrant. The lower pole of the spleen is elevated and adhesions taken down sharply. The peritoneum posterolateral to the spleen is then divided allowing posterior access to the splenic hilum. The surgeon's right index finger is then inserted posterior to the splenic hilum and thumb and finger used to identify the splenic hilar vessels. The assistant's left hand retracts the stomach and transverse colon mesentery to the right, thus exposing the splenic hilum and flattening the folds of the stomach. A window is made in the peritoneum at the splenic hilum superior to the palpated vessels by dissection over the tip of the index finger. The surgeon's left index finger then follows his right as it is withdrawn from behind the hilum. It then guides the insertion of an open Kelly clamp through the created window. The clamp is then applied

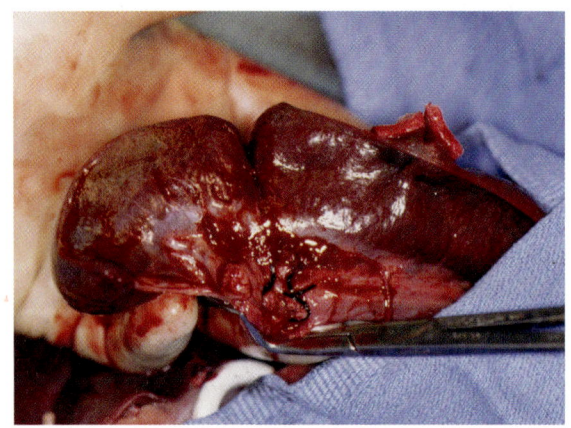

across the hilar vessels as close to the spleen as possible to avoid pancreatic injury. The previously created peritoneal window is then used to separate the stomach from the spleen and tent the short gastric vessels. A second Kelly is then inserted through this window and applied across the short gastrics away from the stomach's greater curve. All bleeding from the spleen stops. The spleen is sharply divided distal to the clamps and removed. The hilar and short gastric vessels are separately identified and ligated. The splenic bed is inspected to identify any bleeding points and assure absence of pancreatic injury. The greater curve of the stomach is inspected to assure ligation of all short gastric vessels and to assure that no gastric injury has occurred during ligation or clamping. With the bleeding stopped, the remainder of the abdomen is inspected. No injuries other than the diaphragm are identified.

Attention is then turned to the diaphragm injury. Long Allis clamps are applied to the points of the laceration, the diaphragm is inverted and the pleural space exposed. All blood and clots are suctioned from the pleural space and the absence of active bleeding from lung parenchyma and intercostal vessels is confirmed. A chest tube is inserted in the pleural space through the fifth intercostal space via a small chest incision. It is positioned under direct vision from the abdomen. It is secured at the chest wall. The diaphragmatic rent is then closed using a nonabsorbable 2-0 or 0 suture in a continuous or interrupted figure of eight fashion. I prefer interrupted sutures especially for stellate lacerations and don't tie them until all are in place. This allows for good traction and better exposure for all sutures.

No abdominal drains are placed unless there is clear pancreatic injury. The abdominal wall is closed with a continuous fascial suture and skin staples.

The patient's chest tube is removed in 48 hours and on postoperative day three, she demands to return to her lobster boat but is told she can't until she receives her vaccinations and fully understands the risks associated with the postsplenectomy state.

TECHNICAL OPERATIVE PROCEDURES:

HOW I DO IT

Burst Wound of Dome of Diaphragm

David G. Burris, MD, FACS, DMCC

Scenario

A 35-year-old man presented after an automobile ran over his abdomen with one tire. He is hemodynamically stable, but has difficulty breathing, and an abnormal chest-ray with air-fluid level seen above the normal level of the diaphragm.

Management

Preoperative antibiotics to cover gram positive and gram negative organisms, and anaerobes should be given intravenously. An exploratory laparotomy is conducted through a generous midline incision. Any active hemorrhage should be controlled, and all injuries identified.

- Débride devitalized tissue

- Attempt to create a single linear defect

- Close with monofilament non-absorbable interrupted horizontal mattress sutures 1 cm apart

- Any leaks closed with running-locking buttress repair

The right diaphragm is inspected with hand traction of the liver while lifting on the costal margin. The falciform ligament may have to be divided to facilitate this. The falciform and triangular ligaments will usually need to be divided to repair an injury to this side. Inspect the left side by lifting the costal margin while using the hand to move the stomach and spleen downward.

Procedure:

Repair of diaphragmatic injury

In this scenario, the stomach, and spleen will be reduced from the chest and a non-bleeding laceration of the spleen identified. A 7 cm x 8 cm stellate laceration of the central portion of the diaphragm is seen. Any devitalized tissue is carefully débrided, with an attempt to create a single linear defect.

This should be closed with # 0 or 1 non-absorbable monofilament sutures in an interrupted horizontal mattress fashion to obtain eversion of the edges. These should not be placed more than 1 cm apart. After closure, water is instilled into the abdomen while multiple pressure breaths are created. Any leaks should be closed by a running or running-locking buttress of the repair. Some will use a running suture to buttress any laceration over 2 cm in length.

If a single linear defect cannot be made from this stellate laceration, or if too much tissue is lost, a soft non-absorbable mesh can be sutured to the margins of the defect. Several arms of the stellate laceration may be closed with interrupted sutures as described above, and then reinforced with a mesh.

A chest tube is placed in the ipsilateral chest cavity after repair. If mesh was used, suction should be limited to that required to keep the thoracic cavity free of fluid, and the lung inflated, and converted to water seal as soon as possible.

If there has been massive spillage of intestinal contents into the chest, adequate cleaning is often not possible through the diaphragm and the chest should be opened after repair to ensure that all spillage is removed.

While the diaphragm can be repaired from the chest, this should not be the primary incision for repair, since the abdominal organs cannot be adequately assessed for injuries through the diaphragm from the chest.

TECHNICAL OPERATIVE PROCEDURES:

HOW I DO IT

Repair of Left Diaphragmatic Laceration

Glen Tinkoff, MD, FACS

Scenario

A 6 cm linear laceration to the left diaphragm is encountered during exploratory laparotomy for trauma. The laceration extends laterally to medially toward the crus of the diaphragm. The esophagus and heart are not injured.

Technical Aspects of the Repair

Placing a hand over the body of the spleen and applying gentle traction caudad and medially attains adequate exposure. With this maneuver, the fundus of the stomach should also be retracted downward exposing the central tendon of the diaphragm, as well as the lateral and posterior margins.

Procedure: *Repair of left diaphragmatic laceration*

The laceration can now be identified in its full extent. If encountered, the edges of the laceration are débrided of devitalized tissue and hemostasis is achieved with electrocautery or suture ligation. Allis or Babcock clamps are utilized to grasp the medial and lateral margins of the defect and define the subsequent suture repair. These clamps are also used on the inferior and superior margins of the laceration and manipulated in order to inspect the hemithoracic pleural space and evacuate any blood and contaminant prior to closure. In most situations, a chest tube will have previously been inserted or it should be inserted prior to the repair of the laceration.

Although a smaller laceration less than 2 cm can be repaired simply with 0 or #1 non-absorbable sutures in simple or figure-of-eight fashion, larger lacerations, such as this, are repaired utilizing a two-layer closure. The initial layer is created from horizontal mattress stitches of 0 or #1 non-absorbable sutures in order to evert the edges toward the abdominal cavity. Care should be taken to avoid injury to the myocardium and branches of the phrenic nerve when placing the medial sutures. Using the previously placed suture as a retractor helps expose the remainder of the wound as the repair proceeds.

- Clamps are used to grasp the medial and lateral margins of the defect

- Inspect the hemithorax through the laceration

- Two layer closure

- Evert the edges toward the peritoneal cavity

Once the row of horizontal mattress sutures are completed and secured, they are then reinforced with a running suture of the same non-absorbable suture material. At completion of the repair the integrity of the suture line should be tested by increasing the intrathoracic pressure by administering a large tidal volume and assessing diaphragmatic motion. This maneuver is then repeated with the suture line covered in sterile saline to ascertain if there is escape of air or pleural fluid through the suture line.

TECHNICAL OPERATIVE PROCEDURES:
HOW I DO IT

Laparoscopic Repair of Diaphragmatic Injury

Rocco Orlando, III, MD, FACS

Scenario

This 24-year-old male sustained a stab wound to the left upper quadrant at the mid-clavicular line. The patient was hemodynamically stable. The wound was 1.5 cm in length and a small portion of the omentum was noted to be protruding from the wound. The primary and secondary survey revealed no other injuries, a chest x-ray was negative and the patient was brought to the operating room for laparoscopic exploration to evaluate for possible intraabdominal injuries.

Operative Procedure

Following the induction of general endotracheal anesthesia, the entire abdomen and chest are prepped and draped with the surgeon standing on the patient's right side and the assistant on the left. A 1 cm vertical incision is made just above the umbilicus and Hasson cannulation of the abdomen is carried out. A carbon dioxide pneumoperitoneum is established to 15 mmHg and video laparoscopy is performed. Initial visual inspection of the abdomen reveals the omentum draped to the anterior abdominal wall where it can be seen entering the stab wound. The presence of the omentum obscures complete visualization of the peritoneal cavity.

A 5 mm incision is then made in the right upper quadrant and a trocar introduced into the abdomen under direct vision. An atraumatic grasping forceps is then used to reduce the omentum from the stab wound. Leakage of carbon dioxide through the stab wound is managed by placing a 12 mm trocar through the stab wound to both eliminate the gas leak and permit two-handed exploration of the abdomen. A fourth trocar, 5 mm, is introduced into the abdomen in the left upper quadrant to allow the first assistant to provide retraction.

- Inspect the upper abdomen completely

- Bowel inspected

- Rent in the diaphragm repaired around a catheter

- Interrupted sutures used for closure

Laparoscopic exploration begins by inspecting the upper abdomen. The assistant applies downward traction to the stomach and transverse colon to visualize the liver and spleen, both of which were free of injury. The surgeon employs atraumatic graspers to adequately visualize these structures. A 2 cm rent was visualized in the mid-portion of the left hemidiaphragm just lateral to the fundus. The stomach is grasped, inspected and noted to be free of injury. Downward traction is applied to the omentum and the anterior surface of the transverse colon is inspected and found to be free of injury. The descending and ascending colon were also uninjured. The patient is then placed in reverse Trendelenburg position, and the triangle retractor is used to apply cephalad traction to the transverse colon. This allows inspection of the posterior aspect of the colon. The ligament of Treitz is now visualized and the small bowel is run by manipulating it carefully with atraumatic forceps to ensure that there is no injury. The bowel is inspected from the ligament of Treitz to the ileocecal valve. No injuries are found. No hematoma or bloodstaining is seen in the retroperitoneum.

Attention now turns to the diaphragmatic injury. Before closing the hole in the diaphragm, a 10 Fr. red rubber catheter is passed through the assistant's 5 mm port and placed through the wound into the left hemithorax to deal with the carbon dioxide pneumothorax which results from the injury. The catheter is clamped so that the pneumoperitoneum will not be lost. The pneumothorax is readily managed by the anesthesia team by increasing minute ventilation without hemodynamic effects. The rent in the diaphragm was repaired around the red rubber catheter with interrupted 2-0 PTFE (Gore-Tex) sutures tied extra-corporeally. Laparoscopic suturing permits closure of the defect with large bites using permanent suture material. Following repair of the diaphragm, all trocars were removed under direct vision. Suction is applied to the red rubber catheter and the lungs are expanded fully by the anesthesiologist and the red rubber catheter is removed. The fascial defects at the umbilicus and the stab wound were closed with 0 Vicryl sutures. The skin was closed with subcuticular 4-0 Monocryl, with the exception of the stab wound, which was left open. A postoperative chest x-ray is obtained. A small to moderate residual carbon dioxide pneumothorax does not require chest tube placement and usually resolves spontaneously within six to twelve hours.

TECHNICAL OPERATIVE PROCEDURES:
HOW I DO IT

Stab Wound to Lower Pole of Spleen

Alasdair K.T. Conn, MD, FACS

Scenario
A stab wound to the spleen was found with significant hemorrhage to the lower pole but with an intact hilum.

Management
Preoperative antibiotics were given to the patient prior to surgery. As this was the only intraoperative finding, this will not be continued into the postoperative period. A generous midline incision is made to allow for full exploration and the identification of any other injuries.

Procedure
With the finding of a lower pole partial injury with an intact hilum but with significant hemorrhage, a lower pole partial splenectomy with splenic preservation is the procedure of choice rather than a complete splenectomy. The secret is to completely mobilize the spleen into the wound to obtain not only vascular control of the splenic hilum but also to be able to provide a good repair under optimal circumstances and good visualization. Adequate mobilization is key. The spleen is rotated medially with the non-dominant hand and then the posterior reflection incised and the spleen then is brought into the abdominal wound. Care must be taken not to injure the pancreas. At the completion of the mobilization, the spleen should be completely in the wound and exposed. Digital pressure may be used to control the bleeding from the splenic hilum. The devitalized and damaged portion of the spleen may now be removed by sharp dissection. I find that one cannot identify individual bleeders by ligation or coagulation, so I complete the splenorrhaphy and the splenic repair using interrupted sutures over pledgets. A running suture has been described. I find that interrupted sutures are easier to control. It is important to take big bites of the splenic parenchyma, otherwise the sutures will pull out. As the sutures are tied down, care must be taken that adequate hemostasis is achieved. At the conclusion of the operation, there should be minimal drainage from the lower pole of the spleen. I am a great believer in the power of omentum and at the conclusion of the operation would pass a portion of omentum firmly into the left upper quadrant. The abdomen should then be closed in layers. Splenic injuries do not require drainage.

- The secret is to completely mobilize the spleen onto the anterior abdomen
- Do not injure the pancreas
- Digital pressure on the hilum
- Interrupted pledgeted splenorrhaphy

Although not many surgeons have seen the complication of overwhelming post-pulpectomy sepsis, it reminds us to make efforts to retain the spleen even though the incidence is relatively low, approximately 1%. These patients often succumb to sepsis within 24 hours if they are asplenic. For this reason, splenic preservation should be attempted in these types of patients.

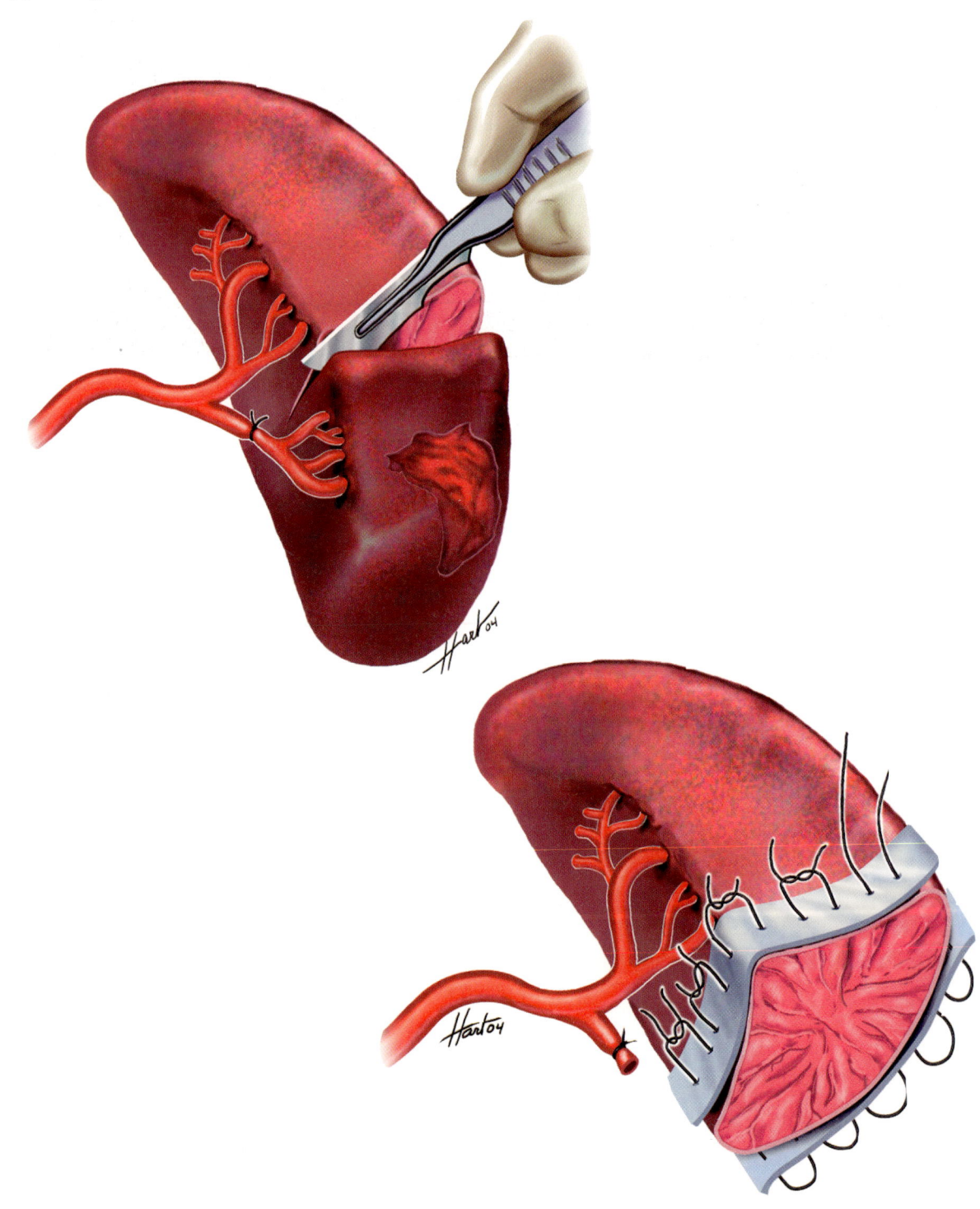

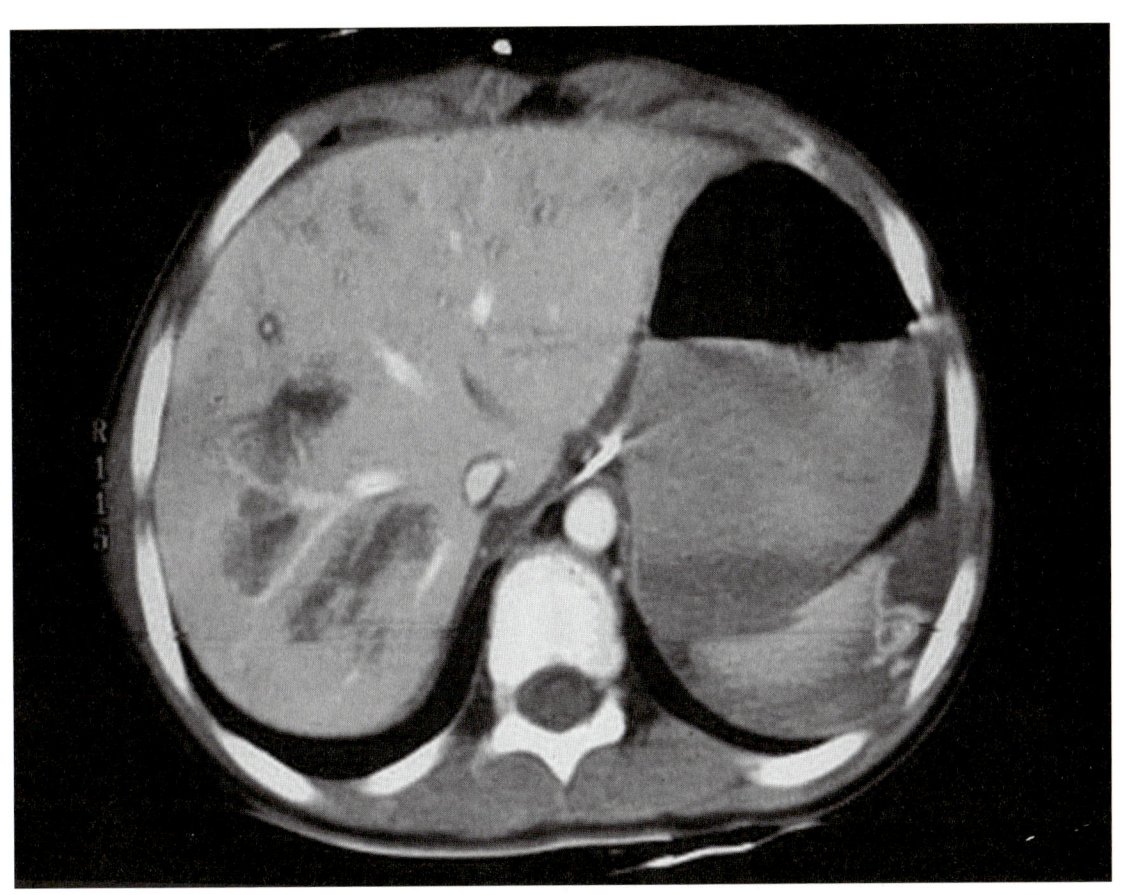

3

The Liver

Liver Injuries

Liver injuries are fairly common following blunt and penetrating traumas. Most of these injuries are minor, require minimal intervention, and have excellent outcomes. More severe liver injuries occur less frequently, but the mortality rate from these injuries is significant. The most significant complication that may develop as the result of severe liver injuries is hemorrhage.

Techniques for managing hepatic injuries vary, depending on the available resources. However, the principles behind the techniques remain the same.

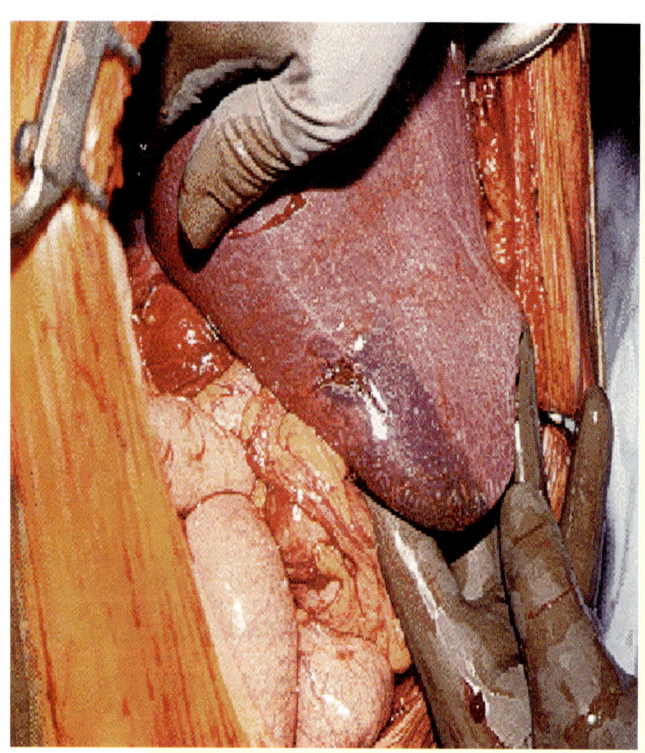

Grade I

- Nonexpanding subcapsular hematoma, < 10% surface area

- Capsular tear, nonbleeding, < 1 cm in depth

- Incidence: common

- Mortality: essentially none

Grade I

Hepatic injuries are graded using the Organ Injury Scale of the American Association for the Surgery of Trauma (AAST-OIS). According to the AAST-OIS, a Grade I hepatic injury can be defined as a nonexpanding subcapsular hematoma that involves less than 10% of the surface area of the liver, or a capsular tear that is not bleeding and has a depth less than 1 cm. This picture shows a small capsular defect less than 1 cm in depth. These lesions are common and seldom require intervention. The mortality rate from isolated Grade I liver injuries is essentially zero.

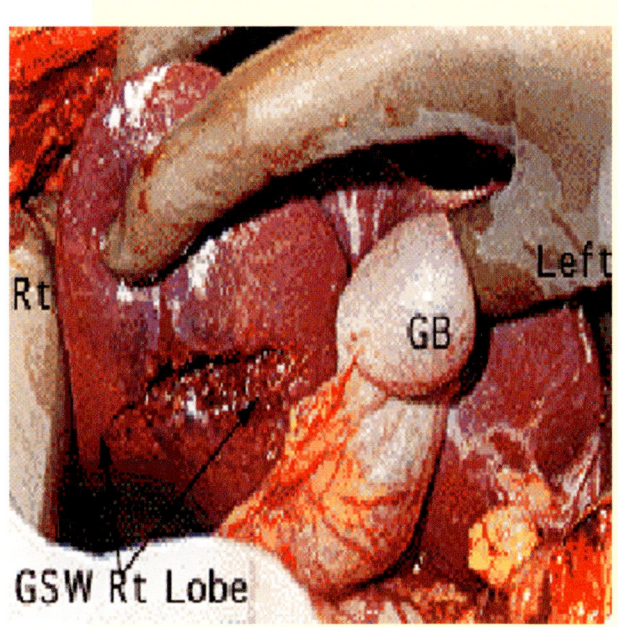

Grade II

- Nonexpanding hematoma, subcapsular or intra-parenchymal, 10 to 50% of surface area or < 10 cm in diameter

- Bleeding capsular tear

- Laceration 1 to 3 cm in depth, < 10 cm in length

- Incidence: 75%

- Mortality: < 10%

Grade II

A Grade II hepatic injury can be defined as a nonexpanding hematoma that is subcapsular or intraparenchymal, and involves 10% to 50% of the surface area of the liver, or is less than 10 cm in diameter. It can also be characterized as a bleeding capsular tear or a laceration 1 cm to 3 cm in depth but less than 10 cm in overall length. These injuries are fairly common, with an overall incidence rate of 75%. The mortality rate from Grade II hepatic injuries is less than 10%.

Grade III

This CT scan image shows a Grade III liver laceration with no extravasation of contrast or blush noted. A subcapsular hematoma involving more than 50% of the surface area of a lobe is a Grade III hepatic injury. The hematoma can be expanding or ruptured with free bleeding or extravasation of contrast on diagnostic studies.

A Grade III hepatic injury can also be defined as an intraparenchymal hematoma that is larger than 10 cm in size, or an intraparenchymal hematoma that is expanding. A liver laceration greater than 3 cm in depth is categorized as a Grade III hepatic injury, regardless of its length.

The incidence of Grade III hepatic injuries is dramatically lower than that of Grade II injuries. The incidence of Grade II injuries is 75%, whereas the incidence of Grade III injuries is 15%. However, the mortality rate from Grade III injuries is higher than that from Grade II injuries. It is 25% in Grade III injuries compared with 10% in Grade II injuries.

Grade III

- Subcapsular hematoma, > 50% of surface area expanding or ruptured with bleeding

- Intraparenchymal hematoma > 10 cm or expanding

- Laceration > 3 cm deep

- Incidence: 15%

- Mortality: 25%

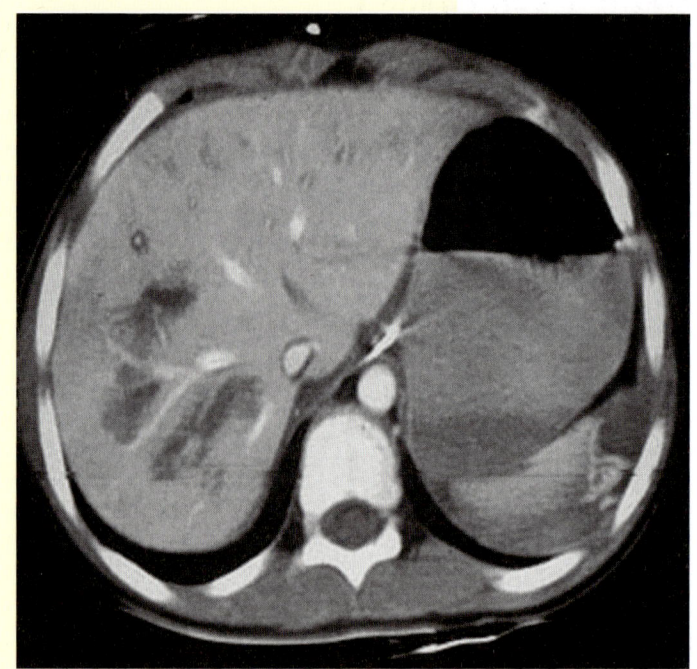

Grade IV

- Ruptured intraparenchymal hematoma with bleeding

- Parenchymal disruption involving 25 to 75% of lobe or 1 to 3 segments

- Incidence: 7%

- Mortality: 46%

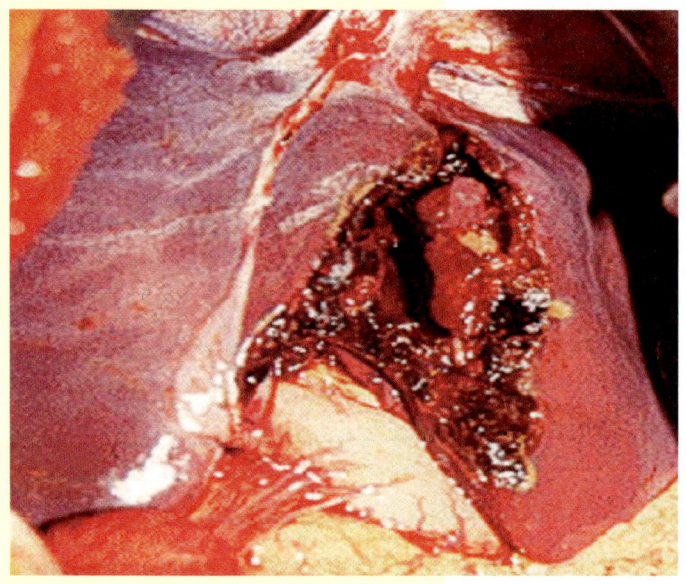

Grade IV

Grade IV hepatic injuries are typically the result of high-energy motor vehicle crashes or high-energy gunshot wounds. A Grade IV injury can be defined as a ruptured intraparenchymal hematoma that is actively bleeding. It can also be defined as a parenchymal disruption involving 25% to 75% of a lobe or one to three segments of a lobe. The photograph shows parenchymal disruption involving almost 75% of the left lobe of the liver. The incidence of Grade IV injuries is approximately 7%, and the mortality rate is about 46%.

Grade V and Grade VI

Mortality increases significantly with severe liver injuries, which are difficult to manage. A Grade V hepatic injury can be defined as a parenchymal disruption of more than 75% of a lobe or more than three segments in a single lobe. A juxtahepatic venous injury is also a Grade V injury. These injuries can be a challenge to diagnose and manage because of their location and massive hemorrhage. Although Grade V injuries are rare, with an incidence of approximately 3%, the mortality rate from them is greater than 80%.

Grade VI liver injuries are lethal injuries. These injuries occur when the liver is completely avulsed from the venous and arterial structures and there is fragmentation of the liver with exsanguinating hemorrhage. There is often very little that can be done to salvage the patient with Grade VI injuries.

Overall, the mortality rates from these injuries have not changed over the past several years. The operative mortality rate for severe liver injuries remains high.

Grade V

- Parenchymal disruption of > 75% of lobe or more than 3 segments
- Juxtahepatic venous injury
- Incidence: 3%
- Mortality: > 80%

Grade VI

- Hepatic avulsion
- Incidence: rare
- Mortality: near 100%
- Take home: no change over time

Hepatic Anatomy

Unless hepatic anatomy is dealt with routinely, review of the anatomy is essential for safe hepatic surgery. The liver can be divided into left and right hepatic lobes by an imaginary line that joins the inferior vena cava (IVC) and the gallbladder.

The hepatic veins define the true anatomy of the liver. The three main hepatic veins are the right, middle, and left veins. These veins divide the liver into four sections: the right posterior lateral, right anterior medial, left anterior, and left posterior sections. The sections are further divided into segments I to IV, which include the left lobe, and segments V to VIII, which include the right lobe and the caudate lobe.

The middle hepatic vein, which usually joins the left hepatic vein, occasionally drains directly into the vena cava. The caudate lobe can also drain directly into the vena cava. The retrohepatic veins that communicate between the liver and the IVC are shown in the illustration. The liver is widely mobilized and the right lobe of the liver is rotated medially to allow this view of the retrohepatic veins and the IVC.

Hepatic Anatomy: Three Arterial Traps

The surgeon must be aware of variations in the arterial anatomy of the liver. These illustrations show a variable takeoff of the middle hepatic artery from the left hepatic artery, a situation where the replaced right hepatic artery is directly coming off the superior mesenteric artery, and an instance where there is a replaced left hepatic artery coming off of the left gastric artery.

Hepatic veins define plane of resection.

The situations described above should be considered upon application of the Pringle maneuver to the portal triad. A window is created in the hepatoduodenal ligament, and a noncrushing vascular clamp is applied across the common bile duct, portal vein, and common hepatic artery. The compression of the porta hepatis should control hepatic inflow and bleeding. In the instance of a replaced left hepatic artery, application of the Pringle maneuver may not control the blood flow from the replaced left hepatic artery because the liver is perfused by a vessel that is not controlled by compression of the porta hepatis.

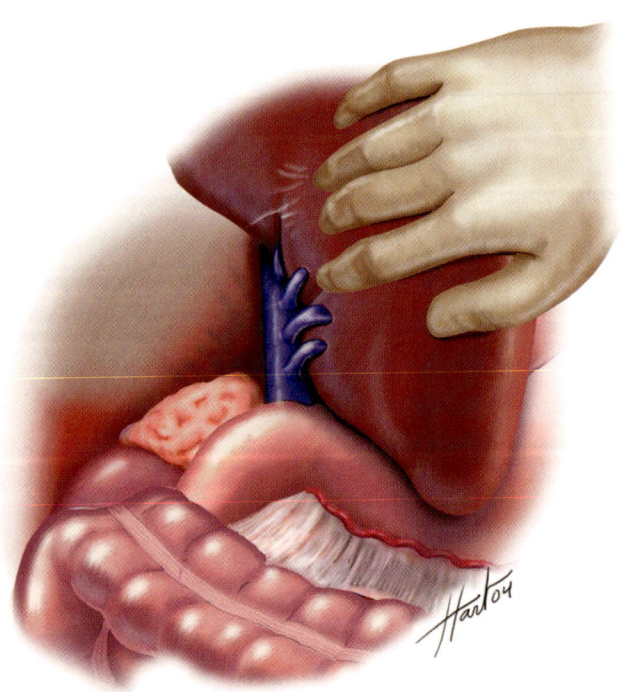

Retrohepatic caval branches are easily avulsed.

Techniques: Operative Management

Operative management techniques for liver injuries include packing and wrapping the liver, hepatotomy and local hemostasis, and resectional débridement. Hepatic artery ligation and vascular control are also options for management of the liver.

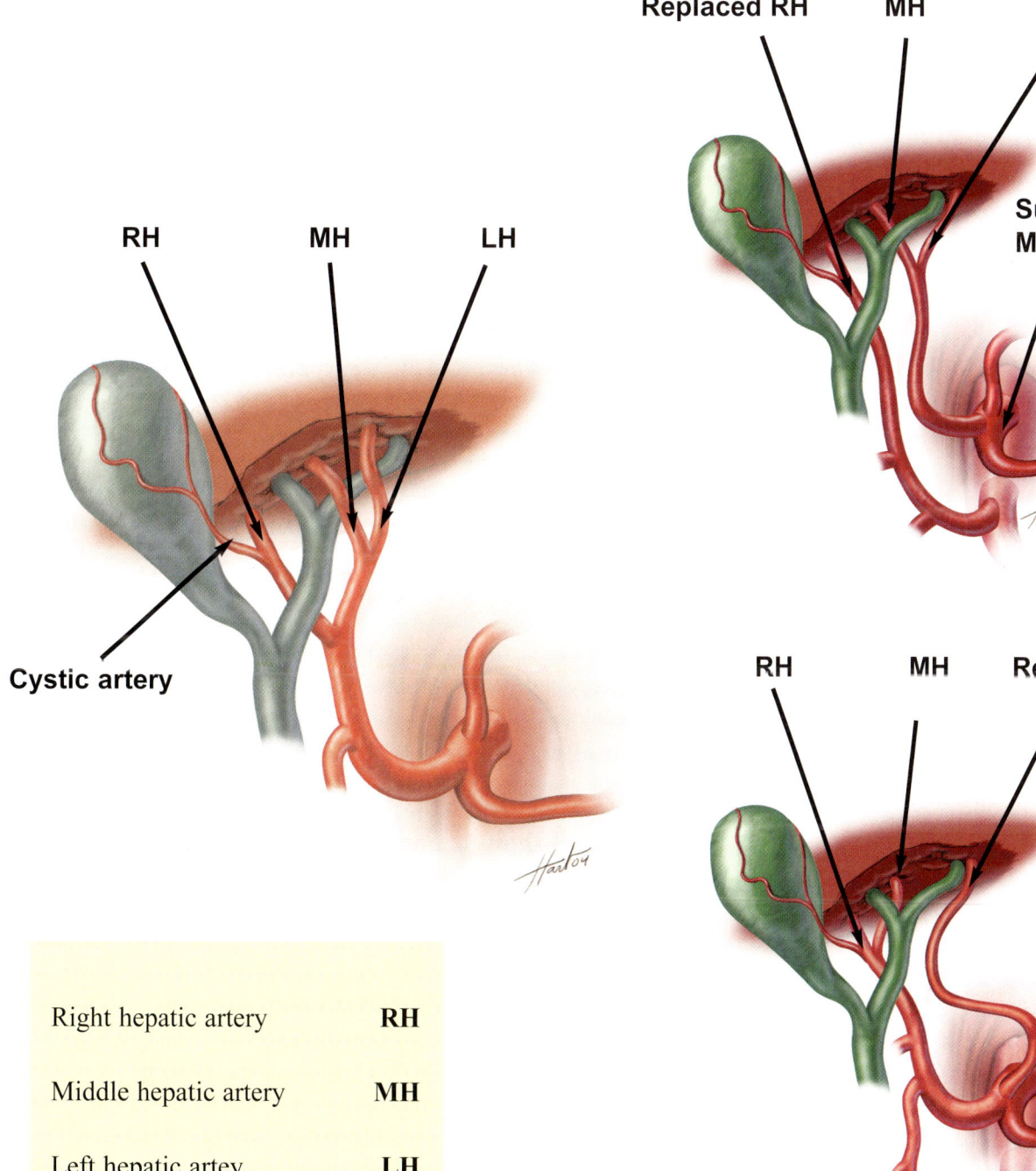

Right hepatic artery	RH
Middle hepatic artery	MH
Left hepatic artey	LH

Best Incision?

In an elective setting, the transplant surgeon may favor a chevron-type incision or a right subcostal incision. A midline incision provides the most expeditious entry and visualization of the abdomen in a trauma patient. The incision should extend from the xiphoid process to the pubic symphysis. This allows complete exploration of the abdomen and its contents. It also allows for the possibility of extension into the chest cavity through a median sternotomy or a lateral thoracotomy as necessary.

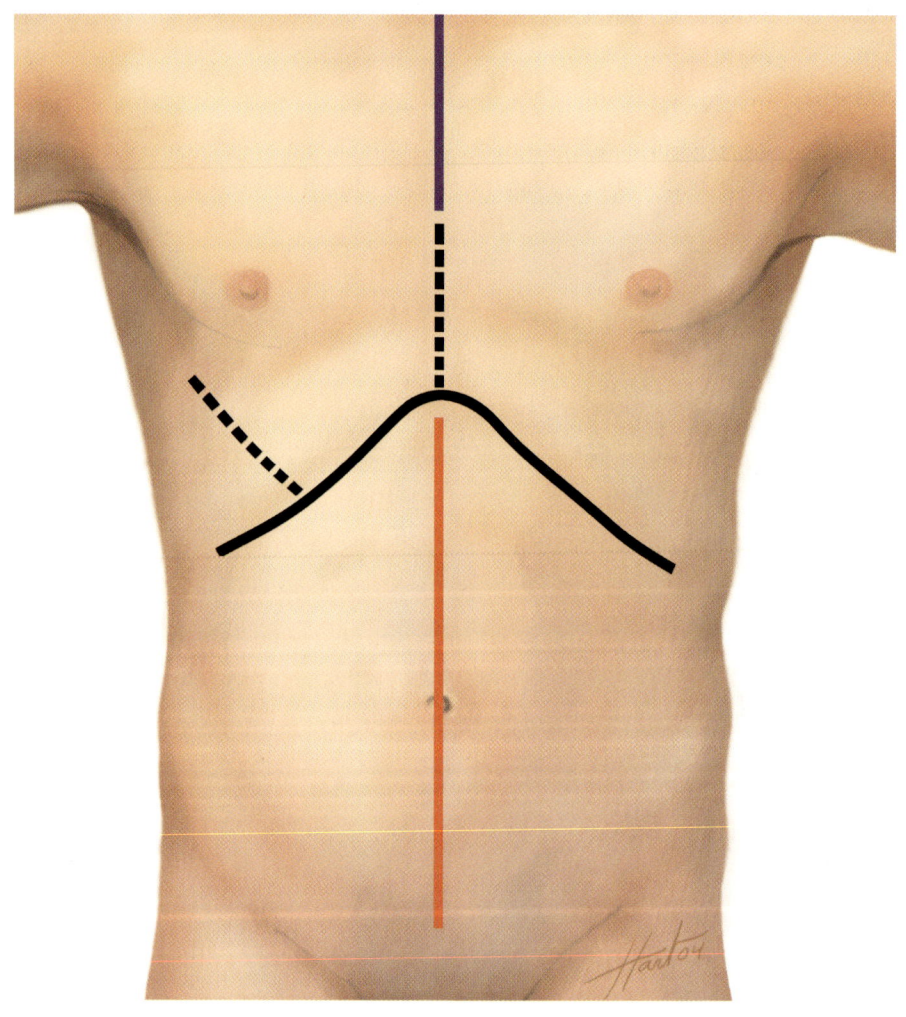

Mobilization and Exposure

William S. Halsted said, "See what you are doing and leave a dry field," more than 100 years ago. This remains essential in dealing with liver injuries today.

The most important point is exposure. The liver must be fully mobilized. Dividing the triangular, coronary, and falciform ligaments mobilizes the entire liver. This exposure facilitates the examination and exploration of the posterior surface of the liver and the retrohepatic vena cava. It is essential that adequate functioning suction and a cell saver suction device are available, as these injuries can hemorrhage at a significant rate. The bleeding site must be adequately visualized in order to identify, control, and repair the bleeding.

Exposure

- Packing/wrapping
- Hepatotomy-local hemostasis
- Resectional débridement
- Hepatic Artery Ligation
- Vascular control

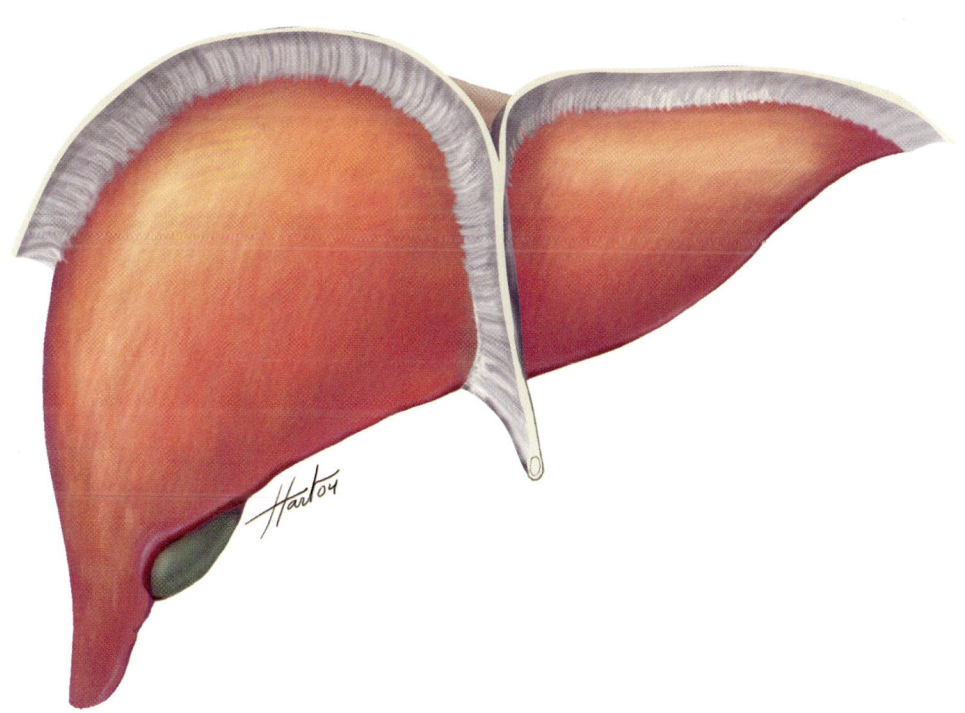

Dividing the triangular, coronary, and falciform ligaments mobilizes the entire liver.

Simple Liver Injuries

- Grade I to Grade III
- Not actively bleeding
- Generally can be treated with pressure, and hemostatic agents

Simple Liver Injuries

Simple hepatic injuries such as Grade I, II, and III injuries that are not actively bleeding can usually be treated by simple application of pressure with or without the application of a hemostatic agent. Hemostatic agents such as a collagen sponge or thrombin with Gelfoam have been utilized to control these injuries. There are various hemostatic agents currently available. Trauma surgeons must know what agents are available at their facilities.

Packing/Wrapping

Packing is one of the most effective and widely utilized methods for temporarily controlling hepatic hemorrhage. Often, after removal of the packing, there is no further hemorrhage and no further treatment is required. If the packing is effective in controlling hemorrhage but hemorrhage recurs on removal of the packs, consideration should be given to leaving the packing in place and performing temporary closure of the abdomen. The patient should be fully resuscitated, normothermic, normalotic, and not coagulopathic before returning to the operating room for packing removal.

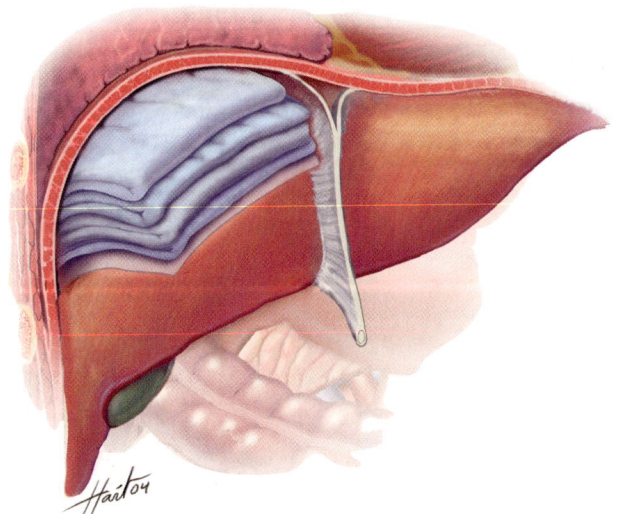
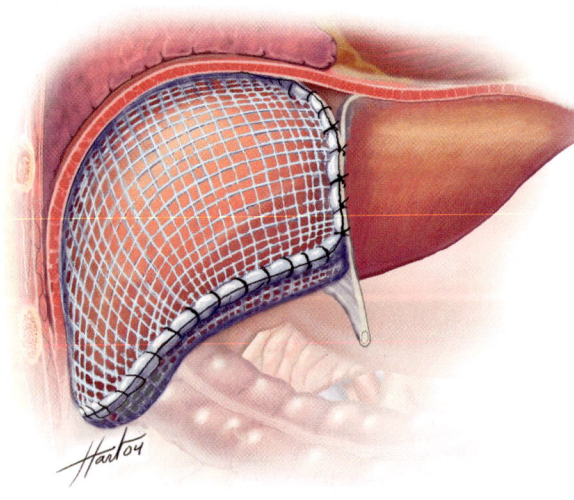

The illustration on the left shows the application of a nonadherent plastic drape next to the liver injury and placement of laparotomy pads over the plastic drape. The laparotomy pads are placed around the liver injury. They compress the liver between the anterior chest wall, diaphragm, and retroperitoneum. The plastic drape prevents the laparotomy pads from adhering to hemostatic liver surface. Packing is more effective with the right lobe of the liver than the left lobe of the liver because the left lobe is not as easily compressed against the diaphragm or anterior chest wall. Application of packing early in the trauma laparotomy is essential for improved patient outcome.

Another technique of hemorrhage control is complete mobilization of the liver and the use of an absorbable mesh wrap that can be fashioned and tightened around the injured portion of the liver to control bleeding. Although it is not widely utilized, this option also controls liver injuries.

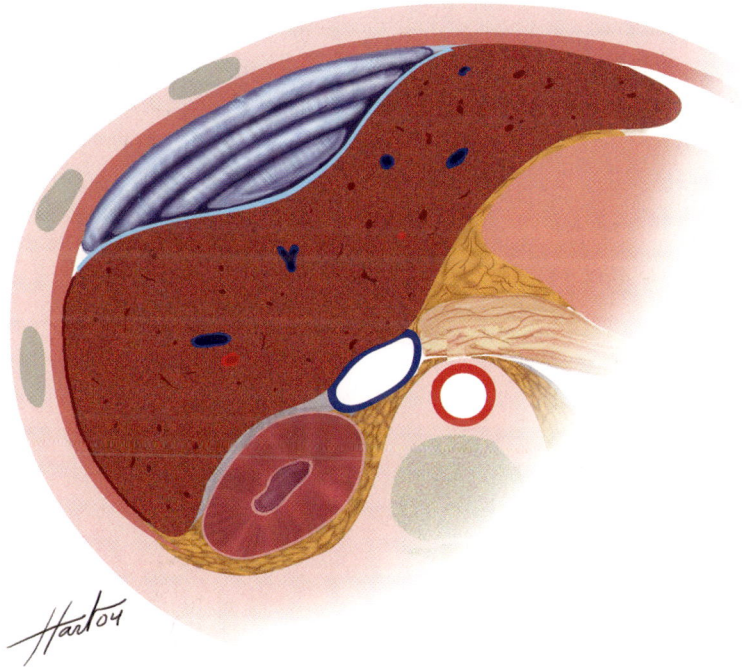

Decreased Vascular Return

Although packing is effective in controlling hemorrhage, its effect is based on application of pressure which can be too high resulting in vena cava compression.

Compromising venous return and portal venous thrombosis and high airway pressure resulting from elevation of the diaphragm.

Packing is also not very effective for major arterial bleeding.

Packing Limitations: Decreased Vascular Return

One of the limitations of packing, which needs to be considered, is that it requires application of pressure in order to effectively control hemorrhage. If too much pressure is applied to the anterior and superior surfaces of the liver, this pressure can be transmitted to the vena cava causing vena cava compression. Excessive compression of the vena cava then leads to decreased venous return and decreased cardiac inflow. In addition, excessive packing of the liver can lead to high peak airway pressures resulting from inability to adequately move the diaphragm. This results in hypoventilation. Although packing typically works very well for venous bleeding, it does not control major arterial bleeding very well.

Hemostatic Agents

Local hemostatic agents are useful adjuncts for controlling hemorrhage. It is important for surgeons to know what agents are available at their facilities.

Fibrin glue, which is a combination of fibrinogen with thrombin and calcium chloride, has been utilized as a hemostatic agent. The components are held in separate syringes and mixed as they are applied to the bleeding surface. This works well on less briskly bleeding surfaces. There have been reports of hypotension with direct intraarterial injection of fibrin glue.

Activated factor VII (factor VIIa) is the newest agent being utilized to control bleeding in the trauma patient. Many centers are still developing protocols and defining the use of factor VIIa, and there are ongoing trials to determine the optimal dose. The initial results of these factor VIIa trials have been promising.

Grade IV and Grade V:

- Collagen/gel preps
- Thrombin
- Fibrin sealant
- Omentum
- Electrocautery
- Argon beam coagulator
- Radiofrequency coagulator
- Factor VIIa

Hemostasis: Argon Beam Coagulator

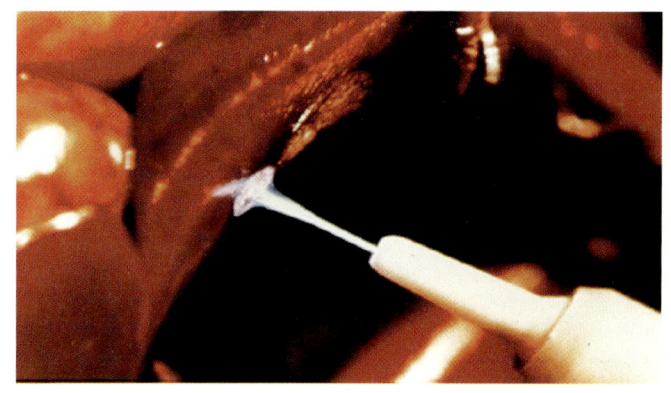

This photograph shows the use of the argon beam coagulator. Rapid coagulation is achieved through several methods. The flow of argon gas clears the liver tissue of blood, and the ionizing energy is transmitted through the argon gas stream. This allows for even application of energy over a broad area, with a maximum temperature of 110°C compared with 205°C with traditional electrosurgical generators. Less energy is needed to create the eschar, and the depth of tissue necrosis is less than conventional spray coagulation. The overall effect is to lessen charring, tissue destruction, and formation of necrotic tissue.

As with any bleeding surface, starting from the top or surface of the injury and working towards the base allows for better visualization. The argon beam clears and controls the bleeding and allows visualization of the tissue and bleeding source during progression to the deeper levels of the injury.

Hemostasis: Radiofrequency Coagulation

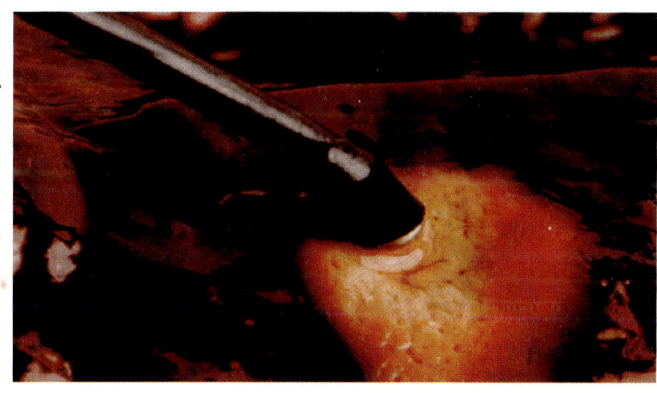

This photograph shows the conductive fluid-enhanced radiofrequency technology used to create hemostasis within the liver. A standard 1liter bag of sterile 0.9% NaCl is hung and dripped though a specialized handpiece that is connected to a standard electrosurgical cautery unit. The normal saline is infused and serves as a conductive fluid at the point of contact via a special ball at the end of the device. This, coupled with the radiofrequency energy, is used to seal tissue.

The energy causes collagen contraction within the tissue. As the collagen shrinks, it causes the vessels to contract and cease bleeding. It does not cut tissue or vessels. The application of saline enhances conduction and cools the tissue and keeps temperatures around 100°C. This has the advantage of minimizing tissue burning, eschar, and smoke production. Its depth of coagulation and area of tissue control can be precisely controlled by altering the level of current, time of tissue contact, and saline flow rate. It has been shown to be effective in elective general and orthopedic surgery cases. However, its application in trauma is not well defined.

Complex Liver Injuries

Grade III to Grade V

- Active bleeding
- Systemically sick patient
- Requires more aggressive intervention
- Damage control measures may be necessary

Complex Liver Injuries

Grade III, IV, and V injuries that are bleeding are classified as complex liver injuries because their severe nature often requires aggressive surgical techniques. Operatively, early application of damage control measures may be necessary, particularly if the patient has received massive transfusions and is acidotic, hypothermic, and coagulopathic.

Portal Triad Occlusion Diagnosis and Treatment

The Pringle maneuver, which was described earlier, is a useful initial technique for hemorrhage control in severe liver injuries. When properly applied, the Pringle maneuver should control hemorrhage from the hepatic artery and portal venous systems. The technique also helps to rule out other sources of bleeding. Continued brisk bleeding after application of the Pringle maneuver suggests other sources of bleeding, for example, the retrohepatic veins and the vena cava or an anomalous hepatic artery.

In an elective situation, the portal triad can be occluded for 90 minutes. The safe duration in the hypotensive trauma patient is not known. However, if possible, intermittent release of the clamp and rapid control of the bleeding should be practiced to limit the total duration of ischemia to the liver.

Use of Pringle maneuver

- Time
  - 90 minutes in elective case
  - unknown in trauma

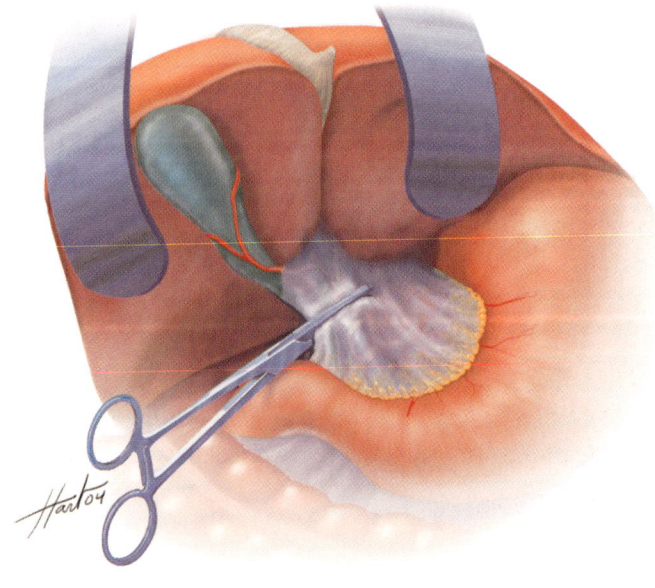

Hepatotomy

A hepatotomy is typically performed after the Pringle maneuver. Vascular inflow allows occlusion and deeper exploration of lacerations by utilizing retractors and suction to enter the liver parenchyma. Bleeding vessels can be controlled using a combination of methods, including surgical clips, sutures, and electrocautery. This technique works reasonably well as long as bleeding is well controlled by the Pringle maneuver and adequate visualization of the wound can be maintained.

Hepatotomy

- Limitations:
  - exposure
  - technical complexity
  - limited visualization

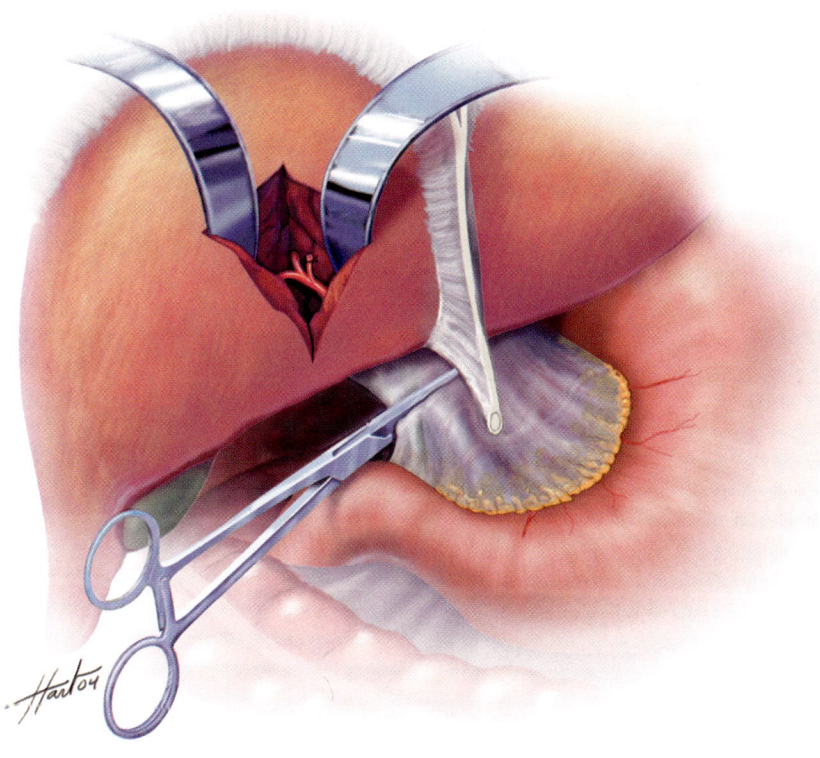

In deeper wounds, it may be necessary to perform a finger-fracture technique to visualize the deeper structures. It should be noted that the finger-fracture technique might increase the amount of hemorrhage from the liver parenchyma. It should be employed only if deep hemorrhage cannot be controlled by the previously mentioned techniques. Hepatotomy and packing are often performed together in the cases of major hemorrhage.

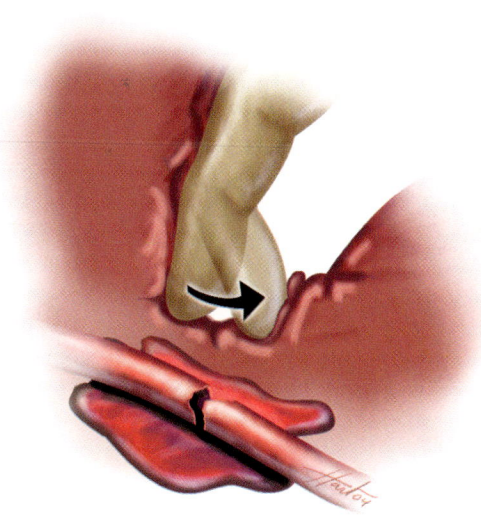

Omental Pack and Drainage

This illustration shows application of flat Jackson-Pratt type drains above and below a liver injury that has been managed with an omental pack. Most surgeons advocate placement of closed-suction drains. Open-suction drainage techniques such as Penrose drains have been shown to increase septic complications and are not recommended.

The application of an omental pack for hemorrhage control is also shown in the illustration. The omentum allows a buttressing suture that may otherwise tear through Glisson's capsule. This has the advantage of eliminating the dead space and the theoretic advantage of bringing living tissue with cellular elements such as macrophages into the wound.

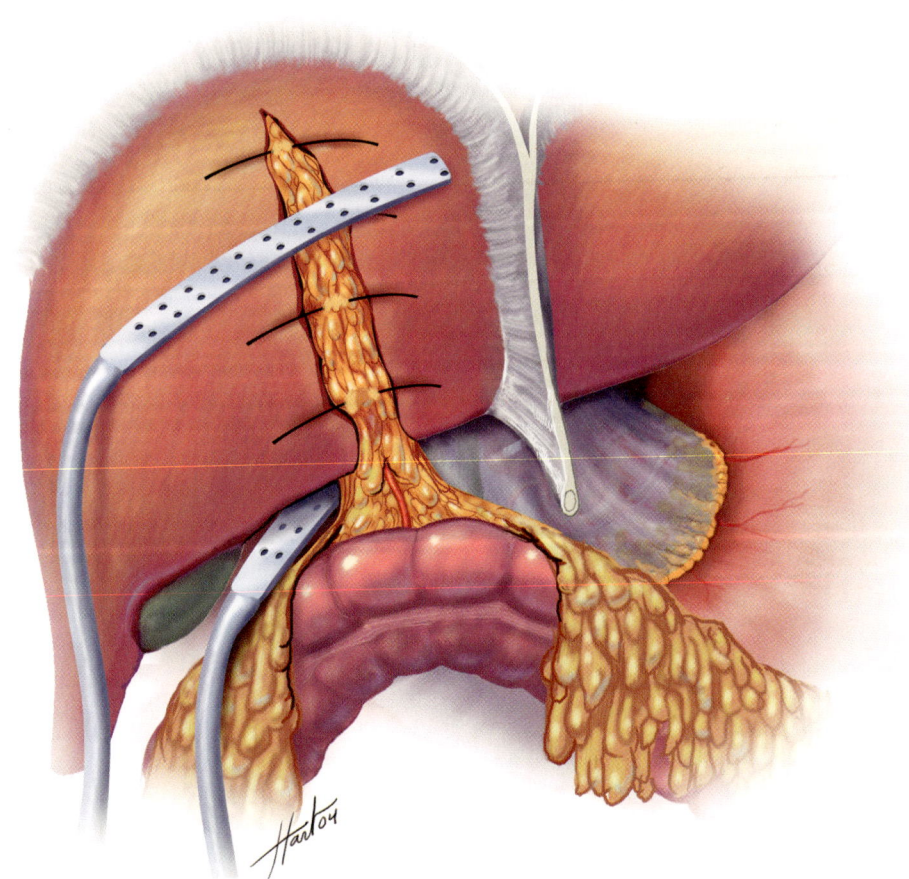

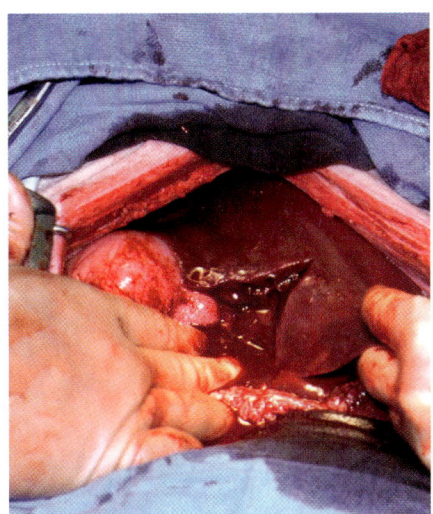 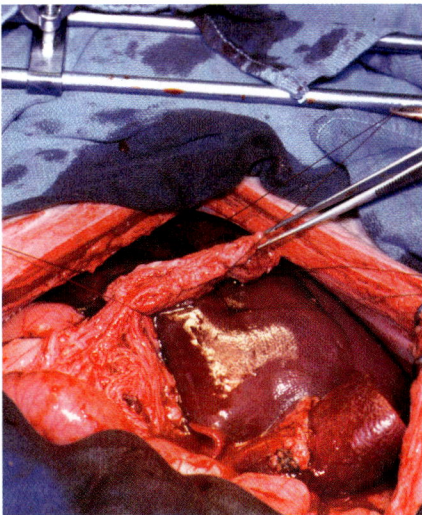 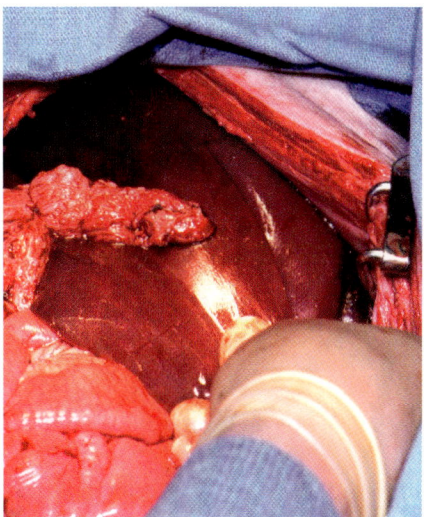

The three photographs depict a large Grade III injury to the left lobe of the liver that is not bleeding. A segment of omentum has been mobilized and placed into the fracture site. The liver has been reapproximated over the omentum.

Resectional Débridement

Formal hepatic lobectomy is usually not necessary in hepatic trauma. Most commonly, resectional débridement is required as directed by the area of injury or necrosis. Typically, this can be accomplished utilizing a combination of the finger-fracture technique, cautery, and sutures and clips. It should be noted that the GIA stapler would work well in some areas, especially the edges of a lobe such as the lateral segment of the left lobe.

> **Resectional Débridement**
>
> Primary vs. delayed

If a patient is hemodynamically unstable, resectional débridement should not be performed at the time of the original operation, especially if further resection will cause further hemorrhage. Following vascular control or arterial ligation, ischemic areas can be allowed to demarcate. The patient should be resuscitated in the intensive care unit and returned to the operating room at a later time for further resection and débridement.

Packing

Limitations: pressure on IVC decreasing vascular return

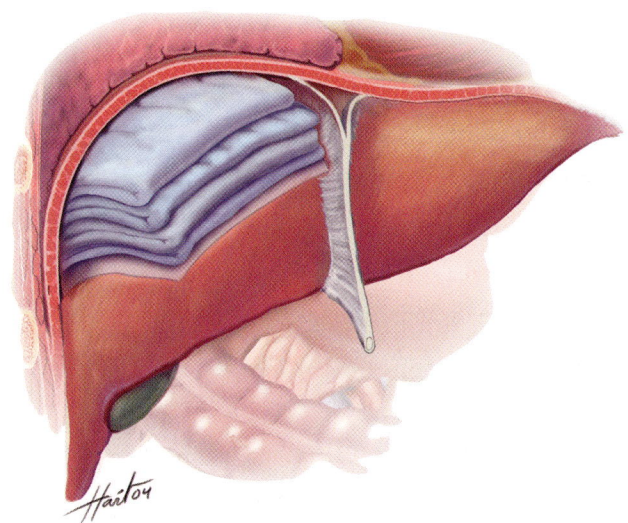

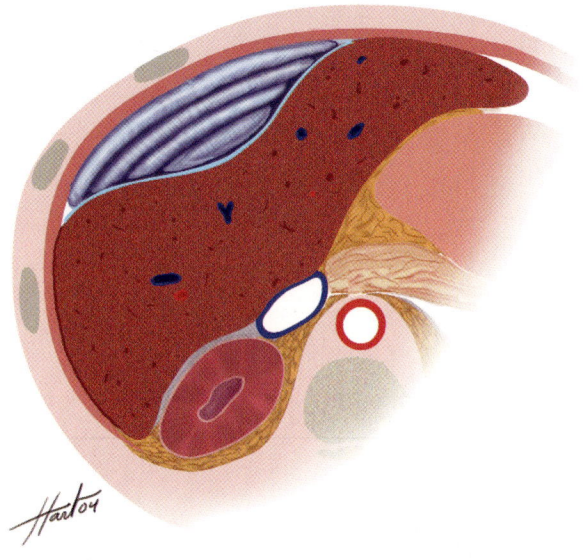

Damage Control: Packing

Packing is the mainstay of damage control. The goal is to control hemorrhage, especially in severely hemodynamically compromised patients who have had massive blood transfusions and are acidotic, hypothermic, and coagulopathic. The application of excessive packing requires caution to avoid compromising diaphragmatic excursion and increasing the airway pressure and decreasing the venous return. After the patient is stabilized and warm and coagulopathy has been reversed, the packing can be removed and the injury reassessed in the operating room.

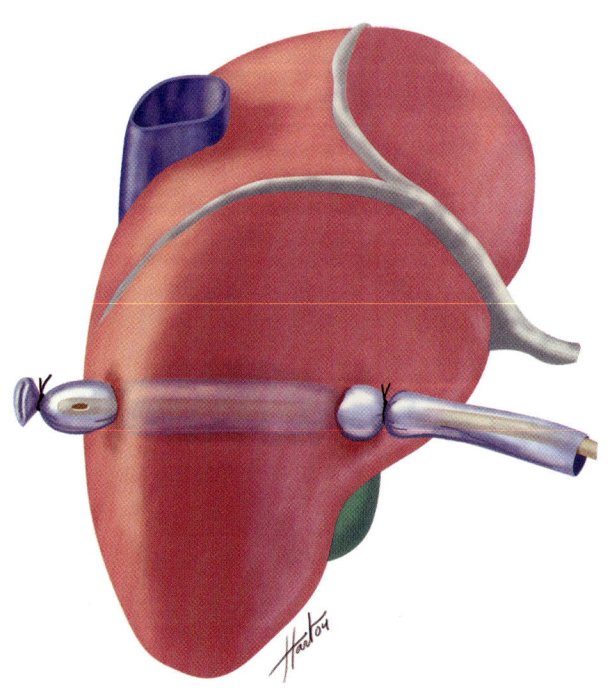

Damage Control: Penetrating Injury

One method of hemorrhage control, particularly for through-and-through penetrating injuries, is to avoid an extensive hepatotomy and utilize an intrahepatic balloon. The illustration demonstrates the creation of an intrahepatic balloon from a Penrose drain that acts as a balloon and hollow catheter. Inflation of the balloon causes a tamponade within the liver parenchyma. Commercial devices that perform a similar function are also available.

Damage Control: Hepatic Artery Ligation

Hepatic artery ligation was first used in 1972 by Truman Mays on a series of six patients, two of whom suffered delayed hemorrhage after trauma.

Variation in arterial anatomy must be considered when performing hepatic artery ligation. Although collaterals have been described via the abdominal wall and diaphragm and between the lobes of the liver, the hepatic arteries are effectively considered end-arteries. It is safe to ligate the artery if clamping the artery results in control of the hemorrhage without major signs of ischemia. Another method for control of the hepatic artery is selective angiographic embolization of the individual bleeding vessel.

> **Hepatic Artery Ligation**
>
> - Hepatic artery - end vessel
>   - ligaments divided
>   - variant anatomy
>
> - Angiographic embolization

Complex Vascular Lesions

Grade VI lesions do not usually respond to typical damage control techniques and packing. It is essential to obtain early proximal and distal control of the hepatic vasculature. Since Grade VI lesions can produce exsanguinating hemorrhage, adequate exposure and suction are vital to allow for visualization. Grade VI injuries are often fatal.

> **Complex Vascular Lesions**
>
> - Grade VI
>
> - Establish proximal and distal control

Vascular Control

The most important concept in vascular control of the liver is to obtain proximal and distal control of all vessels to totally isolate the liver. Proximal control can be obtained by clamping the supradiaphragmatic IVC. Clamping the infradiaphragmatic IVC achieves distal control. This maneuver can be performed through the abdomen, but it may be necessary to extend the midline abdominal incision into a median sternotomy to gain control of the proximal IVC.

The addition of a Pringle maneuver will effectively control hemorrhage of these complex injuries by stopping hepatic inflow through the hepatic artery and controlling the splanchnic inflow through the hepatoportal vein. The maneuver is not well tolerated in a hypovolemic patient because of the sudden decrease in venous return, which can lead to cardiac arrest. It is essential to alert the anesthesiologist prior to the maneuver in order to achieve adequate preload by transfusion through intravenous access.

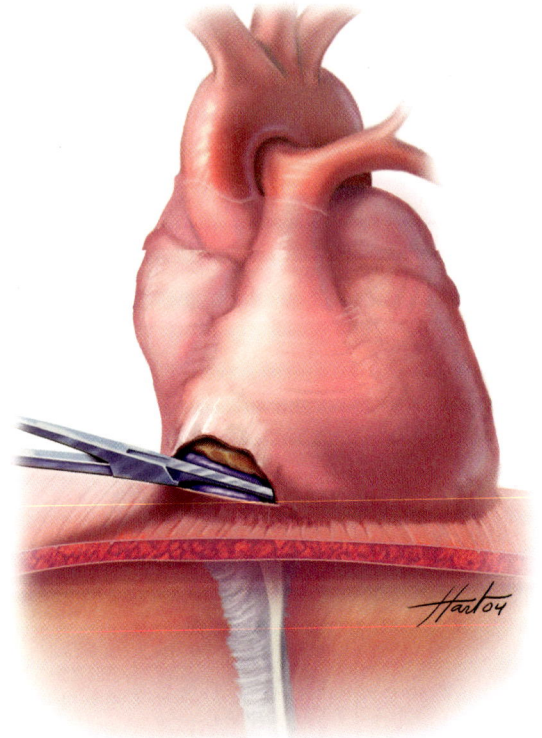

Proximal

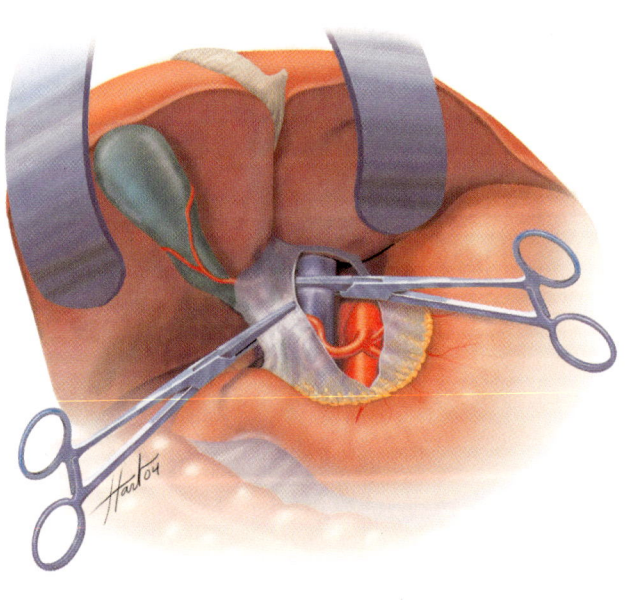

Distal

Atrial Caval Shunt to the Superior Vena Cava

Several different caval shunt techniques have been developed in order to preserve venous return while controlling a retrohepatic caval injury.

The Schrock shunt is an atrial caval shunt that involves placing a large chest tube through the right atrial appendage and advancing it into the IVC to a site distal to the renal veins. The side holes of the chest tube are placed below the renal veins. Additional side holes are cut in the chest tube at the atrial level, and the tube is secured to the atrial appendage with a purse-string suture. Umbilical tapes are tightened around the vena cava at the level of the supradiaphragmatic and suprarenal cava levels. This selectively forces the blood from the lower extremities, abdomen, and kidneys to flow through the shunt and isolates the caval area of injury from blood flow.

Most trauma surgeons do not frequently practice the application of this technique, and the lack of familiarity with the technique limits it use. The shunt should be used early in the operation, and the components should be assembled before laparotomy. If a shunt is indicated, it should be employed early in the operation after the diagnosis of a retrohepatic caval injury has been made.

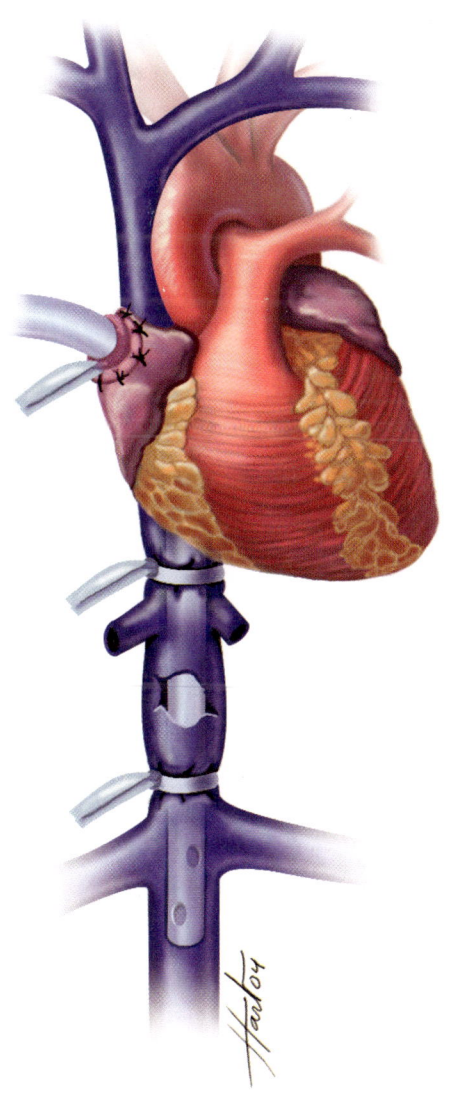

Atrial Caval Shunt To The Superior Vena Cava

Limitations:
- timing
- technical complexity

Hepatic Venous Exclusion

Limitations:
- timing
- technical complexity

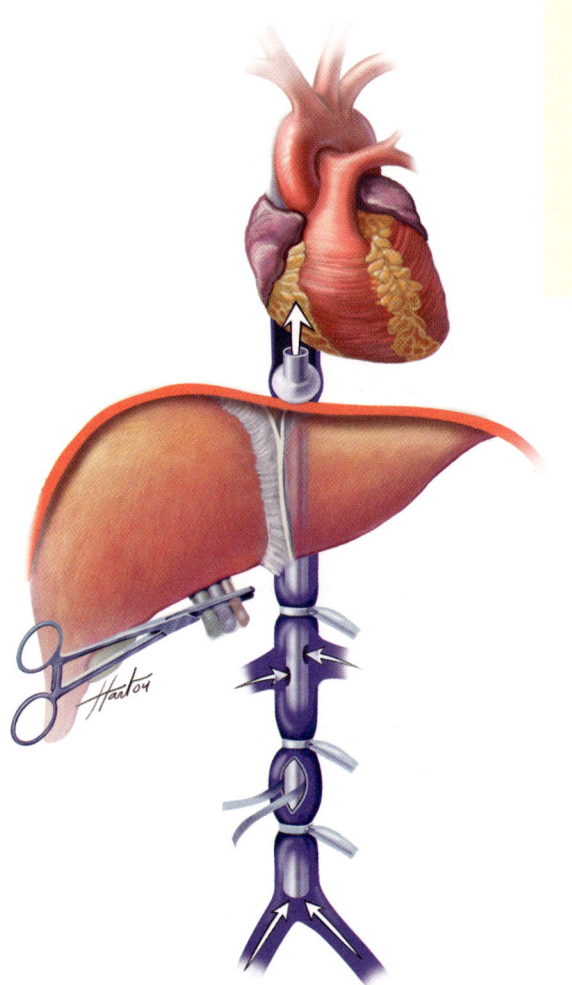

Hepatic Venous Exclusion

Another method of hepatic venous exclusion is introducing a Moore-Pilcher balloon caval shunt through a venotomy. The balloon is advanced past the liver and positioned at the level of the supradiaphragmatic vena cava. Umbilical tapes are placed in the suprarenal position and around the venotomy site. Blood then flows through the hollow tube, draining the lower body and renal veins and excluding the liver from vena caval flow.

Adding a Pringle maneuver provides hepatic artery and portal vein control. It should control most bleeding from the liver injury.

As with the Schrock shunt, this technique requires forethought and planning. Many surgeons have limited exposure to this technique, and this may limit its use.

Hepatic venous exclusion involves a combination of proximal and distal vena caval clamping with the Pringle maneuver and aortic clamping. It results in total vascular exclusion of the liver. The procedure usually requires a median sternotomy to gain intrapericardial control of the superior vena cava, a right medial visceral rotation to gain inferior vena caval control, and the application of a Pringle maneuver and aortic cross-clamping. This allows for complete vascular isolation of the liver.

Hepatic Venous Exclusion and Venovenous Bypass

Venovenous bypass is another method of venous exclusion. This technique borrows from the hepatic transplant experience. A drainage line, which can be placed percutaneously, is inserted into the femoral vein. A similar drainage line is inserted into the inferior mesenteric vein to decompress the bowel. Both catheters are connected to a BioMedicus pump, which has an inline heating element. The warmed blood is returned to circulation via the superior vena cava. The superior vena cava line is percutaneously placed in an internal jugular vein or axillary vein line catheter.

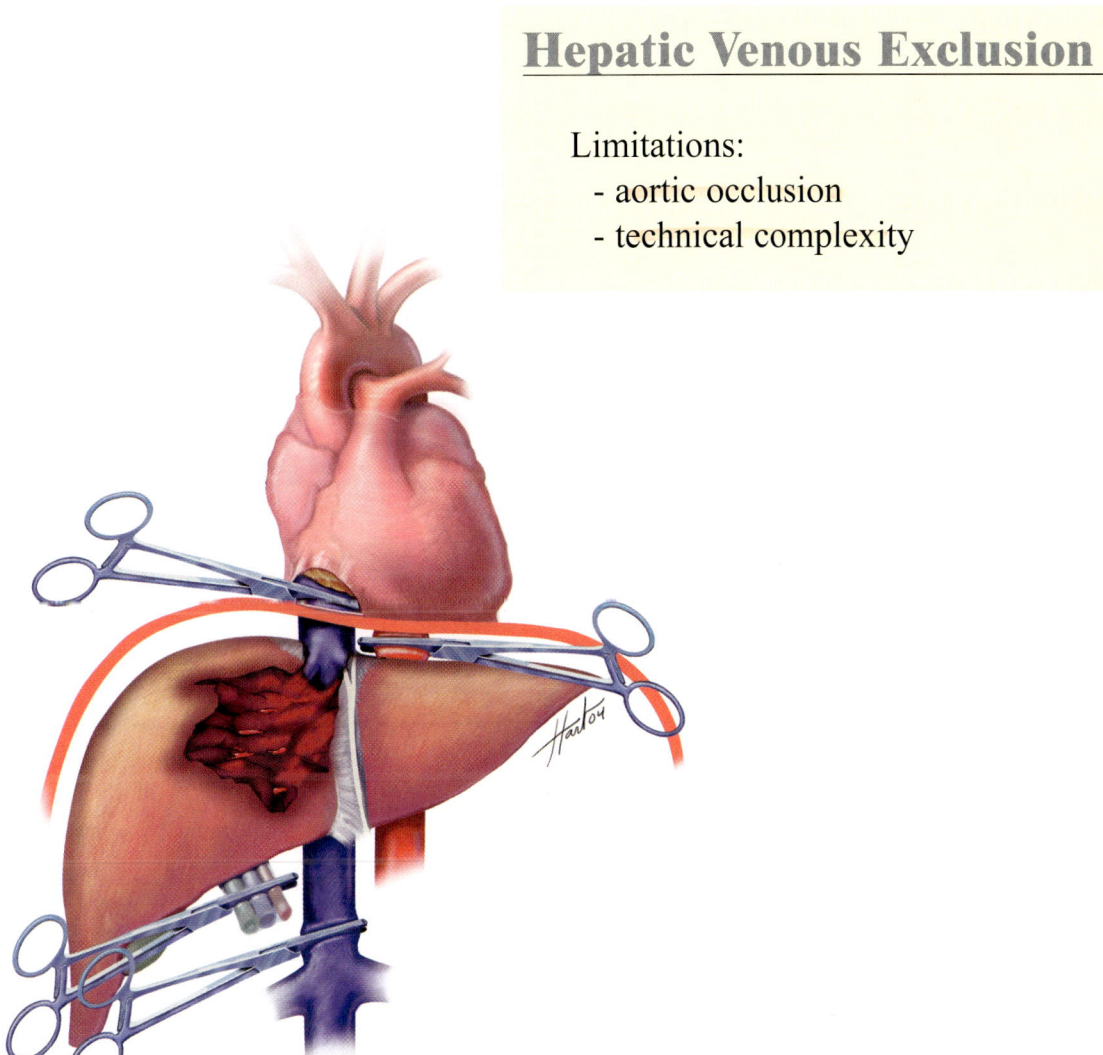

Hepatic Venous Exclusion

Limitations:
- aortic occlusion
- technical complexity

Hepatic Venovenous Bypass

Limitations:
- rarely used
- time consuming
- technical complexity

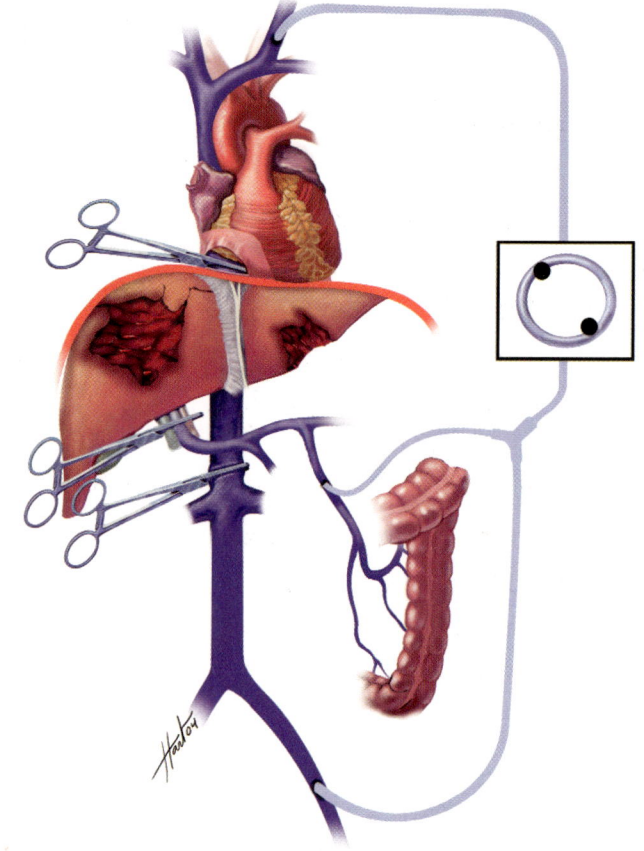

Venovenous bypass can be time consuming and requires the availability of a pump, appropriate circuitry, and a pump technician to operate the pump. It requires familiarity with the anatomy and equipment, and practice before use in the severely injured patient.

Goals of Management

- Physiology drives algorithm
  - unstable patients require celiotomy

- Early, definitive intervention
  - avoid late damage control

- Primary vascular control
  - multiple techniques

- Definitive control, possible repair
  - define the injury

Principles of Management: Goals

Appropriate management techniques are determined by the hemodynamic stability and physiology of the patient. Hemodynamically unstable liver patients require urgent laparotomy. Early intervention before the onset of acidosis, hypothermia, and coagulopathy allows for more definitive management and increases the possibility of a successful outcome. The appropriate and early use of vascular control allows for accurate identification of the injury and control of the hemorrhage.

Principles of Management: Intrinsic Problems

It is important to review the complex vascular anatomy of the liver, as it is essential in managing complex liver injuries. Grade IV and Grade V hepatic injuries are relatively uncommon, and damage control techniques are successful in most patients with severe hepatic injuries. Early primary vascular control is essential if packing fails to control the hemorrhage. The Pringle maneuver and vascular isolation techniques should be performed early in order to adequately identify the characteristics and severity of the hepatic injury.

Intrinsic Problems

- Know the anatomy and physiology
  - complex vascular injury

- Very severe liver injuries are uncommon

- Most patients - damage control mode
  - packing may fail if used late

- Need early primary vascular control
  - portal triad occlusion
  - atrial caval shunt - often employed too late

Technical Summary

For successful treatment of hepatic injuries, the surgeon must know when to employ nonoperative embolic techniques and explore the patient. It is essential to be comfortable and familiar with the techniques used to expose and mobilize the liver, evaluate the injury, obtain primary vascular control of the injury, address these specific injuries, obtain definitive vascular control, and finally, repair these injuries.

Technical Summary

- When to operate

- How to expose and mobilize

- How to evaluate the injury

- How to obtain primary vascular control

- How to address specific injuries

- How to obtain definitive vascular control and repair

Complications

- Recurrent bleeding
  - usually in first 48 hours
  - angiography if hemodynamically stable

- Hemobilia
  - triad of GI bleed, RUQ pain, and jaundice
  - angiographic embolization

- Intraabdominal abscess

- Hyperpyrexia
  - temperatures of 38° to 39°C, mechanism unknown
  - usually resolves in 3 to 5 days

- Biliary fistulae
  - 50 mL/day for more than 14 days
  - drainage and possible ERCP
  - major ductal injury requires operative repair

- Arterial-portal venous fistulae
  - causes portal hypertension
  - usually present with GI bleed
  - angiography for diagnosis and treatment

Complications

Hemorrhage is the most common complication following hepatic injury. Recurrent bleeding typically occurs within the first 48 hours after injury. Angiography can be helpful if the patient is hemodynamically stable. Identification and possible control of the vessels may be accomplished by selective embolization.

Hemobilia can present suddenly in a patient who has undergone liver repair. The incidence of hemobilia is less than 2% in patients who have undergone hepatic injury repair. Presentation following injury is highly variable and can range from days to months. Significant upper gastrointestinal bleeding is often the only symptom. The classic description of hemobilia includes the triad of jaundice, right upper quadrant pain, and gastrointestinal bleeding. Angiography, which is the preferred diagnostic and treatment modality, allows identification of the pseudoaneurysm and embolization of the vessel. Intraabdominal abscesses are common and are usually amenable to percutaneous drainage techniques.

Hyperpyrexia, from 38°C to 39°C, is fairly common. The etiology may be related to the release of tumor necrosis factor and IL-6. Patients with hyperpyrexia develop an elevated temperature and require frequent fever work-ups. The fever typically resolves within 3 to 5 days without identification of an infectious cause for the fever.

A biliary fistula is defined as a bile output of more than 50 cc per 24-hour period for 14 days. It can be diagnosed with a radionuclide hepatobiliary scintigraphy scan, which can demonstrate the leak but may be nonspecific, or with endoscopic retrograde cholangiopancreaticography (ERCP), which can define the leak. An ERCP facilitates some form of controlled drainage of the biliary system. This can be through a sphincterotomy or a biliary stent or biliary drainage catheter. The cause of the biliary fistula will determine the method to be utilized.

Penetrating ductal injuries are typically partial transections. Major ductal injuries should be identified and repaired. Minor partial tears can be repaired primarily. Severe and complete transections and devascularization injuries may require biliary enteric anastomosis. Roux-en-Y hepaticojejunostomy with a cholecystectomy and T-tube drainage has been recommended for reconstruction of ductal injuries.

Although arterial-portal venous fistulas have been reported, they are rare. They can result in portal hypertension and present with gastrointestinal bleeding. Angiography is helpful for the diagnosis and treatment of these fistulas.

Liver Replacement Therapy

Orthotopic liver transplantation may be considered in extreme circumstances at institutions with hepatic transplantation programs. Extracorporeal liver support may be available at research facilities, making liver cell transplantation a possibility for the future.

Liver Replacement Therapy

- Orthotopic liver transplantation
- Extracorporeal liver support
- Cell transplantation

Hepatic Trauma: Summary

The AAST-OIS grading system classifies liver injuries according to their characteristics and severity. Mortality rates and treatment methods differ among the injury grades.

Early diagnosis and prompt vascular control of hepatic injuries should allow for effective definitive treatment of a hypotensive patient. Damage control measures should be instituted if these methods fail. These measures include packing of the liver, confirming the resuscitation in the intensive care unit, and using angiographic embolization.

Hepatic Trauma Summary

- AAST Grades
- Treat shock
- Damage control
- Operative techniques:
  - vascular control
  - definitive treatment

ADVANCED TRAUMA OPERATIVE MANAGEMENT
Selected Readings
Chapter 3 - The Liver

Feliciano DV et al. Intraabdominal packing for control of hepatic hemorrhage: a reappraisal. J Trauma 1981;21:285-290.

Cue JI et al. Packing and planned reexploration for hepatic and retroperitoneal hemorrhage: critical refinements of a useful technique.
J Trauma 1990;30:1007-1013.

Pachter HL, Feliciano DV. Complex hepatic injuries. Surg Clin North Am. 1996;76:763-782.

Renz BM et al. Failure of nonoperative treatment of a gunshot wound to the liver predicted by computerized tomography. J Trauma 1996;40:191-193.

Richardson JD et al. Evolution of the management of hepatic trauma: a 25-year perspective. Ann Surg. 2000;232:324-330.

Buckman RF et al. Juxtahepatic venous injuries: A critical review of reported management strategies. J Trauma 2000;48:978-984.

Carrillo EH et al. Evolution in the treatment of complex blunt liver injuries Curr Prob Surg 2001;38:1-60.

Johnson JW et al. Hepatic angiography in patients undergoing damage control laparotomy. J Trauma 2002;52:1102-1106.

Ascensio JA et al. Operative management and outcomes in 103 AAST-OIS Grades IV and V Complex hepatic injuries: Trauma surgeons still need to operate, but angioembolization helps. J Trauma 2004;54:647-654.

Tips From the Masters

There are a number of safe methods to manage blunt and penetrating trauma in the operating suite. The following technical surgical tips have been successfully used by the authors to deal with difficult or challenging operating situations.

Chapter 3: The Liver

TABLE OF CONTENTS

Exposure & Management of a Grade IV Penetrating Hepatic Injury-The Pachter Pack 136
H. Leon Pachter, MD

Management of Major Hepatic Trauma 138
Donald D. Trunkey, MD

Balloon Tamponade Technique for Through-and-Through Injury to the Liver 142
Kimball I. Maull MD

Grade IV Liver Laceration 144
Fred A. Luchette, MD

Grade IV Liver Injury Without Active Hemorrhage Fibrin Glue Hemostatic Agent 146
David G. Burris, MD

Complex Hepatic Trauma – Grade IV Burst Injury 148
Rao Ivatury, MD

Hepatic Vascular Exclusion 151
George A. Perdrizet, MD

Exposure and Management of a Major Injury to the Right Lobe of the Liver 154
David V. Feliciano, MD

TECHNICAL OPERATIVE PROCEDURES:

HOW I DO IT

Exposure & Management of a Grade IV Penetrating Hepatic Injury - THE PACHTER PACK

H. Leon Pachter, MD

Scenario

A 22-year-old male sustains a gunshot wound 3 cm below the right costal margin which exits 4 cm below the right scapula. His systolic blood pressure is 80 with a pulse rate of 110. Diffuse abdominal tenderness is present.

Management

Two liters of Ringer's lactate are rapidly infused raising his blood pressure to 100 systolic and slowing his pulse rate to 90. A chest X-ray reveals a right pneumo-hemothorax and a right chest tube is rapidly placed which drains 400 cc of blood. He is taken to the operating room.

Procedure

A midline incision is made from the xyphoid to several centimeters below the umbilicus. An auto transfusion device is prepared but not inserted until a colonic injury is excluded. Once excluded the catheter is inserted into the peritoneal cavity. All blood clots are rapidly evacuated and all four quadrants are packed off with multiple lap pads. A large stellate laceration to the right lobe of the liver is found which is actively bleeding. The injury is immediately compressed bimanually between several lap pads and full resuscitation is commenced. No attempts at mobilization of the liver or addressing the injury are initiated until volume replacement has been achieved and metabolic acidosis corrected. Bimanual compression is slowly released and the injury fully evaluated. If active bleeding persists a Pringle maneuver may be required. Cross clamping the porta hepatis can safely be performed for up to one hour providing adequate volume replacement has been achieved. The right triangular and coronary ligaments as well as the falciform ligament (to the IVC) are rapidly incised with an electrocautery device. This maneuver is essential as it allows for maximum mobility of the liver resulting in excellent exposure. The injury can then easily be manually controlled by exerting anterior and posterior pressure on the liver between several lap pads. The liver may also be torqued to the patient's left which can control profuse bleeding, adequately

- Bimanual hepatic compression

- Do not mobilize the liver until volume replacement has been achieved

- Pringle maneuver can be applied for up to one hour

- Place a folded Steri-Drape on the liver first then place abdominal packs assessed, rapidly repaired or resected, if necessary. Short of a juxta-hepatic venous injury, the combination of complete and full mobilization of the liver combined with the Pringle maneuver will virtually arrest all major bleeding. It has been our preference to open the injury tract from entrance to exit and repair or ligate lacerated blood vessels and bile ducts under direct vision. The Pringle maneuver is slowly released, and any further areas of bleeding are oversewn with 3-0 Prolene sutures. Parenchymal bleeding from the raw surface of the liver can be managed in a variety of ways. Particularly useful is the combination of the argon beam coagulator and any one of a variety of hemostatic agents such as microfibrillar collagen. More recently, the application of commercially available biologic glues applied to the liver surface has been especially effective. Once hemorrhage has been controlled, an omental pedicle based on either the right or left gastroepiploic vessels is fashioned and inserted into the hepatic defect and held in place by several 2-0 chromic liver sutures. The injury area is then drained with two closed Jackson-Pratt suction drains anteriorly and posteriorly.

Packing

The indications to pack a liver injury are basically three: 1) the onset of circumstances which pose an immediate threat to the patient's life such as the Triad of Death when acidosis, hypothermia and coagulopathy set in; 2) as part of a damage laparotomy; 3) the inability to control bleeding deep within the liver necessitating rapid closure and bringing the patient from the operating room to the radiology department for angioembolization. Under any of these circumstances, it has been our preference to apply multiple lap pads anterior to the liver injury and inferior to the diaphragm in order to create a tamponading effect. To facilitate this maneuver, and to more effectively enhance the role of these laparotomy pads we place a folded Steri-Drape on top of the liver and then place multiple laparotomy pads on top of the Steri-Drape until the ipsilateral hemidiaphragm is reached. The adhesive drape serves a twofold purpose. Firstly it avoids the inevitable bleeding that ensues when laparotomy pads that were in direct contact with the raw hepatic parenchyma are removed. Secondly, placing the laparotomy pads on a relatively dry surface enhances their efficacy. The need for packing should always be accompanied by rapid abdominal closure by any means available. Multiple towel clip closure of the abdomen is a rapid and simple method of achieving this goal.

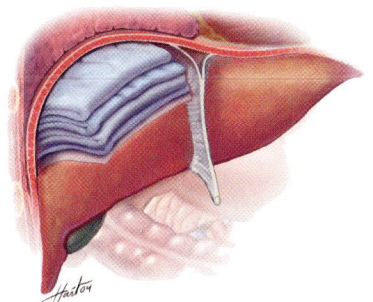

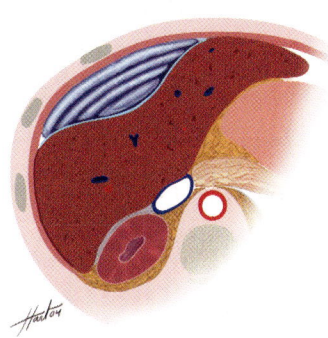

TECHNICAL OPERATIVE PROCEDURES:

HOW I DO IT

Management of Major Hepatic Trauma

Donald D. Trunkey, MD, FACS

Scenario

An 18-year-old male falls asleep and is involved in a motor vehicle crash. He has a seatbelt mark from his left clavicle across the sternum and right chest. Initially, he is hypotensive but responds to fluid resuscitation.

Management

He is taken to CT scan, which shows approximately 1½ to 2 liters of fluid in his abdomen. His injuries are confined to the liver, which demonstrate a Grade IV injury with near complete transsection along the major fissure into the hilar plate. Two cuts show an extravasation of contrast from the left portal vein. The patient is taken from CT scan to the operating room.

Your initial priorities in the operating room are to prep and drape the patient from the mid-neck to the mid-thighs anteriorly and from tabletop to tabletop laterally. In an unstable patient, the preparation and draping optimally should be done before the induction of anesthesia, since the administration of a muscle relaxant may lead to significant drop in blood pressure. The surgeon should be prepared to open the abdomen as soon as possible after the induction of anesthesia.

A generous midline incision is made from the xyphoid to below the umbilicus, often to the suprapubic area. Once the abdomen is open, the surgeon is often met with a large amount of blood within the peritoneal cavity. My initial approach is to immediately evacuate as much clot as possible and then to pack all four quadrants of the abdomen. This will usually temporarily control hemorrhage and allow the anesthesiologist to replace needed volume. The surgeon should make some critical decisions at this juncture. Every effort to keep the patient warm must be done. This includes turning the thermostat in the operating room up to 85°F. There should be adequate blood-warming devices, and the humidifier on the ventilator should be turned to 105° F. If the hospital has a massive transfusion protocol, it should be initiated.

I first remove the packs from the lower abdominal quadrant, checking for associated injuries, particularly those causing fecal contamination. If there is no fecal soilage, the surgeon can then use autotransfusion devices. The packs in the left upper quadrant are removed, and if there is an associated injury to the spleen, it should be promptly removed in order to reduce associated hemorrhage while the liver injury is being addressed. Finally, the packs in the right upper quadrant are removed.

At this point, I do a simple diagnostic maneuver: gently retract the dome of the liver rostrally. If a gush of blood emanates from the central area, this is a presumptive diagnosis of hepatic vein injury. Packs are replaced, and the surgeon must decide what isolation technique is to be used. More often the bleeding is from deep lacerations in the liver substance and blood is coming from the depths of the wound. Another diagnostic maneuver is to apply a vascular clamp across the porta hepatis. If this controls the hemorrhage, it eliminates the hepatic veins as a source of major bleeding and one should presume it is either hepatic arterial or portal venous bleeding. This may lead to further dissection within the distal porta hepatis to isolate the left and right portal vein and left and right hepatic artery in order to selectively control them and determine which is the source of bleeding. Ligation of one of these vessels can be done, but is seldom indicated.

After temporary control of hemorrhage has been achieved by packs or compression, the first priority is to mobilize the liver. This includes sharply dividing the falciform ligament, taking down both leaves of the coronary ligament and dividing the triangular ligament of the left lobe. If not already performed, the lesser sac should be entered by dividing the avascular area of the gastrohepatic ligament. With these ligamentous attachments divided, the surgeon can mobilize the individual lobes in order to compress and get access to the injuries.

The most common major hepatic injury that surgeons will be called upon to treat is deep lacerations into the parenchyma; usually involving the right hepatic lobe or segment IV, quadrate lobe, proximal to the falciform ligament. Controlling the bleeding is best achieved by the assistant, who stands on the left side of the patient. He or she can extend the left hand underneath the right lobe and compress the dome of the uninjured part with the right hand.

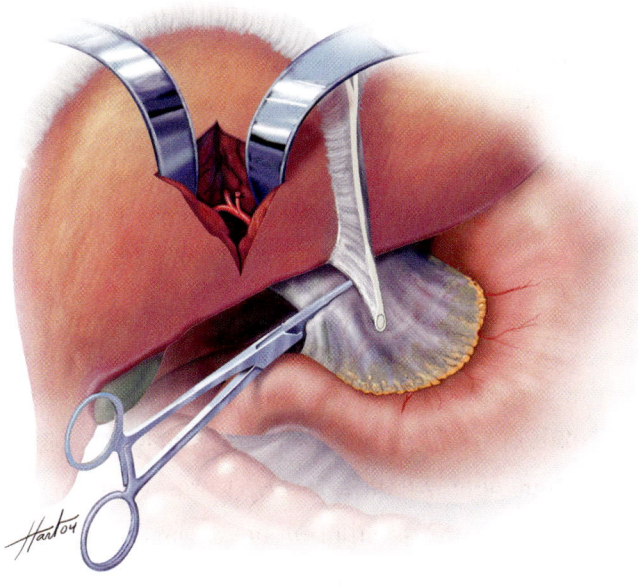

This allows the surgeon to deepen the laceration using finger fracture technique in clamping the bleeding vessels and bile ducts, followed by suture ligation with 3-0 or 4-0 silk sutures. I prefer to use silk ligature since clips often fall off with rostral displacement of the liver during ventilation. Deep liver sutures or mattress sutures are not commonly indicated for control of hemorrhage. These can lead to hemobilia, hepatic necrosis, abscess and hematoma formation within the liver parenchyma. Useful adjuncts include all of the hemostatic agents such as thrombin-soaked Gelfoam, Tisseel, etc. Once hemorrhage has been controlled with suture ligation of the individual vessels, the margins are checked for viability. The use of a viable pedicle of omentum is a useful technique to help with hemostasis and to close the dead space. The omentum also aids wound healing and reduces sepsis.

If compression by the assistant is inadequate to control bleeding from the laceration, a vascular clamp can be placed across the porta hepatis (Pringle maneuver). Once hemostasis is achieved, this clamp should be removed as soon as possible. Although the Pringle maneuver has been used for up to one hour in elective hepatic surgery, it has not been established what is the safe limit for hypovolemic trauma patients. In general, I would prefer to limit warm ischemia time to 15 minutes, but would accept up to 30 minutes.

Resectional débridement is the next most common procedure performed in major hepatic injuries. Resection is not determined by segmental anatomy, but by the extent of injury and liver viability. Most often these injuries are caused by shotgun blasts or large lacerations from blunt trauma which have lateral extensions. The general principles are straightforward: all non-viable liver tissue is resected using a finger fracture technique or the back of the scalpel handle. When resistance is encountered with either technique, this usually indicates the elastic tissue of vessels or biliary ducts. These are doubly clamped, divided and suture ligated.

- Right hepatic lobe bleeding is initially controlled by manual compression

- Finger fracture with digital vessel isolation

- Silk sutures

- Pedicle omental packs aid hemostasis and close dead space

Non-pulsatile oozing from the parenchyma can be controlled with the electrocautery unit or the argon beam coagulator.

Overall, hepatic lobectomy is indicated in 2 to 4% of all liver trauma cases, however, in major liver trauma such as this patient, it is indicated in approximately 15 to 20%. Usually the extent of injury has made it obvious to the surgeon that a formal lobectomy will be necessary to control the hemorrhage. The lobectomy is started by incising the liver capsule with a scalpel or the electrocautery unit in the anatomical plane. The blood loss is minimized by isolation of the liver or by compression of the liver between the assistant's hands. As described above, the liver parenchyma is divided by the finger fracture technique or the blunt end of a scalpel handle. As vessels and bile ducts are encountered, they are individually ligated with 3-0 or 4-0 silk sutures. Knowledge of the liver segmental anatomy is paramount since there are anomalies of the vascular inflow into the hilum and segment four blood supply is a recurrent blood supply after the blood vessels leave the hilar plate.

In very few patients, there may be an injury to the left or right hepatic vein or to the retrohepatic inferior vena cava. As noted above, this is diagnosed by rostral displacement of the liver from the diaphragm. A gush of blood is very presumptive that such an injury exists. These injuries will usually require vascular isolation of the liver. There are at least three methods currently in use: The Heaney maneuver, atrial-caval shunting, and veno-venous bypass. Of these three techniques, I prefer the Heaney maneuver. Atrial-caval shunting has been abandoned by most surgeons.

The Heaney maneuver is performed by clamping both the suprahepatic and infrahepatic inferior vena cava while simul-taneously applying the Pringle maneuver. During the Heaney maneuver, it is crucial that central pressures are monitored by the anesthesiologist and that fluid replacement is adequate when the inferior vena cava is clamped. If the hepatic vein is injured, attempts at isolating the supra-hepatic vena cava may be associated with significant blood loss. In my opinion, it is better to pack the area of injury below the diaphragm, extend the midline incision into a sternotomy and isolate the inferior vena cava within the pericardium prior to exposing the injury at the junction of the right or left hepatic vein into the cava.

Segment one of the liver sends several venous branches directly into the inferior vena cava. Shear injuries may cause these to be pulled out of the wall of the inferior vena cava or avulsed. In order to successfully repair this injury to the cava and to ligate the venous branches, it is necessary to isolate the liver, as noted above.

The second most common method of hepatic vascular isolation is veno-venous bypass using a centrifugal pump, which was initially described by Starzl. The modification of this technique is to simply cannulate the femoral vein in the groin and the axillary vein in the upper arm. Heparin coated tubing connects the two cannulae. The centrifugal pump is used to assist flow. Hepatic vascular isolation can then be accomplished by clamping the suprahepatic vena cava at the diaphragm or above the diaphragm and clamping the suprarenal vena cava and porta hepatis. It is not necessary to place a portal vein catheter as originally described by Starzl.

In this particular patient, the Pringle maneuver controlled most of the bleeding and a left hepatic lobectomy was performed. The left hepatic vein was isolated between the cava and the junction of the middle hepatic vein and the left hepatic vein. This was sutured with 2-0 silk sutures. The left portal vein and the left hepatic artery and left hepatic bile duct were ligated 1 cm from the junction of the their counterparts to the right lobe. Parenchymal bleeding was controlled with 3-0 and 4-0 silk sutures and the electrocautery unit. Drainage was not considered necessary since there was no obvious bile leaks at the end of the procedure.

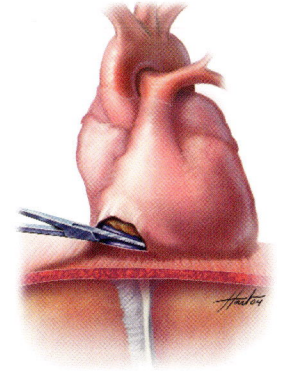 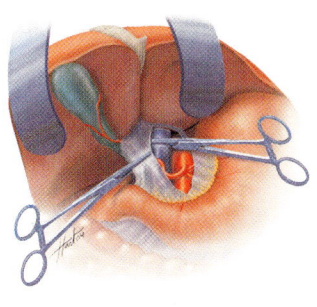

Proximal **Distal**

TECHNICAL OPERATIVE PROCEDURES:

HOW I DO IT

Balloon Tamponade Technique for Through-and-Through Injury to the Liver

Kimball I. Maull MD, FACS

Scenario

A 41-year-old truck driver is shot in an attempted robbery. The entrance wound is in the lower right lateral thorax. The bullet is palpable in the subcutaneous tissue just inferior to the xiphoid. FAST shows fluid around the liver but no pericardial fluid.

Management

The patient is prepared from chin to mid-thighs and draped for an extended midline celiotomy. The bullet is encountered incidentally while opening the abdomen. It is collected and scored with the surgeon's initial on the bullet base. It is then passed from the operative field to police custody. The right upper quadrant is packed with laparotomy pads and compressed manually by the assistant. The remainder of the abdomen is rapidly explored. No other injuries are detected.

Upon careful removal of the packs, a wound measuring approximately 2 cm is discovered along the lateral aspect of the right lobe of the liver, yielding brisk bleeding of combined bright red and dark red blood. A similar wound is identified immediately to the right of the falciform ligament with similar but less profuse hemorrhage. An angled vascular clamp is placed across the gastrohepatic ligament, occluding arterial and portal venous inflow, the Pringle maneuver. Using an angled clamp allows for vascular control without the operative field being obstructed by the clamp handle. Bleeding slows dramatically. Using the long arm of the Army-Navy retractor, both wounds are inspected. No discreet vessels are seen. The vascular clamp is partially released with return of active bleeding. The Pringle maneuver is re-established.

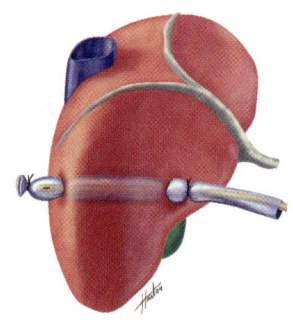

Procedure: *Intrahepatic balloon tamponade*

A half-inch Penrose drain is placed around a size 16 to 18 Levine tube in a manner which includes the distal-most hole of the Levine tube within the confines of the Penrose drain. Using a 2-0 silk suture on a fine round needle, the Penrose drain is anchored to the distal end of the Levine tube. The suture is tied circumferentially around the distal Levine tube, thereby occluding the distal lumen of the Penrose drain.

The right lobe of the liver is rotated medially to allow access to the lateral wound. The combined Levine-Penrose unit is gently passed into the lateral hepatic wound and guided to the medial exit wound. The Levine-Penrose unit is gently extracted for a distance of 2 cm from the lateral wound; the Penrose drain is divided, leaving sufficient length of drain to secure to the Levine tube with circumferential 2-0 silk sutures. The Levine tube is checked to make certain that no holes of the Levine tube are outside the ligated portion of the Penrose drain. The Levine-Penrose unit is gently re-inserted into the tract. The proximal Levine tube is brought out through a stab wound in the right flank, juxtaposed to the site where the liver wound meets the parietal peritoneum when the liver is returned to its normal anatomic position.

The balloon tamponade unit is now ready to be distended. Using a catheter-tipped syringe, saline is injected into the Levine tube, distending the Penrose drain. The Levine tube is crimped and clamped to assure no leakage. The position of the balloon tamponade is re-assessed. The tip of the Levine tube should be visible at the medial wound only with Army-Navy retractor exposure, allowing ample liver tissue for inclusion in closure of the medial wound. Pitfall: if the Penrose is too close to the liver surface, it could be caught with a closing suture.

The vascular clamp is partially, then fully, released. Modest oozing is identified from the medial wound. This bleeding is controlled by closing the medial wound with absorbable sutures over pledgets. I favor making absorbable pledgets at the operating table from

- A Levine tube is placed inside the Penrose drain

- Introduce the unit through the tract

- Distend the Penrose balloon

- Tamponade is maintained for 48 hours

1 cm squares of Gelfoam, wrapped with strips of Surgicel. These pledgets hold sutures well and have intrinsic hemostatic properties. The 2-0 absorbable sutures are placed using horizontal mattress technique.

The lateral wound is re-inspected, and the tension on the balloon is rechecked. Drains are placed dependently and brought out a second separate lateral incision. Closed suction drains are favored although Penrose drains can also be used. The anterior medial wound is not drained.

Tamponade is maintained for 48 hours. Serial hematocrits are checked and sonographic imaging of the liver is performed prior to release of tamponade. If the patient shows no further indication of bleeding, the pressure within the balloon tamponade device can be slowly released over a 30-minute period. The apparatus should not be removed for an additional 24 hours and in the interim the patient should be re-assessed. Reinflation should be considered if there is indication of recurrent bleeding. Following removal of the Levine-Penrose unit, drains remain in place for an additional 24 hours and are then removed.

TECHNICAL OPERATIVE PROCEDURES:
HOW I DO IT
Grade IV Liver Laceration

Fred A. Luchette, MD, FACS, FCCM

Scenario

A 33-year-old restrained female driver crashed into a bridge abutment after losing control on icy roads. There is prolonged extrication time of greater than 20 minutes. She arrives in the emergency department cold and hypotensive. A FAST examination demonstrates blood in all four quadrants with no other obvious source of bleeding.

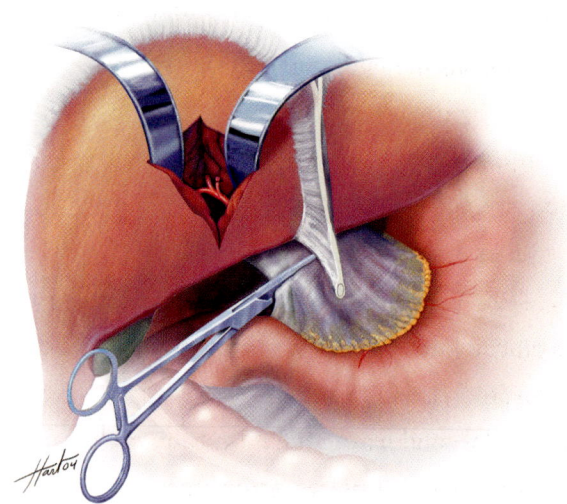

Management

Blood should be sent immediately for type and cross match (8 units) and the massive transfusion protocol initiated for transfusion in the operating room. A generous midline incision is necessary for adequate exposure and exploration of the peritoneal cavity.

The first order of business is to control the hepatic hemorrhage. A quick Pringle maneuver using your thumb and index finger initially or a vascular clamp will help reduce portal venous inflow and hemorrhage from the liver parenchyma or the intrahepatic branches of the portal vein. Continued bleeding after the Pringle maneuver suggest a hepatic venous source. An additional method for reducing hemorrhage while anesthesia continues aggressive resuscitation is to occlude the aorta at the diaphragmatic hiatus. This can be performed

- A self-retaining retractor facilitates exposure by retracting the costal margin

- Avoid manual liver traction

- Mobilize the right lobe to the midline

- Débride devitalized tissue by finger fracture

quickly with digital compression against the vertebral bodies or using various instruments. Once the patient is adequately resuscitated, arterial flow is restored. Use of a blood salvage system is helpful for autotransfusion when there is no evidence of GI tract contamination.

This patient with prolonged extrication and class IV shock has the fatal triad of hypothermia, coagulopathy and acidosis. Once the major venous hemorrhage is controlled, strong consideration should be given to a damage control laparotomy. Perihepatic packing can further reduce bleeding from the liver. Lap pads are placed between the diaphragmatic and visceral surface. On average, 11 to 13 pads are required. The abdomen should be quickly closed with towel clips or temporary skin closure.

The patient is then transported to the intensive care unit for ongoing resuscitation, rewarming and correction of the coagulapathy. After resuscitation is completed, the patient is then returned to the operating room for pack removal and further débridement of the wound.

Procedure: *Control of liver hemorrhage*

Exposure for a Grade IV stellate liver laceration to the dome of the right lobe is facilitated by the use of a self-retaining retractor (Bookwalter, Thompson, or Omni), which allows retraction of the costal margin and lower ribs. Manual traction on the medial liver surface for exposure should be avoided in order to not extend the laceration. Rather, the triangular ligament, coronary ligaments, and falciform ligament should be quickly divided for mobilization of the entire right lobe into the midline. Care should be taken when approaching the posteromedial surface of the liver to avoid injury to the retrohepatic collateral veins feeding directly into the cava. The liver laceration should be digitally explored and gentle retraction will allow visualization of transected vessels. These should be directly ligated with permanent sutures. Releasing the Pringle maneuver restores the portal inflow and arterial bleeders should then be controlled.

At the time of reexploration for packing removal, any devitalized tissue should be débrided by finger fracture technique and ligation of vessels. Omentoplasty may be warranted to help reduce the risk of a significant bile leakage and also to tamponade venous oozing. An alternative is to utilize the argon beam coagulator for cauterizing the raw liver surface. Closed suction drainage is critical to allow adequate drainage for any bile leak. Large sutures placed in an effort to close the laceration have been reported to increase the risk for abscess formation and should be avoided.

TECHNICAL OPERATIVE PROCEDURES:

HOW I DO IT

Grade IV Liver Injury Without Active Hemorrhage Fibrin Glue Hemostatic Agent

David G. Burris, MD, FACS, DMCC

Scenario

A 35-year-old man presented after a horse kicked him in the right upper quadrant. He is requiring fluids to maintain hemodynamic stability and has a tender, distended abdomen.

Management

Preoperative antibiotics to cover gram positive, gram negative organisms and anaerobes should be given intravenously. The patient should be placed on a warming blanket, and care taken to ensure normal body temperature during the procedure. An exploratory laparotomy is conducted through a generous midline incision. Any active hemorrhage should be controlled, and all injuries identified, including inspection of the diaphragm. A Grade IV injury of the right lobe of the liver is identified. There is not active bleeding, but there is significant oozing from the liver surface.

Procedure: *Hepatic local hemostasis*

Division of the falciform ligament and triangular ligaments is performed to give mobilization and visualization of the liver. For massive bleeding, or for a patient who is already cold, coagulopathic and acidotic, the liver is compressed, packs placed over a non-adherent barrier such as plastic surgical drape to compress the liver, temporary closure of the abdomen accomplished, and the patient resuscitated and warmed in the intensive care unit.

For that annoying, persistent ooze in the stable patient, a variety of hemostatic agents are available. Currently, it is not known what the best method is so the surgeon should be familiar with the characteristics of some options, and what is available in their institution. When others are not available, a two component glue mixed separately and sprayed onto the wound through a Y-connector is very effective. The components are fibrinogen concentrate 10 mL in one syringe, and bovine thrombin, reconstituted with calcium containing 10 mL diluent at a concentration of 1000U/mL. The fibrinogen concentrate must be thawed and prepared. This may require 30 minutes to become available.

Commercially available two component systems are now available and are widely used in thoracic and vascular operating rooms. Those with fibrinogen and thrombin require special mixing and warming devices and about

> • A two-component glue sprayed onto the wound is very effective

30 minutes to reconstitute, so they offer no major advantage to the surgeon in the urgent situation, but are effective at controlling this type of oozing. FloSeal is thrombin in a gel matrix without fibrinogen, and requires only a few minutes of mixing in the two syringe system. It is currently the most rapidly available two component system.

A 4 x 4 inch hemostatic bandage made of chitose, the physiologic glue that holds shrimp shells together, adheres to such wounds and is absorbable. There appears to be some anti-microbial effect from this substance. It would be a good choice. The rigidity of this bandage leads to some challenge in deep or irregularly shaped bleeding surfaces.

A granular powder of aluminum silicate (Quik Clot) is not approved for internal use. There are anecdotal reports of use for overwhelming internal hemorrhage with some success. However, due to an exothermic reaction that may cause some local tissue damage it is not recommended for the situation in this scenario.

Electrocautery used on high settings, and other hemostatic meshes and powders have been used to some success, but this author has not been as pleased with the results.

TECHNICAL OPERATIVE PROCEDURES:

HOW I DO IT

Complex Hepatic Trauma – Grade IV Burst Injury

Rao Ivatury, MD, FACS

Scenario

A 25-year-old man involved in a motor vehicle crash sustained a Grade IV liver laceration. He was hypotensive and has been resuscitated. He is now in the operating room.

Management

Burst injuries due to blunt trauma and large caliber missile wounds cause greater destruction of the parenchyma of the liver, often involving both lobes and require more complex repairs. These are the kind of injuries that will require a coordinated effort by a team. You must warn the anesthesiologist for the need for such ancillary techniques as autotransfusion by a cell-saver, blood warmers to combat hypothermia and timely replacement of clotting factors before embarking on such major hepatic repairs.

The next step is to mobilize the liver adequately by dividing its ligamentous attachments. This will enable the organ to be delivered into the operative wound. The assistant can then manually compress the liver to temporarily staunch hemorrhage.

Occlusion of the portal triad (Pringle maneuver): In order to reduce vascular inflow to the liver and consequently reduce bleeding from the liver laceration, the Pringle maneuver is an important adjunct. It consists of sliding the operator's hand into the lesser sac and occluding the free edge of the lesser omentum and its contained portal and hepatic vessels between the fingers. If the procedure is effective in slowing the hemorrhage from the liver laceration, a vascular clamp may be applied across the free edge of the omentum.

Hemostasis by finger-fracture technique or débridement or resection: With reduction in the rate of bleeding by portal occlusion, the liver laceration is evaluated and an effort is made to control bleeding vessels by direct visualization and ligation. Deeper lacerations may be explored by the finger-fracture technique. The parenchyma of the liver is teased between the surgeon's fingers so that the hepatic vessels are exposed as threads traversing the teased liver substance. These can then be individually ligated. The process is continued until the entire laceration is explored and hemostasis is achieved.

- A vascular clamp occludes hepatic vascular inflow across the porta hepatis

- Viable omentum fills dead space and controls venous bleeding

- Perihepatic packing is an important advance

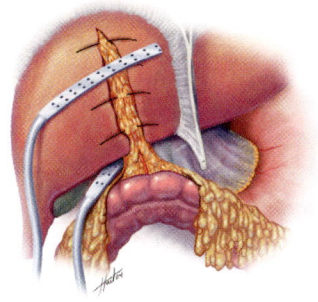

The viable omental pack: In patients with large stellate fractures or deep lacerations of the liver, the finger-fracture technique of hemostasis and débridement of non-viable liver tissue inevitably results in large defects in the hepatic lobes. Minor bleeding, usually of venous origin, may persist from the raw surfaces of the divided liver. A graft of viable omentum with an intact vascular supply can be used to fill in this dead space and control the venous bleeding. The omentum may be sutured in place. I make sure that the omental graft is well vascularized. Using devascularized pieces of omentum will only necrose the graft and increase the chances for an abscess.

Internal tamponade of the liver lacerations, missile tracts: In patients with missile wounds of the liver that traverse the entire thickness of the lobes, control of the hemorrhage may involve an extensive tractotomy and débridement. In such patients a method of internal tamponade by a Penrose pack may be employed. It involves passage of a red rubber catheter through the missile tract. A pack made of a number of Penrose drains is tied to the end of the catheter and pulled back through the tract and left in the laceration. The Penrose pack acts as a tamponading plug and controls the bleeding. The drains, brought to the exterior through the flank, also serve to drain the laceration. This technique facilitates hemostasis and helps to avoid a tractotomy or major resection under difficult circumstances. The Poggetti pack is a similar method of tamponading the tracts by a balloon. We have achieved intrahepatic balloon tamponade of missile tracts by using a sterilized Sengstaken-Blakemore tube. The long esophageal balloon may be inflated with saline and placed in the tract for tamponade. This may be brought out by a small incision. Postoperatively, the balloon may be gradually deflated over days and removed in 5 to 7 days.

Despite these various techniques, in a small number of patients, approximately 2% to 5%, profuse bleeding persists and may relate to the onset of coagulopathy. Massive red cell transfusions, hypothermia and acidosis contribute to the development of coagulation defects. The liver injury, which might have stopped bleeding, may start to bleed diffusely without controllable points of hemorrhage. Perihepatic packing has emerged as an important advance to control this non-mechanical bleeding.

The generally accepted indications for packing are: coagulopathy from extensive hepatic injuries after hepatotomy or hepatorrhaphy; diffuse bleeding from the resected liver after non-anatomic resectional débridement and extensive subcapsular hematomas with diffuse bleeding; and as a temporary measure prior to transfer of the patients to a definitive care center. Perihepatic packing may be employed at the primary operation or at a reoperation for continued bleeding from the injured liver. The goal is to produce mechanical pressure to minimize or abolish low pressure, venous bleeding.

The technique of packing consists of using Kerlix rolls or laparotomy pads to pack the crevices of the liver injury and the raw areas of the resected liver. Additional packs are placed around the liver and between the organ and the diaphragm and the lateral abdominal wall. Feliciano et.al. described an interesting modification of using a Surgidrape between the liver surface and the packs to facilitate the subsequent removal of the packs.

A combination of these techniques usually achieves hemostasis. We generally refrain from hepatic wrap with absorbable mesh because it is too involved a procedure in a hemorrhaging patient. Similarly, vascular isolation of the liver is very difficult in inexperienced hands. In these cases, temporary packing will give good results. For packing to be successful: do not mobilize the liver extensively of its natural ligamentous envelope and do not peek repeatedly to see what is bleeding. If packing slows down the bleeding, it is best to undertake damage control celiotomy and resuscitate the patient.

TECHNICAL OPERATIVE PROCEDURES:

HOW I DO IT

Hepatic Vascular Exclusion

George A. Perdrizet, MD, PhD, FACS

Scenario

A 45-year-old male, unbelted driver was invloved in a motor vehicle crash. He lost control at highway speeds and hit a telephone pole head-on. There was significant intrusion into the passenger compartment, the steering wheel was deformed, the windshield starred. The patient underwent a prolonged extrication as he was pinned across the mid-abdomen by the dashboard. Following extrication, the patient was initially hypotensive in the field, however he responded to 2-liters of crystalloid en route to the trauma resuscitation suite where a FAST examination revealed a large amount of free intraperitoneal fluid. During the study, the patient once again became hypotensive and was given two additional liters of warm crystalloid and 2 units of uncrossmatched type O blood. He was then intubated and large intravascular lines were placed in the left groin and the left internal jugular vein. The patient was taken to the operating room for emergent exploratory laparotomy.

Management

Upon arrival to the operating room, the patient once again became hypotensive and an additional three units of type specific blood were infused. Upon opening the abdomen, a large hemoperitoneum was encountered. All four quadrants were packed with laparotomy sponges. An initial survey revealed that the

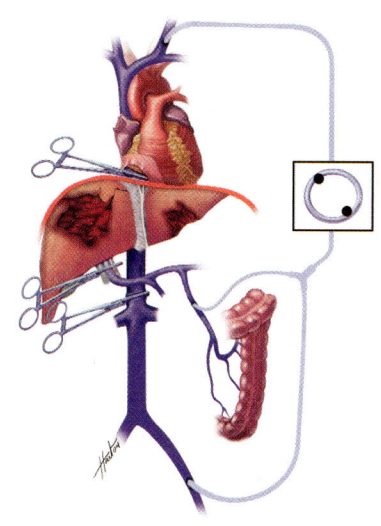

hemorrhage was due to an extensive hepatic laceration. The remainder of the abdominal organs were quickly examined; the spleen was found to be intact as were the kidneys and large and small bowel and infrahepatic vena cava. Despite the right upper quadrant packing the liver continued to hemorrhage and with each assessment additional blood loss was encountered. A Pringle maneuver was performed and despite this, there was copious venous blood welling up from the posterior-superior aspect of the liver. The liver laceration extended through the entire right lobe of the liver and a laceration was noted at the origin of the right hepatic vein. Given the nature of this injury and risk for additional hepatic hemorrhage and possible air embolization, it was decided to perform hepatic vascular exclusion to establish surgical hemostasis.

Procedure: *Hepatic vascular isolation*

A non-crushing vascular clamp was applied to the portal triad through the foramen of Winslow. Next, the left groin central venous catheter was changed over a wire using the Seldinger Technique and venous dilators; a #9 Gott shunt was placed by way of the femoral vein to the level of the common iliac vein. This was then primed with normal saline. The left internal jugular central venous line was changed over to a #7 Gott shunt in a similar manner. The cannulae were then attached to the hemoperfusion pump with an inline heat exchanger. The infrahepatic, suprarenal inferior vena cava was dissected and then occluded with a Satinsky clamp to control the inferior vena caval inflow. Given that the suprahepatic inferior vena cava had a large tear at the site of the takeoff of the right hepatic vein, a transdiaphragmatic approach to the extrapericardial inferior vena cava was performed and a Satinsky clamp was used to occlude the inferior vena cava for control of back bleeding and prevention of air embolization.

The portal venous system did not appear to require decompression as there was minimal bowel edema at this point. To do this, a #4 Gott shunt is placed directly into the inferior mesenteric vein at the level of the ligament of Treitz. The pump was adjusted to deliver 3-liters/minute flow. Adequate venous return was confirmed by adequate cardiac output. Having now adequately excluded the liver, an examination in a bloodless field could then be carried out. The right lobe was found to have been torn from the right triangular ligament and a venous laceration extending from the right hepatic vein proximally for one centimeter along the suprahepatic cava was identified. This was repaired with a 5-0 Prolene suture in a running fashion. Next, the clamp was transiently released from the portohepatic ligament to identify visible vascular disruptions, both arterial and portal. These were controlled using vascular clips.

- The portal triad is occluded through the foramen of Winslow

- A femoral venous shunt is placed

- A left internal jugular shunt is connected to a hemoperfusion pump

- The infrarenal and suprarenal inferior vena cava are occluded

- The portal venous system may require decompression using the inferior mesenteric vein

Then, to confirm adequate hemostasis, the suprahepatic caval clamp was removed, followed by the portal triad clamp to permit repeat evaluation of liver parenchyma for any unaddressed sites of hepatic arterial and portal venous bleeding. Having restored adequate hemostasis to the injured liver parenchyma, the infrahepatic vena cava clamp was then removed to establish native vena caval venous return. The suprahepatic caval repair was re-inspected to ensure adequate hemostasis and having confirmed this, the Gott shunt cannula were then removed and closed with a purse string nylon suture to provide venous tamponade. The liver was then irrigated with warm saline and the damaged parenchyma superficially coagulated using the argon beam coagulator. Several abdominal packs were used to compress this hepatic injury and then the remainder of the abdomen was irrigated with saline and re-inspected for other injuries.

Given that the patient had received 12 liters of crystalloid and 10 units of blood and had significant bowel and tissue edema, the abdominal cavity was left open and a vacuum pack-type closure was performed. The patient transported to the intensive care unit for further monitoring and resuscitation. The patient will be brought back to the operating room in 24 to 48 hours for a second look, at which time devitalized liver parenchyma will be removed.

TECHNICAL OPERATIVE PROCEDURES:

HOW I DO IT

Exposure and Management of a Major Injury to the Right Lobe of the Liver

David V. Feliciano, MD, FACS

Overview

The liver has a blood supply of 1500 mL/minute, and exsanguination can occur rapidly from a Grade IV or Grade V injury. This is particularly true with blunt hepatic ruptures in which a large number of intrahepatic vessels are ruptured at varying levels and in different planes. Such complex lobar injuries often require multiple techniques of hemostasis which should be known by surgeons taking trauma call.

All patients undergoing an emergency laparotomy for abdominal trauma have their arms placed at their sides to allow for the attachment of large self-retaining retractors, particularly for perihepatic exposure, and for easy access to all thoracic incisions.

Procedure: *Mobilization of the injured hepatic lobe*

After the long midline incision has been completed, free blood and gastrointestinal contents are removed using laparotomy pads, warm saline irrigation and a suction device. Rapid manual palpation above and below both lobes of the liver will determine whether a Grade III to Grade V hepatic injury is present. If so, a Pringle maneuver is performed using a noncrushing vascular clamp. I prefer an angled Glover or DeBakey clamp. In patients with blunt trauma, a rapid inspection of the spleen and mesentery of the small bowel is performed to see if active hemorrhage from these areas must be controlled. In patients with penetrating trauma, rapid inspection of the upper right retroperitoneum is performed to see if active hemorrhage from the right kidney or inferior vena cava is present.

With the Pringle maneuver in place, the injured lobe is mobilized into the midline incision by division of the triangular and anterior coronary ligaments right at their junction with the liver. Division of the posterior coronary ligament should be performed with care as the retrohepatic venous structures are much more anterior than expected as the liver is rotated medially. All of these maneuvers are performed with the surgeon using a long Metzenbaum scissors as the assistant applies traction inferiorly and anteriorly. After the injured lobe is mobilized, a quick visual inspection will confirm that neither a hepatic vein nor the retrohepatic vena cava is injured.

Procedures: *Repairs of the injured lobe*

Injuries to the hepatic parenchyma can generally be classified as laceration-avulsion, central burst, subcapsular hematoma, and through-and-through missile tract.

> - Always place arms at patient's side to facilitate use of large self-retaining retractors
>
> - Medial rotation of liver brings retrohepatic venous structures more anterior than expected
>
> - Perihepatic packing appropriate only if Pringle maneuver is effective
>
> - Bleeding from bullet tract in coagulopathic patient controlled by localization with, then tamponade with Foley balloon catheter

Laceration or avulsion often occur at the falciform ligament and involve hepatic segments II and III or through the right lobe and involve segments V, VI, and/or VII. With the Pringle maneuver in place, a new fracture line is marked on the injured lobe inside of the area of frayed tissue. Using the electrocautery and metal clips a resectional débridement is performed on this line, thereby removing all devitalized tissue laterally. When the débridement is complete, the Pringle maneuver is removed, and selective vascular ligation of bleeding vessels in the new edge of the liver is performed with absorbable sutures. In coagulopathic patients, figure-of-eight sutures may be used to compress the anterior and posterior surfaces of the new edge. An omental pedicle around the new raw edge of the liver is not used as it traps bile and blood. Drainage is mandatory because of the 8 to 10% incidence of postoperative biliary fistulae and is accomplished using two 10 mm Jackson-Pratt drains placed in the subphrenic and subhepatic areas. Insertion of a nasojejunal feeding tube is appropriate in the patient with blunt multisystem injuries or a penetrating hepatic injury with 5 to 10 units or more loss of blood.

A central burst injury is treated with resectional débridement as described above, a formal hepatic lobectomy if a trained hepatic surgeon is present, or the insertion of perihepatic packs above and below the injured lobe if a coagulopathy is already present. In the 3 to 5% of patients who require a lobectomy, moving the gallbladder-to-retrohepatic vena cava line of resection just off the middle hepatic vein so that this vessel is not injured is appropriate. Perihepatic packing is appropriate only if reasonable hemostasis is achieved once the Pringle maneuver is performed. Jackson-Pratt drains may be left under or outside perihepatic packs to allow for scavenging of subphrenic blood in the postoperative period.

A large subcapsular hematoma that is stable is treated with the insertion of perihepatic packs for two to three days. If the subcapsular hematoma is ruptured or expanding rapidly, a Pringle maneuver is applied and selective vascular ligation of parenchymal bleeders is performed. The avulsed capsule is replaced with absorbable mesh that can be sewn to the capsular remnant with 3-0 absorbable sutures.

A through-and-through missile track that is not bleeding from either end in the normotensive patient is usually left alone, and perihepatic drains are placed beneath the injured lobe. Should there be a large amount of blood in the abdomen from an isolated gunshot or stab wound to the liver, but the entrance and exit sites are not currently bleeding, intraoperative observation of these sites is appropriate for 15 to 30 minutes before inserting drains and closing the incision. Active hemorrhage from one end of the track mandates application of the Pringle maneuver and a hepatotomy starting at the involved end. Using electrocautery and metal clips, the hepatic parenchyma is divided until the bleeding vessel is identified. Should bleeding be noted from both entrance and exit sites in a coagulopathic patient, a long hepatotomy connecting entrance and exit sites is inappropriate. A Foley balloon catheter is inserted into the track and inflated every 2 cm to 3 cm to see if balloon tamponade controls the bleeding. If one balloon does not do this, a Penrose drain over a red Robinson catheter is tied down proximally and distally to the holes in the Robinson catheter. The Penrose drain over Robinson catheter combination is inserted into the track, and saline inflation of the Penrose drain through the Robinson catheter creates a long tamponading balloon catheter. Balloon tamponade that is effective in controlling hemorrhage acutely can be released and removed at 48 hours in non-coagulopathic patients.

Perihepatic Jackson-Pratt drains and nasojejunal feeding catheters are inserted in all patients undergoing repair or tamponade of Grade III to Grade V hepatic injuries as previously noted.

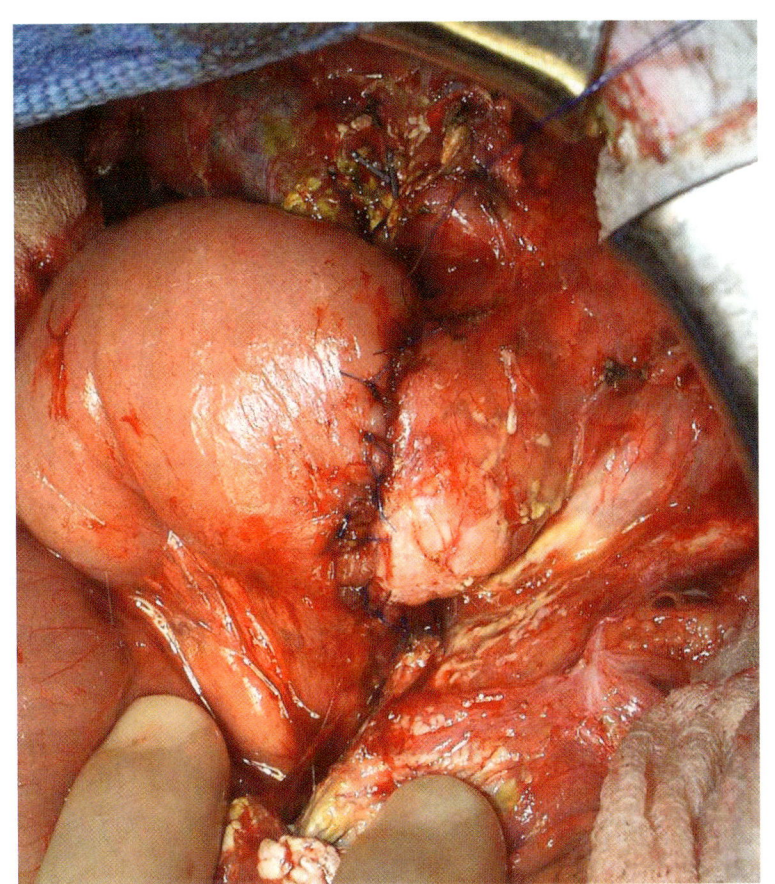

The Pancreas and Duodenum

4

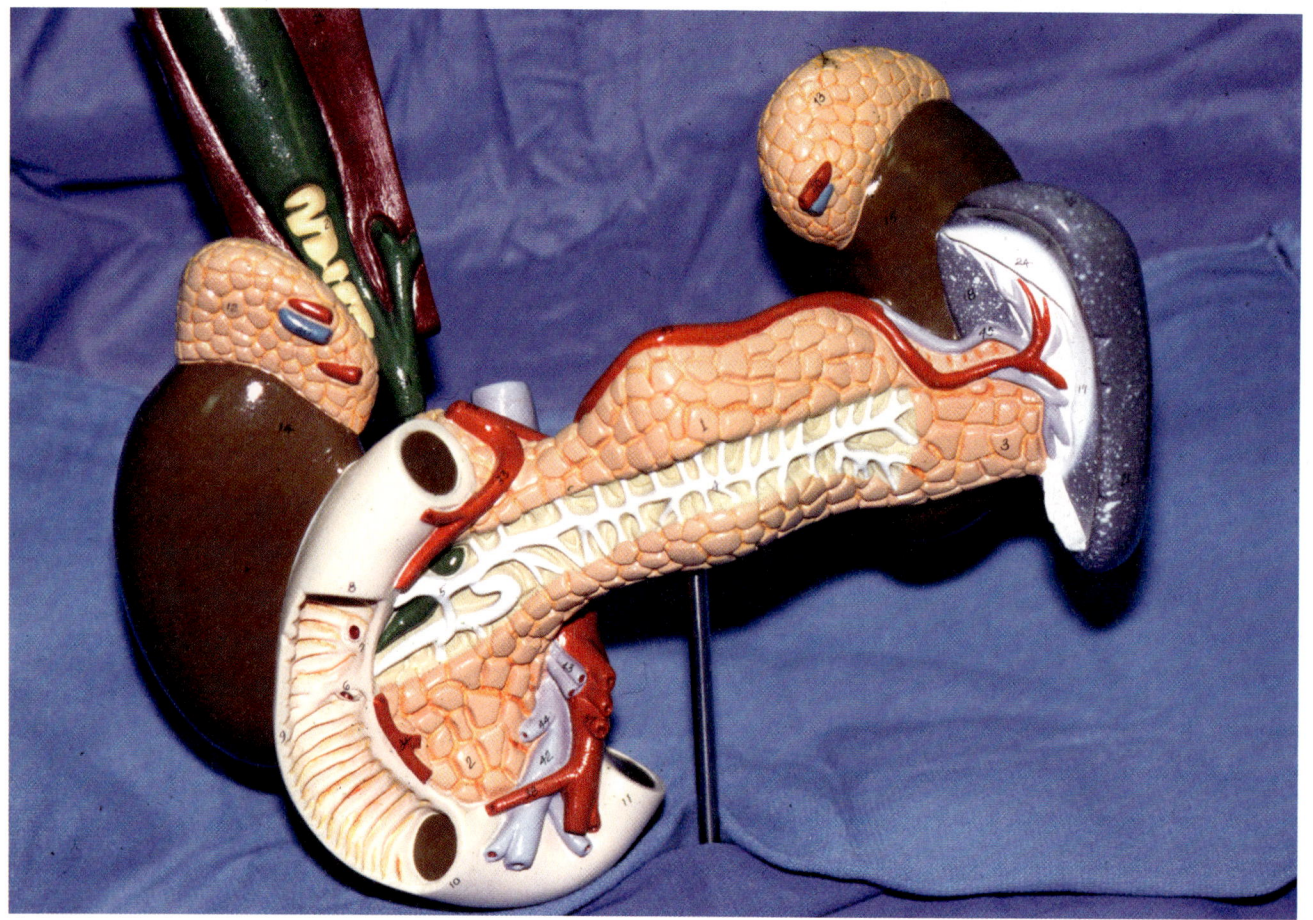

The Nature of the Problem

Injuries to the pancreas and duodenum are considered to be the most perplexing and difficult injuries to deal with, regardless of whether the mechanism of injury is blunt or penetrating trauma. The retroperitoneal location of these injuries makes them practically inaccessible on physical exam, even in the best of hands. The diagnosis of injury to these organs requires sophisticated diagnostic measures, the least sophisticated and least invasive of which is the abdominal CT scan. Patients with injuries to the pancreas and duodenum will have the best outcomes when the injuries are diagnosed, and if necessary, operated on early on in their course. Delay in diagnosis of an injury to the pancreas or duodenum is often associated with high morbidity and markedly increased mortality. This is due to the retroperitoneal location of these organs and their intimate contact with other retroperitoneal structures.

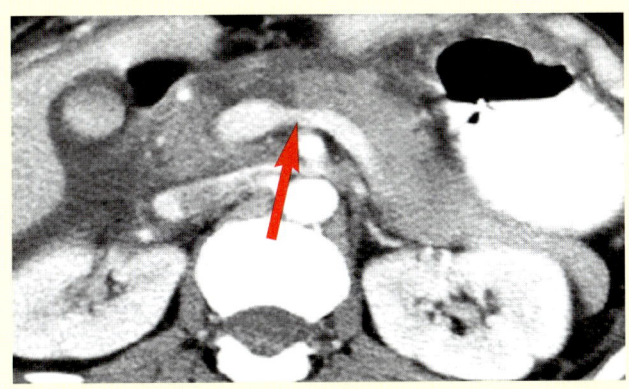
Transected Neck of the Pancreas

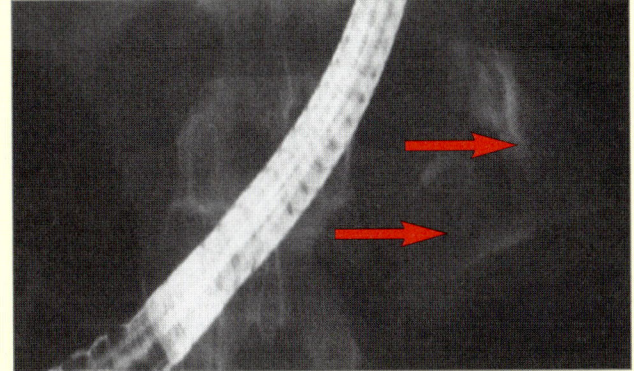
Extravasation of contrast with pooling in the lesser sac

Blunt Pancreatic Injury

- High index of suspicion
- Minimal findings or equivocal exam
- Serial enzymes
- "Normal" CT scan
- Repeat CT scan
- Ductal integrity
  - ERCP
  - MRCP

Blunt Pancreatic Injury

Evaluation of patients with possible blunt pancreatic injury is challenging. It requires a careful assessment of the location of injury, the energy transfer of the impact, and any other associated injuries. The high incidence of associated intra-abdominal injuries results in a significant number of patients demonstrating clear-cut indications for laparotomy. These indications include shock, a positive diagnostic peritoneal lavage (DPL), a positive FAST exam, and clear-cut peritonitis. Direct examination of the pancreas and duodenum is imperative for patients with any of these indications.

Patients who have sustained blunt abdominal injury and are likely to have blunt pancreatic or duodenal injury often have minimal or no findings on physical exam. In these cases, a high index of suspicion is the physician's best tool for diagnosis. In addition to a normal or equivocal physical exam, patients with blunt pancreatic injury may not show any abnormalities on initial enzyme determinations or on the initial abdominal CT scan. Serial enzymes must be followed, and a repeat abdominal CT scan may be needed.

Although they should not be used in an unstable patient or in a patient who requires immediate celiotomy, endoscopic retrograde cholangiopancreatography (ERCP) or magnetic resonance cholangiopancreatography (MRCP) can be helpful in evaluating the integrity of the pancreatic duct. If ERCP is available, it can be performed in the operating room in a stable patient. In a study published in 1982, Berni and colleagues reported that intraoperative pancreatography and accurate determination of the status of the pancreatic duct resulted in a decrease in postoperative complications, from 55% to 15%.

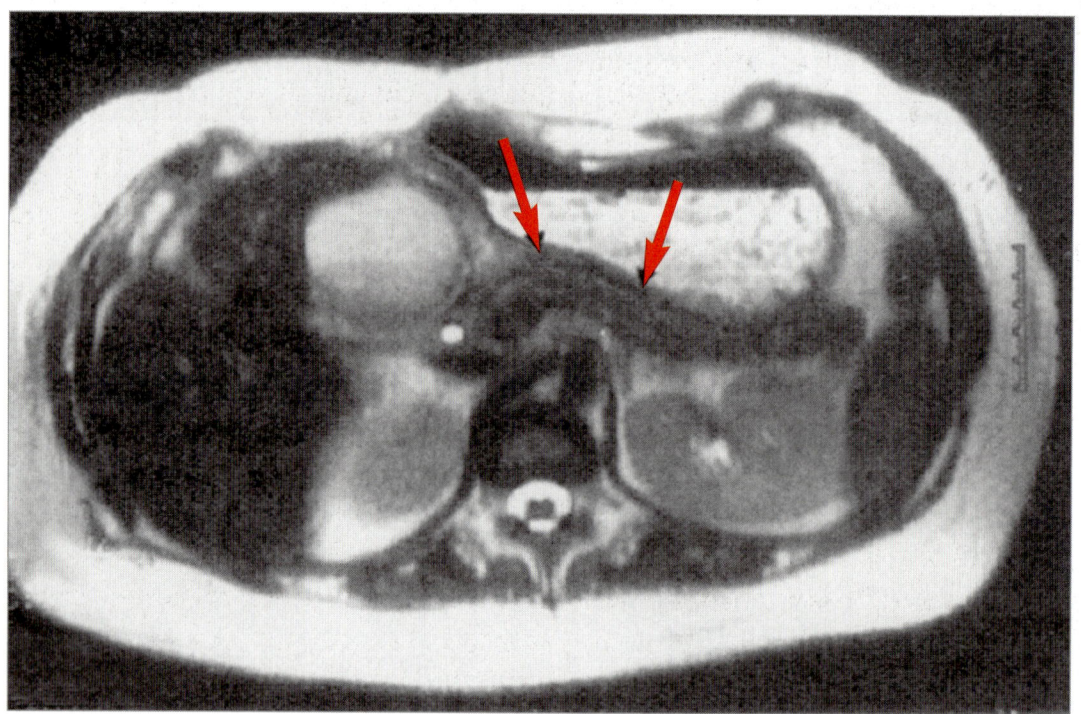

Normal Duct

MRCP and the Diagnosis of Pancreatic Ductal Injuries

This CT image nicely illustrates a normal pancreas. The arrows point to the pancreatic duct, which is nicely demonstrated on the MRCP scan.

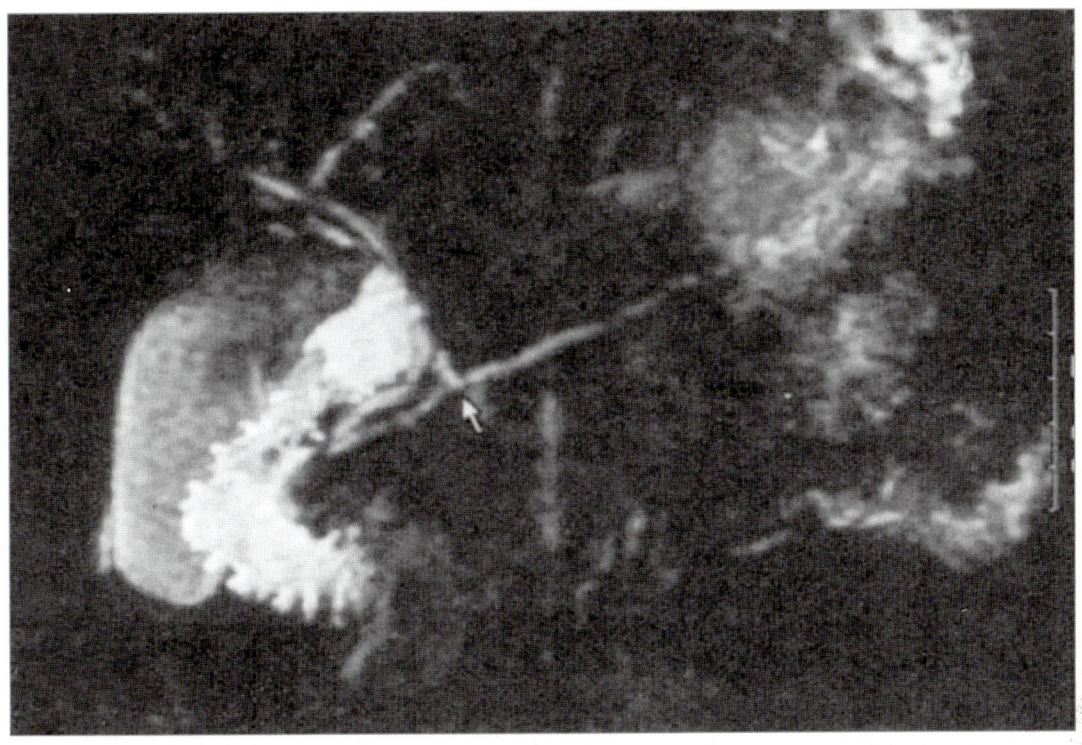

Extravasation

MRCP and the Diagnosis of Pancreatic Ductal Injuries

The use of MRCP to diagnose pancreatic ductal injuries has been demonstrated to be effective, but its utility remains questionable. A relatively recent study found that MRCP is a reliable noninvasive diagnostic tool to determine the status of the main pancreatic duct in patients with pancreatic injury. However, MRCP is applicable only to those patients who are hemodynamically stable and have minimal or no other serious injuries.

A well-performed MRCP is very useful because a normal pancreatogram assures the physician of ductal integrity. Extravasation of contrast from the pancreatic duct on an MRCP, as is illustrated in this image, provides clear-cut evidence of pancreatic ductal injury. The degree of extravasation and the location of the ductal injury dictate the management of the patient.

Blunt Duodenal Injury

Blunt duodenal injury requires a high index of suspicion for early diagnosis. The retroperitoneal location of the third and fourth portion of the duodenum tends to obscure physical findings, giving the clinician an equivocal exam in the early course of these injuries. As with pancreatic injuries, the initial laboratory tests and abdominal CT scans may be normal on admission. In addition, plain abdominal x-rays of the abdomen that include the kidney, ureter, and bladder (KUB) may also be normal. However, early clues to diagnosis are frequently present on plain film. Presence of a psoas stripe, which results from retroperitoneal

Blunt Duodenal Injury

- High index of suspicion
- Equivocal exam
- Serial enzymes
- Abdominal CT scan
- Plain films
- Contrast duodenography
- Diagnostic laparotomy

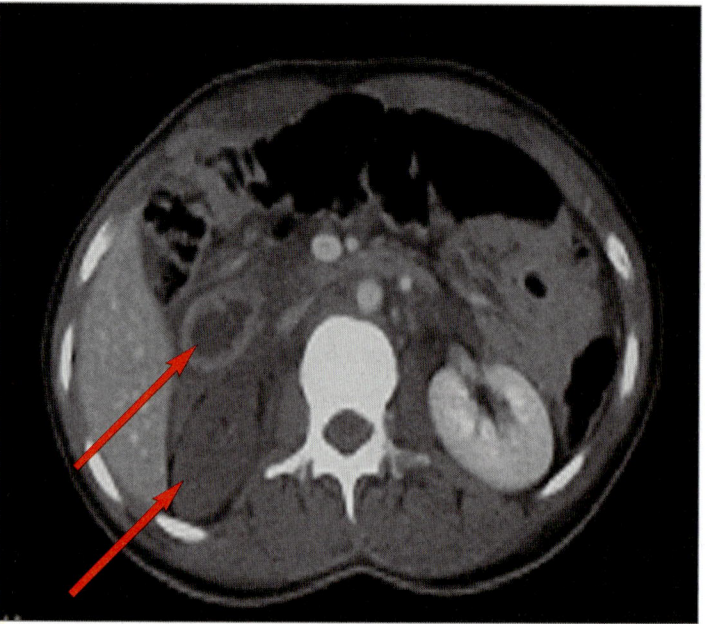

- **Thickened second portion of duodenum**
- **Avascular right kidney**

air highlighting the lateral border of the psoas muscle, indicates duodenal injury unless proven otherwise. Periduodenal fluid collections and a thickened duodenal wall on abdominal CT should also alert the clinician to the possibility of duodenal injury. Early suspicion of retroperitoneal duodenal rupture is best confirmed or excluded using contrast duodenography, with both oral and intravenous contrast on a CT exam, or an upper gastrointestinal series using water soluble contrast medium followed by barium if the initial exam is negative. Either study should be considered normal only if contrast passes through all portions of the duodenum without delay, and there is no extravasation.

In a study published in 1998, Allen and colleagues reported that 83% of patients with delayed diagnosis of blunt duodenal injury had subtle CT findings that were dismissed on initial readings. These findings included pneumoperitoneum, unexplained fluid, and unusual bowel appearances.

In patients requiring exploratory laparotomy for other abdominal injuries, the duodenum should be carefully examined, especially when the mechanism of injury requires a high suspicion for injury to the retroperitoneal organs. Diagnostic laparotomy is indicated in patients when unequivocal preoperative evaluation has not been successful and a high index of suspicion remains.

Penetrating Injuries

Unlike injuries to the pancreas and duodenum resulting from blunt trauma, injuries resulting from penetrating trauma are usually diagnosed at exploratory laparotomy. Most patients with these injuries have nonspecific indications requiring laparotomy, such as shock, peritonitis, a positive DPL, and positive findings on an abdominal CT scan. In some cases, the mechanism of injury itself, for example a transperitoneal gunshot wound, may necessitate immediate exploratory laparotomy without any preoperative workup.

Penetrating Injuries

- Usually diagnosed at exploratory laparotomy

- Nonspecific indications for exploratory laparotomy

- Mechanism alone
  - transperitoneal gun shot wound
  - shock
  - peritonitis
  - positive DPL
  - positive findings on CT scan

Kocher Maneuver

Successful diagnosis and management of pancreatic and duodenal injuries requires direct visual inspection of both organs. The C-loop of the duodenum, the pancreatic head, and the intrapancreatic portion of the common bile duct can best be visualized after performing a Kocher maneuver. The peritoneal lining over the lateral aspect of the duodenum is divided sharply with Metzenbaum scissors, starting at the proximal aspect of the second portion of the duodenum and extending distally on the duodenum as far as possible. The entire duodenal sweep, pancreatic head, and distal common bile duct can then be mobilized from their retroperitoneal position using a combination of sharp and blunt dissection. This enables the surgeon to inspect both the anterior and posterior aspects of all structures. Mobilizing the hepatic flexure of the colon can enhance visualization.

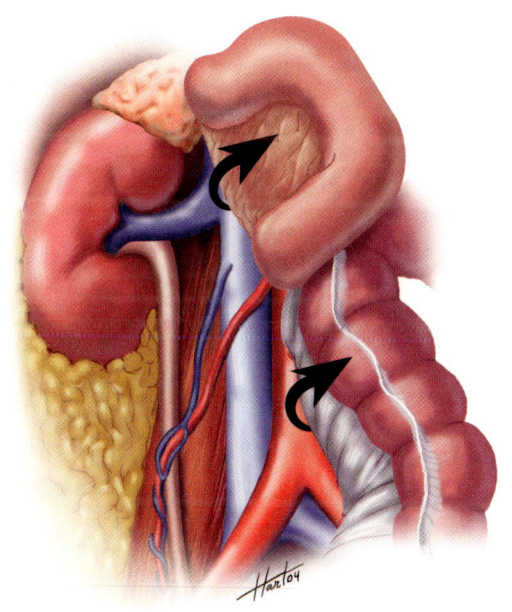

Surgical Exposures

- Kocher maneuver:
  - medial rotation of duodenum, pancreatic head, distal CBD

Cattel Braasch Maneuver

Performing the Cattel Braasch maneuver provides further exposure of Zone I in the abdomen. The white line of Toldt is sharply incised with Metzenbaum scissors. This dissection is carried from the cecum up to and including the hepatic flexure, onto the transverse colon. Once this has been completed, the entire right colon and small bowel can be mobilized medially. This exposes the third and fourth portions of the duodenum, as well as all structures within the right Zone II and Zone I regions of the abdominal cavity.

The Cattel Braasch maneuver and the Kocher maneuver provide excellent visualization of the entire duodenum, from the pylorus down to the ligament of Treitz.

Aird Maneuver

Exposure of the pancreatic tail and distal body of the pancreas is best accomplished using the Aird maneuver. The lienophrenic and lienorenal ligaments are taken

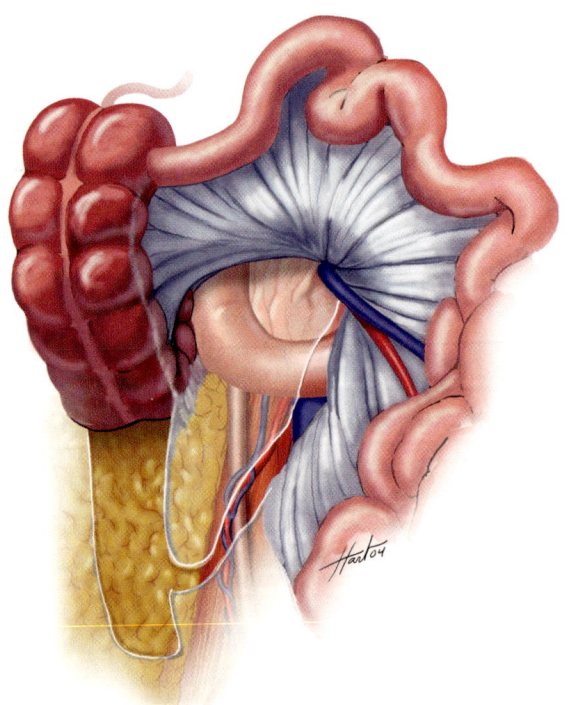
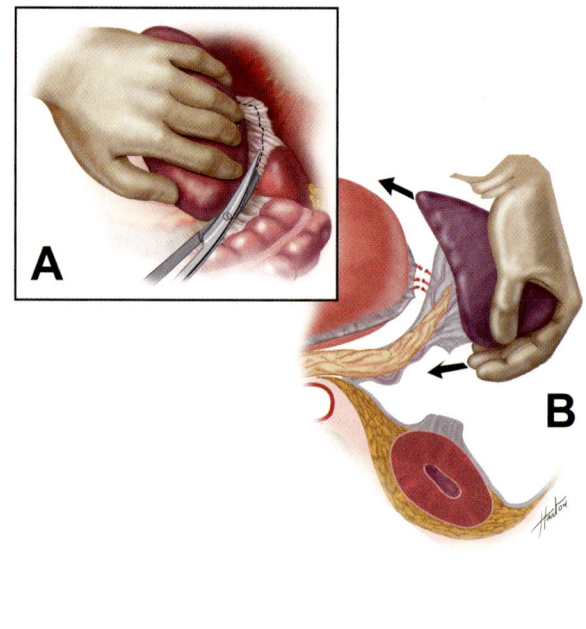

Surgical Exposures

- Cattel Braasch maneuver:
  - right abdominal visceral rotation
  - technique for exposure of 3rd and 4th portions of the duodenum

Surgical Exposures

- Aird maneuver:
  - medial rotation of spleen and tail of the pancreas

Chapter Four - The Pancreas and Duodenum

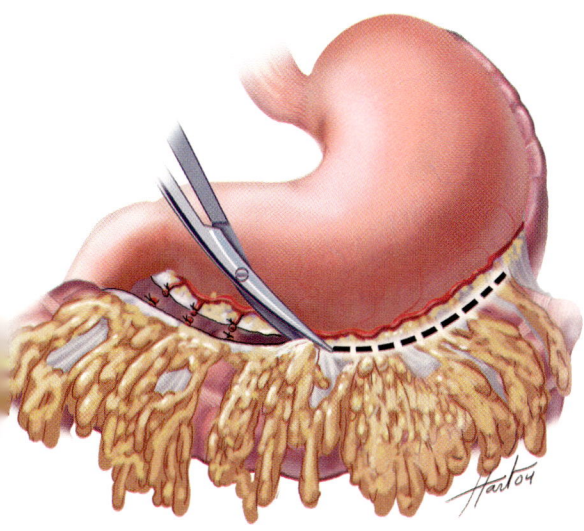

down sharply using Metzenbaum scissors. The surgeon's hand is then placed posterior and medial to the spleen in front of Gerota's fascia. The spleen can then be delivered from its posterior lateral position within the abdominal cavity to a much more medial position, along with the entire pancreatic tail. This provides visualization of the distal aspect of the pancreatic body and tail both anteriorly and posteriorly. The Aird maneuver also facilitates visualization of all structures within the lateral aspect of Zone I and the left Zone II regions of the abdominal cavity.

Surgical Exposures

The body of the pancreas is entirely retroperitoneal, and lies within Zone I of the abdominal cavity. The retroperitoneum must be entered in order to successfully examine it. In order to do this, the gastrocolic omentum is divided. Since this is not an avascular plane, the dissection should be performed using clamps and ties, or stapling devices. The pancreas can be seen within the retroperitoneum once the gastrocolic omentum has been taken down. The retroperitoneum is then sharply divided with Metzenbaum scissors. Next, the inferior aspect of the body of the pancreas can be mobilized using a combination of sharp and blunt dissection. Great care must be taken to ensure meticulous hemostasis.

Once these maneuvers have been performed, the entire pancreas can be inspected from the duodenopancreatic juncture at the head, to the tail of the pancreas sitting at the hilum of the spleen.

Surgical Exposures

- Opening lesser sac
- Opening retroperitoneum
- Elevating the body of the pancreas

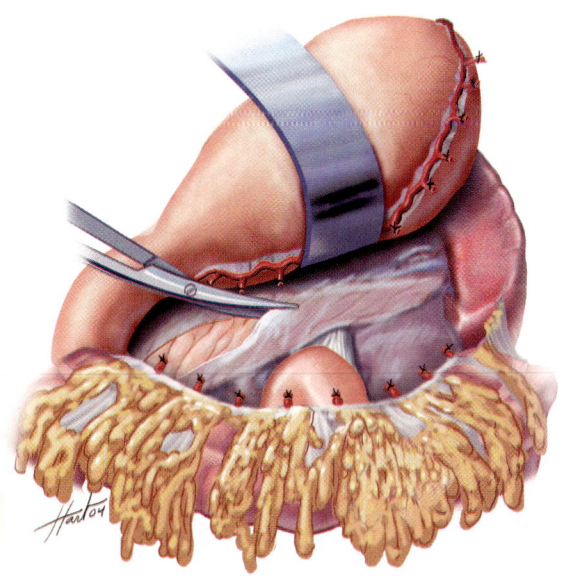

Surgical Exposures

- Divide the gastrohepatic omentum

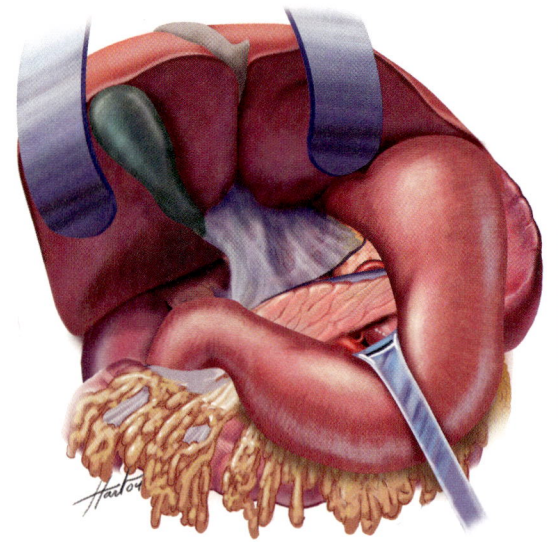

Surgical Exposures

- Transection of ligament of Treitz

- Exposure of the 4th portion of the duodenum and duodenojejunal junction

Surgical Exposures

As previously discussed, the duodenojejunal junction can be freely mobilized by sharply dividing the ligament of Treitz. This illustration nicely demonstrates the medial mobilization of the juncture once the ligament has been divided.

Ligament of Treitz

The last segment of the duodenum that remains unexposed is the fourth portion of the duodenum. The duodenojejunal junction occurs at the level of the ligament of Treitz. Exposure of the entire fourth portion of the duodenum and the duodenojejunal junction can be accomplished by dividing the ligament of Treitz. This freely mobilizes the fourth portion of the duodenum and allows complete and thorough inspection of the duodenum, proximal jejunum, and duodenojejunal junction.

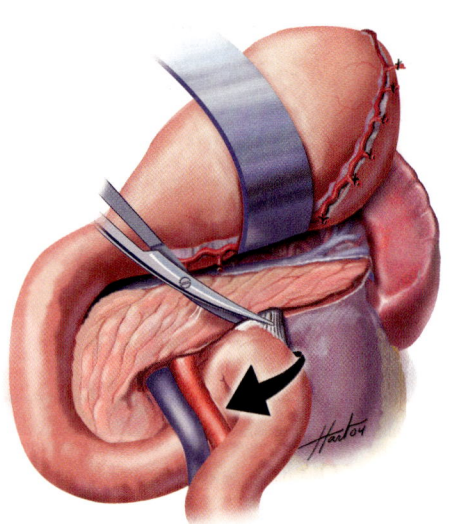

Divide ligament of Treitz

Surgical Exposures

A combination of the Kocher maneuver, the Aird maneuver, division of the ligament of Treitz, and division of the gastrocolic omentum provides excellent visualization of the entire duodenal sweep and pancreas. The only remaining structures that prevent complete mobilization of the duodenum and the pancreas are the superior mesenteric artery and vein, which obviously need to be left intact.

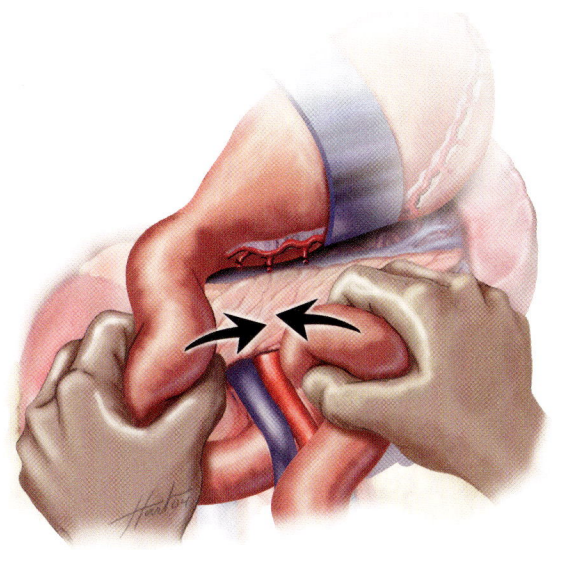

Beware of Missed Pancreatic and Duodenal Injuries

- Emphasize that duodenal and pancreatic injuries may be missed at laparotomy

- The anterior and posterior aspects of the duodenum and pancreas must be visually inspected.

- Emphasize the importance of the exploration of all periduodenal and peripancreatic hematomas.

Beware of Missed Pancreatic and Duodenal Injuries

Regardless of the mechanism of injury, all efforts must be expended to avoid missing pancreatic and duodenal injuries. All peripancreatic and periduodenal hematomas must be entered and the involved areas of the pancreas and duodenum meticulously inspected. Injury should be ruled out definitively.

Pancreas Organ Injury Scale

Pancreatic and duodenal injuries are graded according to the Organ Injury Scale of the American Association for the Surgery of Trauma (AAST-OIS). The scale for grading pancreatic injuries focuses on the presence or absence of ductal injuries.

Grade I and Grade II injuries have subdivisions to include both hematomas and lacerations. Grade I injuries are characterized by the presence of a minor contusion hematoma with no ductal injury, or a laceration that is superficial and does not involve ductal injury. Grade II pancreatic injuries are characterized by major contusions or lacerations to the pancreatic parenchyma. In both cases, the duct has been spared, and there is no major tissue loss.

Grade III pancreatic injuries are characterized by distal pancreatic lacerations involving pancreatic tissue transection without major tissue loss or injury to the duct. A Grade IV pancreatic injury is a proximal transection of pancreatic tissue, or pancreatic injury involving the ampulla of Vater. A Grade V injury is characterized by a laceration with massive disruption of the pancreatic head, including ductal injury. The grade of injury goes up one grade when an organ is injured multiple times.

Grade*		Injury Description
I	Hematoma	Minor contusion without duct injury
	Laceration	Superficial laceration without duct injury
II	Hematoma	Major contusion without duct injury
	Laceration	Major laceration without duct injury or tissue loss
III	Laceration	Distal transection without duct injury or tissue loss
IV	Laceration	Proximal transection or parenchymal injury involving ampulla
V	Laceration	Massive disruption of pancreatic head
		*Advance one grade for multiple injuries to same organ

Operative Strategy

- Stop hemorrhage
  - damage control

- Exposure

- Location of injury

- Selective debridement

- Exocrine function
  - control of activated enzymes

- Endocrine function
  - preservation of insulin and glucagon

Operative Strategies for Pancreatic Injuries

Operative strategies for patients with pancreatic injury begin as they do for all other injuries. The top priority for operative intervention in the trauma patient is to stop bleeding. Hemorrhage control and control of intraabdominal soilage from visceral perforations are the initial steps in any trauma laparotomy. Once these steps have been successfully accomplished, previously placed laparotomy pads can be removed one at a time in order to identify the injured organs.

Pancreatic injuries must be precisely located before attempting selected débridement. Both exocrine and endocrine function should be preserved whenever possible. Exocrine function in the form of activated enzymes must be carefully controlled in order to prevent postoperative fistula formation and peripancreatic tissue destruction, as well as the sequelae known to occur when these complications do develop. The devastating effects of the loss of insulin and glucagon production make it essential to preserve endocrine function whenever possible.

Pancreas: Injury Grading & Operative Management

The AAST-OIS can be used as a guide for the intraoperative management of pancreatic injuries. Grade I injuries, characterized by small peripancreatic hematomas or superficial pancreatic tissue lacerations, can be managed conservatively with evacuation of the hematoma obtaining hemostasis, and placement of closed-drainage systems. Similarly, Grade II pancreatic injuries, characterized by large hematomas or deep lacerations to the pancreatic tissue without tissue loss, can be managed conservatively. There is no ductal injury in either grade of injury. This simplifies management dramatically.

These CT scan images show a Grade III injury, which is characterized by distal ductal transection and transection of the distal pancreatic tissue. Grade III injuries of this nature are best treated with distal pancreatectomy and splenectomy.

Injury Grading & Operative Management

- Grade I
  - small hematoma
  - superficial laceration

- Grade II
  - large hematoma
  - deep laceration
  - no tissue loss

- NO DUCTAL INJURY

- Evacuation

- Hemostasis

- Closed drainage

Distal pancreatectomy with splenic preservation may be considered in the stable trauma patient with a Grade III pancreatic injury and a normal spleen. This procedure should be performed only in the hemodynamically stable trauma patient with minimal, or no other, concurrent injuries. In addition, the patient must be able to tolerate the additional 60 to 90 minutes of surgery required to perform this procedure.

Pancreatectomy with splenic preservation requires careful dissection of the pancreas off of the splenic vein. This can be technically challenging due to the many venous connections from the body of the pancreas to the splenic vein. All connections must be individually ligated in order to prevent postoperative hemorrhage.

Distal Pancreatectomy

A distal pancreatectomy is shown in these illustrations. Although it is often not possible, the pancreatic duct should be located within the pancreatic remnant and suture ligated. This is generally of less concern when a stapler has been used to perform the pancreatic resection.

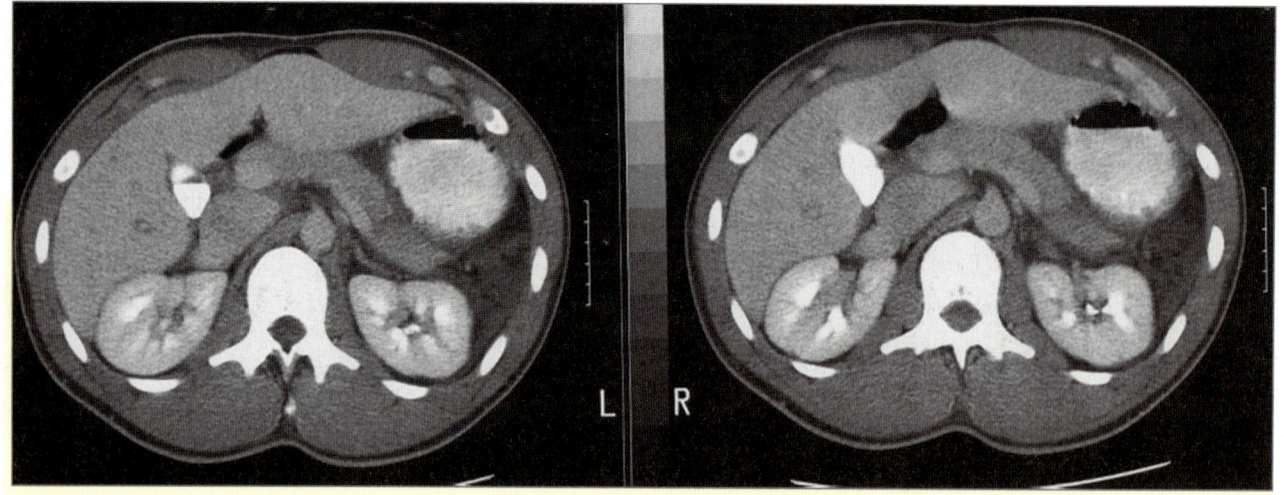

Pancreas: Injury Grading & Operative Management

- Grade III: distal transection or ductal injury

    -distal pancreatectomy and splenectomy

    - splenic preservation

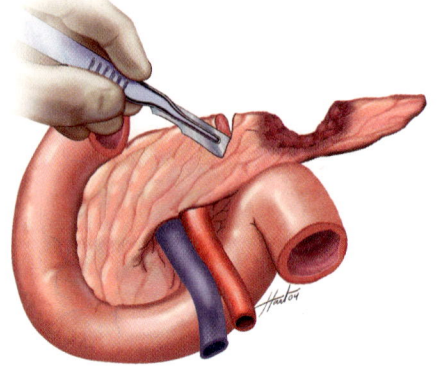

Regardless of whether or not the duct has been ligated, liberal use of closed-suction drainage systems is required. This allows wide drainage of the pancreatic remnant and the retroperitoneal peripancreatic tissue bed.

Pancreas: Injury Grading & Operative Management

This CT scan shows a pancreas that has been transected at the level of the superior mesenteric artery. This is a Grade IV injury, which is characterized by proximal pancreatic transections with ductal injury or ampullary injury. These are very severe injuries that require near-total pancreatectomy.

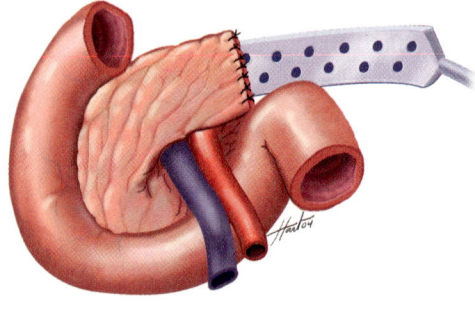

Once the pancreatectomy has been completed, the surgeon must decide how to deal with the distal end of the pancreatic remnant. Some surgeons prefer to place the distal end of the pancreas back into continuity with the gastrointestinal tract, either by using a roux-en-Y pancreaticojejunostomy or performing a pancreaticogastrostomy. Proponents of each procedure feel that the rates of morbidity and mortality are lower than those of other procedures. However, morbidity and mortality rates will be affected by the frequency with which the surgeon performs the procedure, and the surgeon's comfort level with the procedure used.

A third method of placing the distal end of the pancreas back into continuity with the gastrointestinal tract includes ductal ligation and drainage of the distal pancreatic tissue without a pancreaticoenteric anastomosis. This option can be used in patients who require pancreatectomy but are not stable enough for a definitive surgical procedure. Damage control is the initial operative procedure of choice in these patients.

Intraoperative Diagnosis of Pancreatic Ductal Injury

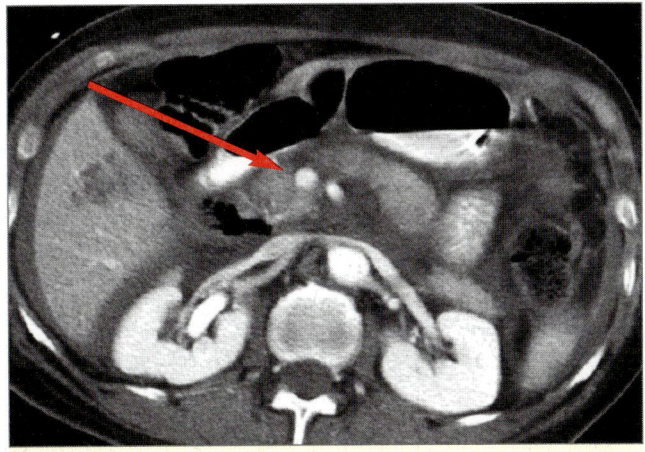

Injury Grading & Operative Management

- Grade IV: proximal transection, ductal injury or ampullary injury

- Near total pancreatectomy
  - roux-en-Y pancreaticojejunostomy
  - pancreaticogastrostomy
  - ductal ligation and drainage

The intraoperative diagnosis of pancreatic injuries can be difficult. Although direct inspection is usually sufficient to determine the status of the pancreatic duct, most surgeons advocate the use of pancreatography when direct inspection is questionable. It is important to exclude a pancreatic ductal injury because the presence of injury to the duct alters the therapeutic course. Although the majority of pancreatic ductal injuries are seen as a result of penetrating injury, blunt impact to the pancreas can result in major ductal transections without complete transection of the gland. This makes imaging the gland especially important.

The simplest technique for imaging the pancreatic duct is intraoperative fluoroscopic cholecystocholangiography. This is most easily performed by inserting an 18-gauge angiocatheter into the gallbladder. In patients who have had previous cholecystectomies, the common bile duct can be used as the site of insertion for the angiocatheter. About 20 cc to 30 cc of water-soluble contrast material is then injected. Intravenous morphine may enhance pancreatic ductal visualization by promoting contracture of the sphincter of Oddi.

Intraoperative Diagnosis of Pancreatic Ductal Injury

WHAT TO DO
- Correlate injury location and ductal anatomy
- Fluoroscopic cholecysto-cholangiography
- IV opiates

WHAT NOT TO DO
- Open the duodenum
- Transect the tail of the pancreas to cannulate the duct

OPTIONAL
- Secretin stimulation
- Intraoperative ERCP

Some researchers have suggested the use of intravenous secretin to stimulate pancreatic function and enhance the diagnostic reliability of cholangiography. The use of intraoperative ERCP has also been advocated. However, ERCP must be restricted to the hemodynamically stable patient and may be technically impossible due to patient positioning. The addition of methylene blue to the contrast material used for cholangiography or during the course of intraoperative ERCP is helpful. It gives the surgeon a direct visual cue to the presence of pancreatic ductal injury.

In the past, researchers have suggested that pancreatograms could also be obtained by opening the duodenum and cannulating the ampulla of Vater or by transecting the tail of the pancreas in order to directly cannulate the pancreatic duct. These procedures are mentioned only for historical context and should not be used. In both cases, an injury is created where there was none previously, creating another suture line not required by the original injury.

Intraoperative Diagnosis of Pancreatic Ductal Injury

This illustration is presented to emphasize what should not be done to assist in the intraoperative diagnosis of a pancreatic ductal injury. The duodenum should not be opened in order to cannulate the ampulla of Vater. The distal pancreas should not be transected in hopes of identifying and cannulating the duct, because the distal pancreatic duct is usually extremely small.

General Principles: Complete Transection

- Débride to viable tissue

- Primary repair with spatulation

- Interrupted absorbable suture

Cholecystocholangiography

This intraoperative photograph provides an excellent demonstration of a pancreatogram utilizing both intravenous radiographic contrast material and methylene blue. The gastrocolic omentum has been divided, the stomach mobilized cephalad, and the retroperitoneum explored. A transection of the pancreas was clinically evident on exploration, and ductal disruption was demonstrated not only fluoroscopically, but also visually, with the use of methylene blue. This assists the surgeon in locating the precise level at which to perform a distal pancreatectomy.

Cholecystocholangiography

- Lessor sac is open to visualize the pancreas

- Radiographic contrast material and methylene blue is injected into gallbladder or the common bile duct.

- X-ray is taken looking for extravasation

- Pancreas inspected for extravasation of methylene blue.

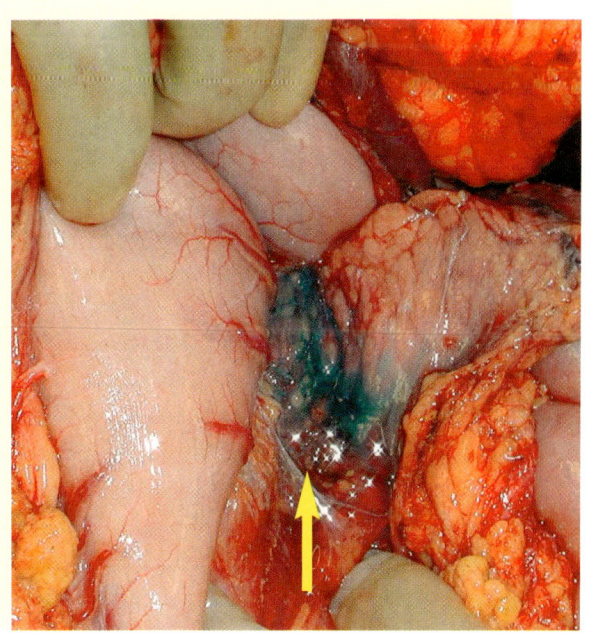

Neck of Pancreas

Treating the Pancreatic Ductal Injury: A Balancing Act

PARENCHYMAL PRESERVATION	PARENCHYMAL RESECTION
• Risky anastomosis	• Pancreatic insufficiency

• Activated fistula	• Malabsorption
	   - diabetes mellitus
	   - > 80% resection

• Secondary hemorrhage	
• Wound complications	

Treating the Pancreatic Ductal Injury: A Balancing Act

Intraoperative decision-making for treating pancreatic ductal injuries is complex and not always clear-cut. It involves a balancing act between the risks of pancreatic preservation and the complications associated with pancreatic resection.

Although pancreatic preservation maintains glandular endocrine and exocrine function, pancreaticoenteric anastomoses are risky, have a high leakage rate, and result in activated fistulas. In addition, secondary hemorrhage and wound complications after fistula formation are common because of the destructive enzymatic activity of the activated fistula.

On the other hand, parenchymal resection of the pancreas is not without complications. Major pancreatic insufficiency associated with pancreatic resection results in malabsorption. When more than 80% of the pancreas has been resected, the loss of endocrine function results in the development of type I diabetes.

Conservative treatment for pancreatic injuries

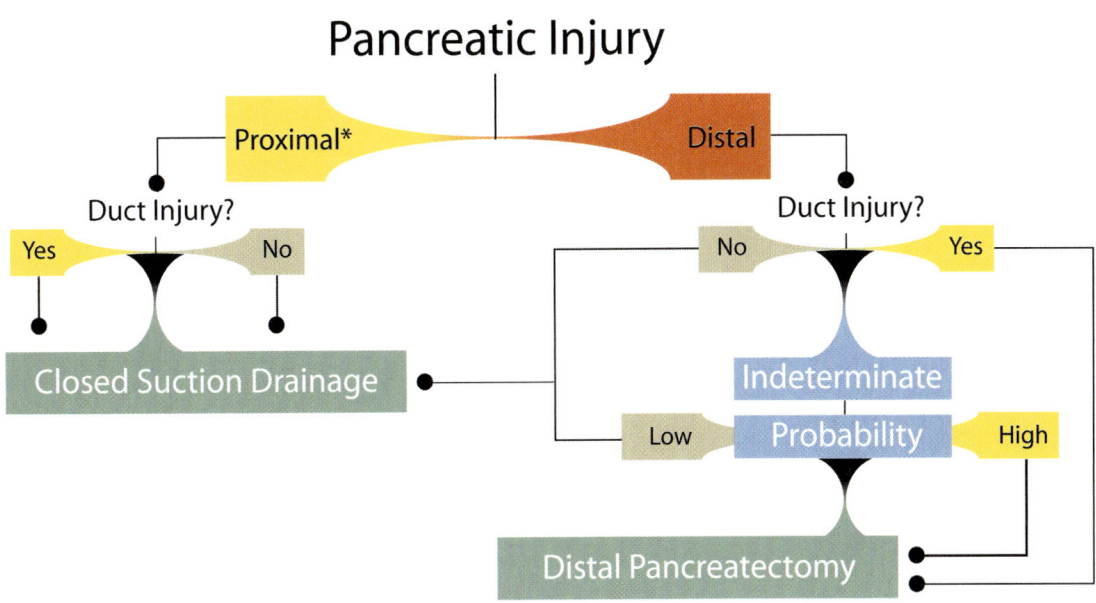

Management algorithm for pancreatic injuries
*Rare devitalizing, destructive injuries may require pancreaticoduodenectomy

From: Patton: J Trauma, 1997

Conservative Treatment For Pancreatic Injuries

The decision-making process can be somewhat simplified by creating a management algorithm for pancreatic injury. The ultimate goal should be conservative therapy and pancreatic parenchymal conservation. It can be helpful to determine operative management based on the location of the ductal injury.

Pancreatic preservation would be the goal in the presence of proximal pancreatic injury, where pancreatectomy would almost certainly result in endocrine and exocrine insufficiency. Following in this logic, conservative therapy with closed-suction drainage should be performed whether or not there is ductal injury. However, injuries resulting in extensive pancreatic or duodenal destruction may require a staged pancreaticoduodenectomy.

Distal pancreatic injuries without ductal injury should be treated with closed-suction drainage alone after débridement of devitalized pancreatic tissue. In the presence of ductal injury, however, a distal pancreatectomy should be performed. In these cases, the distal location of the parenchymal and ductal injuries allows a pancreatectomy with preservation of the major portion of the pancreas.

Grade*		Injury Description
I	Hematoma	Involving single portion of duodenum
II	Laceration	Partial thickness, no perforation
	Hematoma	Involving more than one portion
III	Laceration	Disruption <50% of circumference
	Laceration	Disruption 50-75% circumference of D2
IV	Laceration	Disruption 50-100% Circumference of D1, D3, D4
		Disruption >75% circumference of D2
		Involving ampulla or distal common bile duct
V	Laceration	Massive disruption of duodenopancretatic complex Vascular Devascularization of duodenum

*Advance one grade for multiple injuries to the same organ

Duodenum Organ Injury Scale

Duodenal injuries are graded similarly to other organ injuries graded by the AAST-OIS. A Grade I duodenal injury is characterized by a hematoma involving a single portion of the duodenum, or a partial thickness laceration to the duodenum without perforation into the lumen. A Grade II injury is characterized by a duodenal hematoma involving more than one portion of the duodenum, or a full thickness laceration that has disrupted less than 50% of the duodenal circumference. Grade III injuries are full thickness lacerations that have disrupted 50% to 70% of the circumference of the second portion of the duodenum, or 50% to 100% of the circumference of the first, third, or fourth portions of the duodenum. Grade IV injuries are characterized by lacerations of the duodenum that have disrupted more than 75% of the second portion of the duodenum and that involve the ampulla or the distal common bile duct. Grade V injuries are those characterized by massive disruption of the duodenum pancreatic complex with devascularization of the duodenum. As mentioned for pancreatic injury grading, the grade of injury goes up one grade when an organ has multiple injuries.

Duodenal Injuries Operative Strategy

As with other injuries, the main priority when dealing with duodenal injury is to arrest hemorrhage and achieve hemodynamic stability as quickly as possible. In some cases, this may require damage control procedures, with definitive surgical management of the duodenal injuries at a later time.

Once the decision to proceed with the procedure has been made, exposure is essential. The entire duodenum must be mobilized and inspected as described earlier. The location of the injury must be determined, and whenever possible, primary repair of the injury should be the surgeon's goal.

Unlike surgical repairs to other locations in the gastrointestinal tract, one must consider the need to protect the repair to an injured duodenum. It is important to consider how to control potential fistula formation, as it is a recognized and not uncommon complication of duodenal and pancreatic surgical interventions.

General Principles: Complete Transection

- Stop hemorrhage

- Exposure

- Location of injury

- Primary repair

- Protection of repair

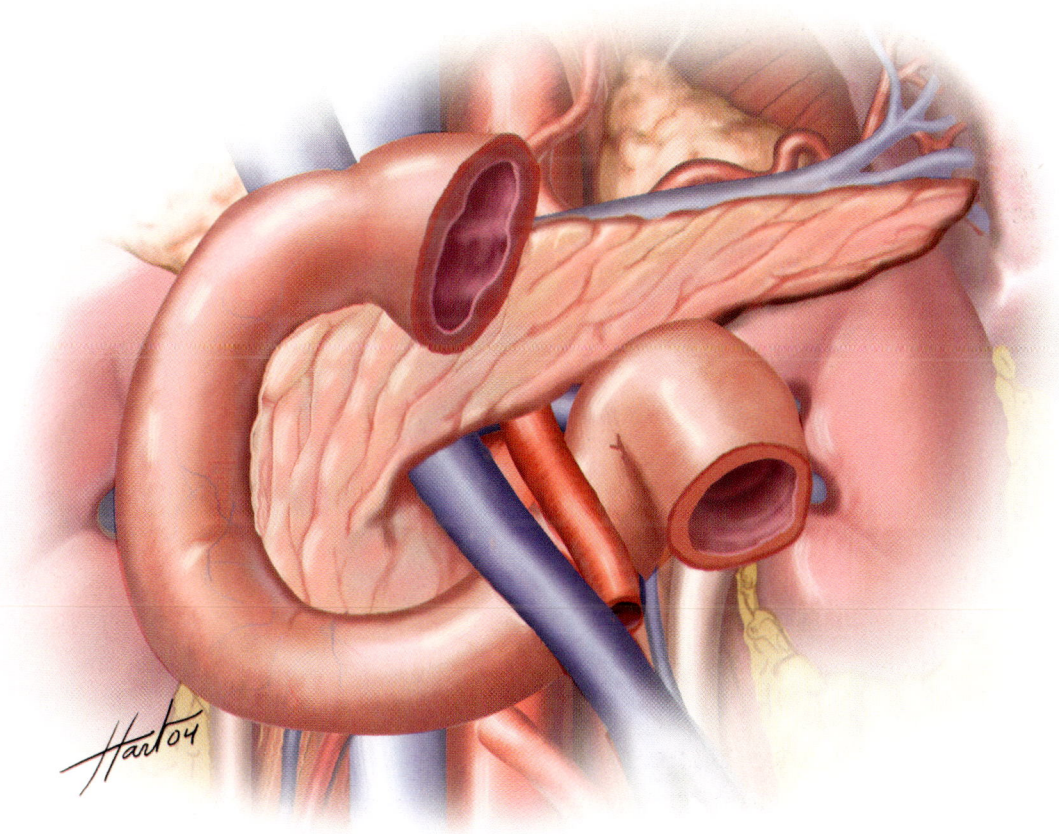

Injury Grading & Operative Management

- Grade I or Grade II hematomas single or multiple segments

- Non operative
    - nasogastric tube for one to two weeks

- Surgical evacuation and seromuscular repair of Grade I or Grade II lacerations
    - primary repair
    - stapled, double layer or single layer as per surgeon's preference

Duodenum: Injury Grading & Operative Management

Grade I or Grade II duodenal hematomas should be managed nonoperatively, regardless of whether they are single or seen in multiple segments. The patient is placed on nasogastric suction for 1 to 2 weeks. Contrast duodenography is performed, and the patient may be fed when there is no further evidence of duodenal obstruction secondary to the hematomas.

Grade I or Grade II lacerations should be repaired primarily. The repair can be done using a single-layered technique, a double-layered technique, or staplers, according to the surgeon's preference.

Duodenum: Injury Grading & Operative Management

- Grade III or Grade IV laceration
    - large
    - very large
    - injured ampulla
    - injured distal CBD

- Management
    - primary repair
    - resection anastomosis
    - roux-en-Y duodenojejunostomy

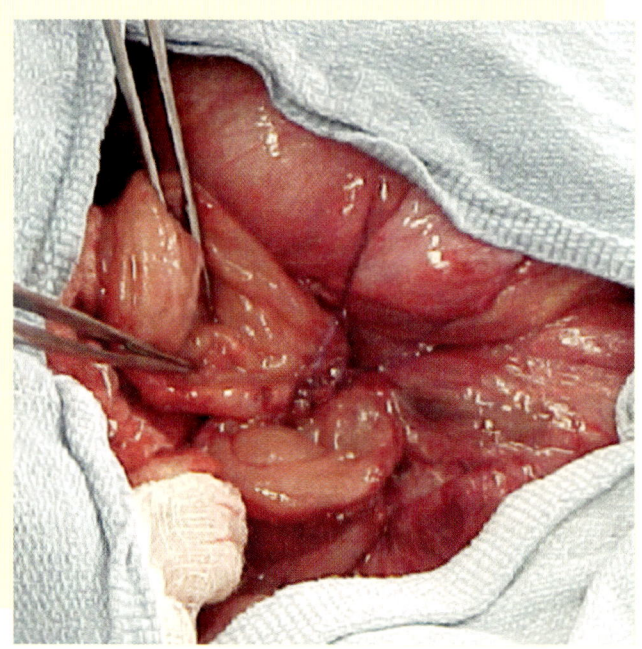

Treating the Pancreatic Ductal Injury: A Balancing Act

MILD	**SEVERE**
• Secondary to stab wound	• Blunt or gun shot wound
• < 75% circumference	• > 75% circumference
• 3rd or 4th portion	• 1st or 2nd portion
• Injury to repair interval < 24 hr	• Injury to repair interval > 24 hr
• No associated biliary or pancreatic injury	• Associated biliary or pancreatic injury
• NO	• YES

Grade III and Grade IV lacerations involve a significant portion of the duodenum. They may involve the ampulla of Vater or injury to the common bile duct distally. Management of these injuries is determined by the mechanism of injury and the degree of destruction of the duodenal tissues.

Injuries caused by stab wounds can most often be repaired primarily but should be hand-sewn. When the duodenum has been devitalized, devitalized tissue should be resected, and a primary anastomosis should be performed between the healthy ends. If this requires extensive duodenal resection, a roux-en-Y duodenojejunostomy may be necessary.

Snyder Duodenal Severity Scale

Approximately 80% of all duodenal injuries can be safely repaired primarily. Before the near-universal acceptance of the AAST-OIS, a study by Snyder and colleagues described factors that determined whether or not a duodenal wound should be primarily repaired, and if the repair required protection. Duodenal injuries were categorized as mild or severe.

Mild injuries were those secondary to stab wounds or those that involved less than 75% of the circumference of the third or fourth portion of the duodenum. In addition, the time interval from injury to repair was less than 24 hours, and there were no associated biliary or pancreatic injuries. The study investigators reported that protection of the duodenal repair was not necessary in these patients.

Decompressive Procedures

- Three tube technique
  - gastrostomy or gastroduodenostomy
  - retrograde duodenostomy
  - feeding jejunostomy

- Tube duodenostomy

- External drainage

Diversionary Procedures

- Duodenal diverticularization

- Pyloric exclusion

- Temporary GI disconnection

- External drainage

Injuries caused by blunt mechanisms or gunshot wounds were categorized as severe injuries if more than 75% of the circumference of the duodenum was involved, the first or second portions of the duodenum were injured, the interval from injury to repair was greater than 24 hours, and there was associated biliary or pancreatic injuries. The study investigators reported that protection of the duodenal repair was necessary in patients with severe injuries, regardless of the mechanism of repair.

Protecting the Primary Duodenal Repair: Decompressive Procedures

Primary repair of extensive duodenal injuries should be protected. Many techniques have been described to protect duodenal repairs. An early technique, which was described as the three tube technique, involved inserting a gastrostomy or gastroduodenostomy tube, a retrograde duodenostomy tube placed through a jejunostomy, and a second jejunostomy tube, placed distally, to be used initially for decompression and subsequently as a feeding tube.

Currently, most surgeons do not recommend tube duodenostomy because it involves creating another injury in an already injured duodenum. Closed-suction drainage should routinely be used after repair.

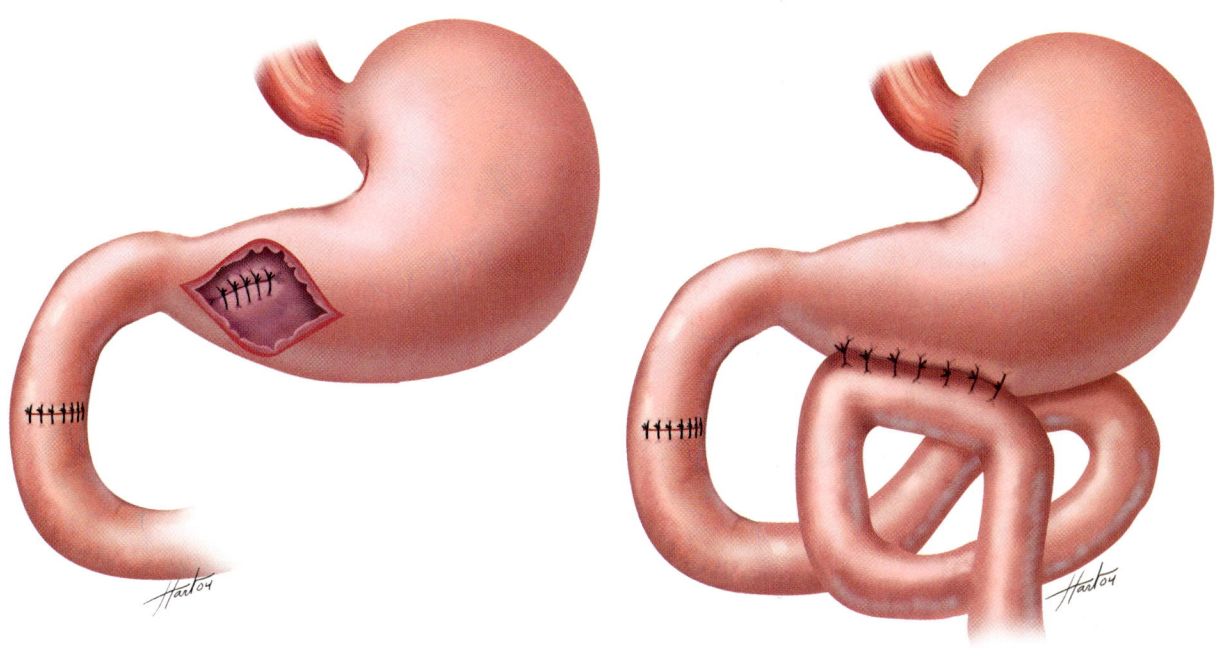

Protecting the Primary Duodenal Repair: Diversionary Procedures

Other techniques to protect duodenal repair have utilized the concept of diversion rather than decompression. Duodenal diverticularization involves diversion of biliary and pancreatic secretions using T-tube drainage, and gastric drainage and decompression using a gastrostomy tube.

Pyloric exclusion is another technique used to protect duodenal repair. This procedure involves a gastrostomy. The pylorus is sutured closed with a nonabsorbable suture, and a gastrojejunostomy is performed. This provides the duodenal protection necessary for adequate healing by completely rerouting the gastric stream. The pyloric closure can also be accomplished by applying a TA-50 to the pylorus. In either case, the pylorus spontaneously opens in about four to six weeks. Again, external drainage should be provided.

Pyloric Exclusion

This diagram illustrates a gastrostomy through which a pyloric exclusion has been completed in order to protect the duodenal repair. Diversion is accomplished by constructing a gastrojejunostomy.

Whipple for Trauma

- Grade V pancreatic injury
  - massive disruption of pancreatic head

- Grade V duodenal injury
  - massive disruption of duodenopancreatic complex
  - duodenal devascularization

- Non reconstructable injury to pancreas, duodenum and distal common bile duct

Whipple for Trauma

Very well suited for staged procedure:

1. Control of hemorrhage & resection débridement

2. Resuscitation in the ICU

3. Gastrointestinal reconstruction

   - Achilles heel: pancreatic remnant anastomosis

   - Alternatives:
     - ductal ligation
     - pancreaticogastrostomy
     - total pancreatectomy
     - islet cell auto transplantation

Whipple for Trauma

Grade V pancreatic and duodenal injuries are devastating injuries. They involve massive disruption of the pancreatic head and the duodenopancreatic complex, and duodenal devascularization. These injuries are so severe that they preclude any repair of the pancreas, duodenum, or distal common bile duct. The surgeon faced with these massive injuries is, therefore, forced to perform a pancreaticoduodenectomy, or a trauma Whipple. Even as an elective procedure, the Whipple procedure is an extensive surgical intervention with known postoperative complications. Although the procedure is necessary in the unstable trauma patient, it can rarely be completed during the initial exploratory laparotomy.

A trauma Whipple can be performed as a staged procedure. As mentioned earlier, the priorities of the initial trauma laparotomy are control of hemorrhage and stabilization of the patient. If the clinical situation permits, surgical débridement and/or resection of devitalized tissue should be accomplished during the initial trauma laparotomy. Restoration of gastrointestinal continuity should not be considered at that time.

Débridement and resection should not be attempted in patients who are acidotic, cold, and coagulopathic. In these patients, the gastrointestinal tract should be isolated from the abdominal cavity through the use of staples or sutures, the abdominal cavity packed, and if possible, the abdominal wall closed. The patient should be brought to the intensive care unit for stabilization, resuscitation, and restoration of normal circulatory and metabolic parameters.

In patients who are successfully resected during the initial surgical procedure, gastrointestinal reconstruction can be accomplished with a second surgery. Patients who are too unstable to undergo an initial resection will require a second procedure for surgical resection of the damaged and devitalized tissue. They may also require a third procedure to complete the gastrointestinal reconstruction. In either case, the pancreatic remnant anastomosis presents a challenge when completing gastrointestinal reconstruction.

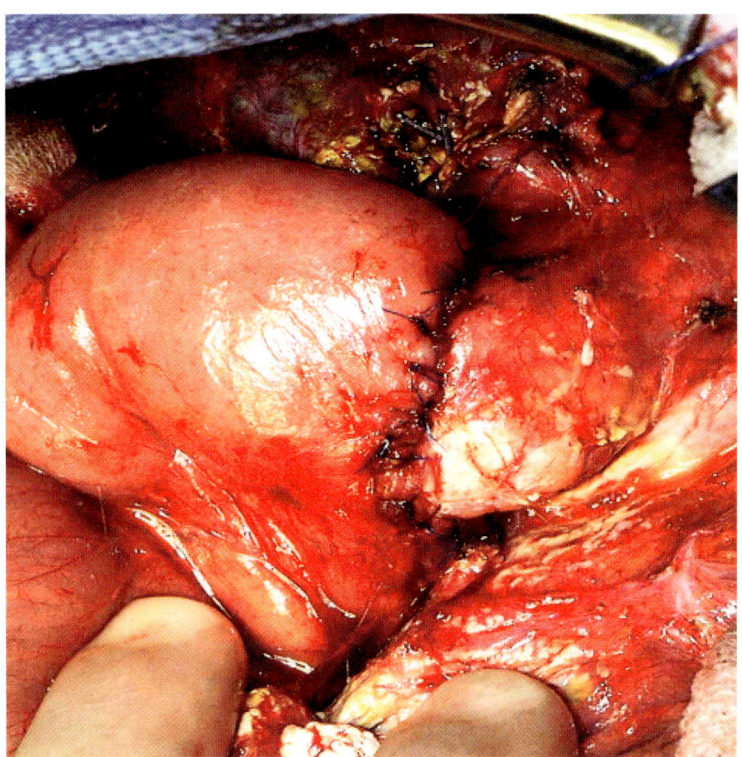

Most surgeons choose to preserve the pancreatic remnant by performing either a pancreaticojejunostomy or pancreaticogastrostomy. As discussed earlier, the success of this procedure is likely not related to the procedure itself, but rather to the surgeon's familiarity with and comfort when performing the procedure.

Alternatives to pancreaticoenteric anastomosis include ductal ligation with preservation of the isolated distal pancreas and total pancreatectomy with islet cell autotransplantation. Although total pancreatectomy is an option available to all surgeons, islet cell autotransplantation is available only to those in transplant centers that have developed the required expertise.

A completed pancreaticojejunostomy can be seen in the picture. The proximal end of the pancreatic remnant has been implanted into the open jejunum.

Nonabsorbable interrupted sutures should be used to sew the mucosa of the jejunum to the pancreatic capsule. A second layer of nonabsorbable sutures is added, imbricating the initial suture line and placing sutures from the capsule of the pancreas to the serosa of the jejunum. This anastomosis must be widely drained using large closed-suction drains in order to protect the perianastomotic tissues from the devastating effects of a potential anastomotic leak.

Pancreatic & Duodenal Trauma

MORBIDITY

- Early hemorrhage
- Late hemorrhage
- Pancreatic pseudocyst
- Pancreatic fistula
- Duodenal fistula
- Intraabdominal abscess
- Obstruction
- Malabsorption
- Diabetes

MORTALITY

- Early
  - hemorrhage

- Late
  - hemorrhage
  - duodenal fistula
  - pancreatitis
  - uncontrolled sepsis
  - multisystem organ failure

Pancreatic & Duodenal Trauma

Severe pancreatic and duodenal trauma injuries are devastating, and postoperative complications are common. The morbidity and mortality associated with these injuries can be categorized as early or late. Early morbidity and mortality is often due to hemorrhage, but hemorrhage can also be seen later on due to tissue destruction caused by anastomotic leaks and the subsequent autodigestion by pancreatic secretions. Other postoperative complications include the development of pancreatic pseudocysts, pancreatic and duodenal fistulas, intraabdominal abscess formation, intestinal obstruction, malabsorption syndromes, and diabetes in patients requiring extensive pancreatic resection.

As previously mentioned, death can result early in patients who have sustained pancreatic and duodenal trauma. This is most often due to hemorrhage, either from the pancreatic or duodenal trauma itself or from injuries frequently associated with this type of devastating trauma. Late complications leading to death in patients with duodenal and pancreatic trauma include hemorrhage, uncontrollable duodenal fistulas, necrotizing pancreatitis, uncontrollable sepsis, and multisystem organ failure.

ADVANCED TRAUMA OPERATIVE MANAGEMENT

Selected Readings

Chapter 4 - Pancreas & Duodenum

Berne CJ et al. Duodenal "diverticulization" for duodenal and pancreatic injury. Am J Surg 1974;127:503-507.

Berni G et al. Role of intraoperative pancreatography in patients with injury to the pancreas. Am J Surg 1982;145:602-605.

Feliciano DV et al. Management of combined pancreatoduodenal injuries. Ann Surg 1987;205:673-680.

Pachter HL et al. Traumatic injuries to the pancreas: The role of distal pancreatectomy with splenic preservations. J Trauma 1989;29:1352-1355.

Carrillo EH et al. Evolution in the management of duodenal injuries. J Trauma 1996;40:1037-1046.

Koniaris LG et al. Two stage trauma pancreaticoduodenectomy: delay facilitates anastamotic reconstruction. J Gastrointest Surg 2000;4:366-369.

De Kerpel W et al. Whipple procedure after blunt abdominal trauma. J Trauma 2002;53:780-783.

Asensio JA et al. Pancreaticoduodenectomy: A rare procedure for the management of complex pancreaticoduodenal injuries. J Am Coll Surg 2003;197:937-942.

Jurkovich JJ, Bulger EM. Duodenum and pancreas. In: Moore EE, Feliciano DV, Mattox KL, eds. Trauma. 5th ed. 2004 McGraw-Hill:709-734.

Feliciano DV et al. Trauma Damage Control. In: Moore EE, Feliciano DV, Mattox KL, eds. Trauma. 5th ed. 2004 McGraw-Hill:877-900.

Tips From the Masters

There are a number of safe methods to manage blunt and penetrating trauma in the operating suite. The following technical surgical tips have been successfully used by the authors to deal with difficult or challenging operating situations.

Chapter 4: The Pancreas and Duodenum

TABLE OF CONTENTS

Exposure of the Entire Pancreas 188
Charles E. Lucas, MD

Exposure of the Pancreas, Duodenum, Common Duct 190
Norman McSwain, MD

Pancreaticoduodenectomy for Trauma to the Pancreas and Duodenum ...192
Ronald I. Gross, MD

Timing of Reconstruction After Pancreaticoduodenectomy Secondary to Severe Blunt Trauma to the Pancreas and Duodenum 195
Robert T. Brautigam, MD

Partial Pancreatic Transection 197
Thomas M. Scalea, MD

Operative Management of Combined Duodenum and Pancreas Injury 199
Patricia M. Byers, MD

Laceration of the Second Portion of the Duodenum 202
David B. Hoyt, MD

Laceration of the Third Portion of the Duodenum 204
Alasdair K.T. Conn, MD

Laceration of the Third Portion of the Duodenum 206
Rao Ivatury, MD

Exposure and Repair of the Third and Fourth Portions of the Duodenum ..208
Erwin F. Hirsch, MD

Methylene Blue Pancreatography 209
Vicente Cortes, MD

Penetrating Duodenal Injury to the Second Portion of the Duodenum 211
Peter Rhee, MD

Pyloric Exclusion for Tenuous Complex Duodenal Injury 213
Edward Cornwell, MD

Pyloric Exclusion 214
Michael Rhodes, MD

Stapled Pyloric Exclusion 216
Orlando Kirton, MD

Management of Injury to the Common Bile Duct 218
Jameel Ali, MD

Stab Wound to the Pancreas with Ductal Injury 221
Margaret Knudson, MD

**Stab Wound to the Pancreas with Ductal Injury
Splenic Preserving Distal Pancreatectomy** 224
Aurelio Rodriguez, MD

TECHNICAL OPERATIVE PROCEDURES:

HOW I DO IT

Exposure of the Entire Pancreas

Charles E. Lucas, MD, FACS

Scenario

A 36-year-old man stabbed in the epigastrium. The knife lacerates the mid body of the pancreas. There are no other injuries.

Procedure: *Exposure of the pancreas*

Exposure to the anterior surface of the pancreas is best achieved by entering the lesser sac between the colon and stomach just outside the arcades of the right and left gastroepiploic vessels. The small crossing vessels between these arcades and the transverse colon are contained by electrocoagulation. The dissection through this plane continues on the patient's right side to the duodenum where the perivascular fat and lymph tissues terminate about three centimeters beyond the pylorus. The dissection to the patient's left continues until all omental attachments covering the splenic flexure have been divided. The thin but ever present membranous attachments along the middle third of the anterior pancreas margin are now easily seen; division of this membrane must be performed on the pancreatic surface to avoid injury to the branches of the lesser curve gastric arcades. Division of this membrane permits complete examination of the anterior surface of the pancreas from the duodenum to the splenic hilum.

Examination of the inferior pancreatic surface requires that the transverse mesocolon attachments to this surface be severed adjacent to the pancreas. The superior leaf of the transverse mesocolon ascends to this inferior border of the pancreas from the duodenum to the splenic hilum. Careful division of this membrane unroofs the mid-colic vessels, the superior mesenteric vein, and the inferior mesenteric vein as they course posterior to the pancreas. The inferior surface and a portion of the posterior pancreatic surface can now be visualized.

The superior border of the pancreas is accessed by severing the lesser curvature mesenteric leaf which extends posteriorly from the lesser omentum to the superior border of the pancreas. Once this membrane has been severed close to the pancreas, one can examine the superior border and the adjacent posterior surface of the pancreas. The splenic artery which descends from the celiac axis and curves to the left as it courses posterior to the pancreas toward the spleen can now be identified. Careful examination of both the superior and inferior pancreatic surfaces, in conjunction with gentle retraction, allows the surgeon to verify that there is no posterior injury in most patients. When a potential posterior injury requires better visualization, the entire posterior surface can be visualized by mobilizing the body and tail of the pancreas along with the spleen anteriorly and medially. When mobilizing the pancreas with the spleen, one must not pull the spleen but should gently push the pancreas anteriorly and medially as the fingers of the right hand are passed posterior to the spleen and pancreas. The spleen will atraumatically move with the pancreas. Excessive force applied to the spleen leads to avulsion of the hilar vessels and often necessitates a splenectomy. Once safe mobilization has been accomplished, the surgeon can completely assess the body and tail of the pancreas to the level of the superior mesenteric vessels. Postoperative problems with the pancreas can be assessed endoscopically.

Mobilization of the splenic flexure of the colon in its precise anatomic plane helps elevate the body and tail of the pancreas with spleen. The retroperitoneal line of Toldt terminates at the beginning of the descending colon. Inadvertent splenic injury or avulsion of the lower pole vessels during splenic flexure mobilization occurs when the dissection from this point to the transverse mesocolon is performed too far from the colon wall. The avascular plane which separates the splenic flexure mesocolon from the perinephric fat lies only two cm from the border of the colon. Dissection more peripherally where no anatomic plane exists leads to bleeding which, in turn, makes the likelihood for splenic hilar injury more likely. Once the splenic flexure has been mobilized, one can quite easily identify how the superior leaf of the transverse mesocolon mesentery attaches to the inferior margin of the pancreatic tail.

- When mobilizing the pancreas with the spleen, gently push the pancreas anteriorly and medially

- Do not pull on the spleen

- Careful examination of both superior and inferior surfaces verifies that there is no posterior pancreatic injury

The posterior portion of the pancreatic head is examined after doing an extended Kocher maneuver. This maneuver should begin at the pylorus and extends to the ligament of Treitz. The common bile duct passes posterior to the proximal duodenum before entering into the pancreas; the proximal mobilization should begin just lateral to the bile duct. Mobilization of the lateral duodenum is almost always safe except when an accessory right hepatic artery courses posterior to the pancreas and duodenum as it ascends from the superior mesenteric artery to the portal triad where it lies to the right common bile duct. This aberrant right hepatic artery may be the only arterial inflow to the right lobe of the liver. The remaining distal duodenal dissection is completed by separating the superior leaf of the transverse mesocolon from the fourth portion of the duodenum in this same avascular plane. The duodenum with the pancreatic head can then be mobilized anteriorly and medially as the posterior plane is freed to the superior mesenteric artery. All of the pancreatic head and the uncinate process can then be examined.

TECHNICAL OPERATIVE PROCEDURES:

HOW I DO IT

Exposure of the Pancreas, Duodenum, Common Duct

Norman McSwain, MD, FACS

Scenario

A 27-year-old sustained a gunshot wound to the head of the pancreas and the second portion of the duodenum, including the distal common bile duct.

Management

As in any hypotensive patient, resuscitation is initiated in the resuscitation bay and continued in the operating room. This process is not described here as it is well addressed in other parts of the course. However the cell saver should be ready before the abdomen is opened.

The management of the wound to the pancreas and duodenum is predicated on the associated injuries. The very high mortality rate associated with duodenal and pancreatic injuries has nothing to do with the pancreatic injury itself, but has to do with the associated vascular injuries. In this area are the aorta, the vena cava, the portal vein, the hepatic artery, the branches of the celiac axis and the branches of the superior mesenteric artery which supply the head of the pancreas and second and third portions of the duodenum.

The initial management of these patients is directed at the initiation of resuscitation of the hypovolemic patient and the initial control of hemorrhage once the abdomen is opened. Once all of these more rapidly fatal injuries have been managed then the surgeon can turn the attention to the management of the pancreas and the second portion of the duodenum. Such management may occur in 24 to 48 hours if damage control procedure is required for the hemorrhage.

Procedure: *Exposure of the pancreas and duodenum*

The critical steps in defining how the pancreas and duodenum should be managed are three-fold.

Step 1: Determination of the viability of the head of the pancreas and the duodenum by assessing the blood supply. Recognition that blood supply comes from two sources, the superior mesenteric artery and the celiac axis, assist in this determination.

Step 2: Identification of the pancreatic duct and the injuries of this structure. Patients with and without injuries to the duct are approached differently.

Step 3: Extent of the injury to the duodenum and the location of the injury. Determine the extent of the duodenum injury, and assess whether the nonperitoneal portion of the duodenum is injured.

Exposure

The abdomen is opened rapidly from xiphoid process to the symphysis pubis. The incision is started at the xiphoid and continues down with one motion to the symphysis pubis. Multiple cuts are not made as they are time consuming. The initial cut goes through the skin, down to the linea Alba. The surgeon's tactile perception indicates when the curve of the blade is on the linea Alba but not cut. The second stroke again begins at the xiphoid and cuts through the linea Alba. This motion goes through the linea Alba, but not the peritoneum.

As the linea Alba is opened and the peritoneum is visualized, one gets the initial impression as to whether there is a large amount of blood in the abdominal cavity or not. The peritoneum is then opened using blunt dissection with the fingers or sharply using the Metzenbaum scissors.

In penetrating injuries, the surgeon suspects that the hemorrhage will be along the pathway that the bullet has followed through the abdominal cavity. Therefore, this area is inspected first. Time is not wasted by placing laparotomy pads in the abdomen. The specific sites of hemorrhage are identified and compression is achieved by direct pressure of the hand or fingers. Only after all homeostasis has been achieved can attention can be turned to the pancreas and duodenum.

The entire pancreas and duodenum must be examined. Both the lesser sac and the free abdominal cavity portions of the pancreas and duodenum must be examined.

The head of the pancreas is mobilized using a Kocher maneuver. The peritoneum is incised just lateral to the duodenum. The head of the pancreas and the second and third portions of the duodenum are exposed by blunt dissection with the fingertips. The forefingers are passed posterior to the pancreas and duodenum. The thumb is placed on the anterior portion of the pancreas so that the entire organ can be felt. The three components of potential pancreatic and duodenal injury are assessed.

The fourth portion of the duodenum is addressed by passing the index finger of the right hand under the ligament of Treitz and along the fourth portion of the duodenum. The index finger of the left hand is passed from the third portion of duodenum along the posterior aspect of this organ until the fingertips meet. This allows either palpation or visualization of the entire fourth portion of the duodenum. The lesser sac is opened and the rest of the aspects of the pancreas are assessed.

Management is addressed based on the extent of the injury which may range from nothing more than simple closure of the duodenum to isolation of the duodenum with the diverticulization procedure or total removal with a Whipple procedure.

- Determine the viability of the head of the pancreas and the duodenum by assessing the blood supply

- Evaluate the pancreatic duct

- Determine the extent of the duodenal injury

TECHNICAL OPERATIVE PROCEDURES:

HOW I DO IT

Pancreaticoduodenectomy for Trauma to the Pancreas and Duodenum

Ronald I. Gross, MD, FACS

Scenario

A 19-year-old male was struck in the abdomen by a jet ski. He was pulled out of the water by bystanders after reportedly being face down for three to four minutes.

Management

The patient is taken to a Level II trauma center where a CT scan of the head, chest, abdomen and pelvis revealed multiple punctate intracerebral and brainstem bleeds. A Grade V splenic laceration, and a Grade IV or Grade V pancreatic and duodenal injury were identified.

While in the operating room, arrangements were made to transfer the patient to a Level I trauma center. The patient underwent a damage control procedure and a splenectomy was performed. The duodenum was stapled at the level of the ligament of Treitz and the common bile duct, and the abdominal cavity was packed. The patient's vital signs remained stable throughout his workup and surgery.

Upon arrival at the Level I trauma center, the patient was hypotensive and acidotic. My initial goal in the management of this patient's injuries was to normalize the patient's hemodynamic and metabolic parameters. The destruction of the pancreatic head and duodenal sweep that necessitated the damage control procedure would require a return trip to the operating room to débride dead tissue.

The patient was brought to the surgical intensive care unit, where he was aggressively resuscitated, correcting his blood pressure, pulse, and temperature to normal range within three hours. In addition, his acidosis was reversed as indicated by a normal pH and a normalized lactate, and his coagulation profile normalized. A follow-up head CT scan was performed to determine the evolution of his intracranial hemorrhages and their potential effect on the management of the patient. There was no change in his intracranial findings.

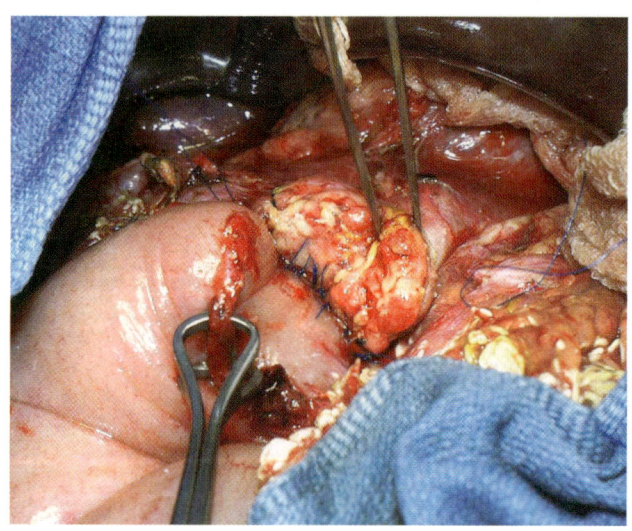

Procedure: *Damage control pancreaticoduodenectomy*

The operative findings upon reexploration included a shattered pancreatic head extending laterally to the superior mesenteric vessels, complete disruption of the second and third portions of the duodenal sweep, a staple line across the duodenum at the level of the common duct, and a second staple line across the duodenum approximately 3 cm proximal to the ligament of Treitz. The devitalized pancreatic head and duodenal sweep were still in situ. A nonbleeding subcapsular hematoma of the lateral aspect of the right lobe of the liver was discovered. A pancreatic duodenectomy was completed, extending from staple line to staple line on the duodenum and to healthy pancreatic tissue approximately 2 cm lateral to the mesenteric vessels. The common bile duct was ligated at the level of the pancreatic head, a cholecystectomy was performed, and the abdomen was then copiously irrigated and repacked.

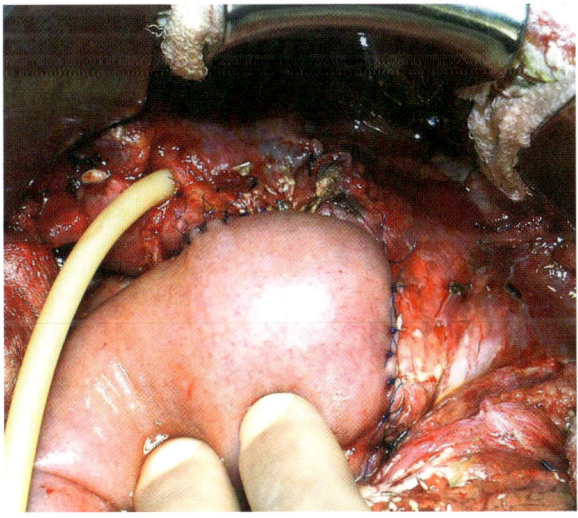

Seventy-two hours after injury, it was felt that the patient was stable enough to undergo his third exploratory laparotomy, in hopes of completing the staged Whipple procedure. Upon re-exploration, it was found that the common bile duct had dilated to approximately 1.3 cm. There was no evidence of peripancreatic edema or tissue necrosis. I felt that restoration of gastrointestinal continuity was indicated. The distal duodenum was carefully mobilized and resected after dividing the ligament of Treitz, and the proximal jejunum was mobilized so that an end jejunopancreatic anastomosis could be performed. The proximal jejunum was mobilized, and a two-layered invaginating pancreaticojejunostomy was created using 3-0 Prolene sutures to sew the jejunal mucosa to the pancreatic capsule. The anastomosis was then invaginated and a second layer of 3-0 Prolene sutures was used to sew the pancreatic capsule to the jejunum taking seromuscular bites of the jejunum. The pancreatic duct could not be identified. Hemostasis was achieved and the anastomosis accomplished. A hand sewn two-layered posterior gastrojejunostomy was performed. A choledochojejunostomy was performed as an end-to-side anastomosis. The anastomosis was accomplished using interrupted 4-0 Prolene sutures to sew the duct to the antimesenteric surface of the jejunum. The choledochojejunal anastomosis was stented with a 16 Fr. T-tube, with the distal limb left long, and crossing the anastomosis. The posterior aspect of the T-tube was removed prior to placement to facilitate its eventual removal. Although choledochojejunal anastomoses are not routinely stented, given the extensive tissue disruption, the presence of bowel wall edema at the anastomotic site, and the possibility of a postoperative leak, a T-tube was used to initially decompress, and subsequently study the anastomosis. A red rubber catheter jejunal tube was placed 10 cm distal to the pancreatico-jejunal anastomosis. It was placed on straight drainage with orders to irrigate the tube with 15 mL of normal saline every eight hours. A second jejunal tube was placed 10 cm distal to the first to be used as a feeding jejunostomy when clinically appropriate.

Finally, I placed a Moss gastrojejunostomy tube through the gastrojejunostomy, with the intent of decompressing and draining both the stomach and the jejunum. The entire operative field was now extensively drained with 10 mm Jackson-Pratt drains. Four drains were placed with two above and two below the pancreaticojejunostomy with the tips extending to the region around the choledochojejunostomy. The abdominal wall was then closed with 0 Prolene horizontal mattress sutures. The patient was then returned to the intensive care unit. The patient did well postoperatively, and was discharged from the hospital approximately six weeks after his injury.

- The duodenal sweep and the head of the pancreas were stapled and removed

- The common bile duct was ligated at the pancreatic head

- 72 hours later the common bile duct had dilated facilitating the anastomosis

- The choledochojejunal anastomosis is stented

TECHNICAL OPERATIVE PROCEDURES:

HOW I DO IT

Timing of Reconstruction After Pancreaticoduodenectomy Secondary to Severe Blunt Trauma to the Pancreas and Duodenum

Robert T. Brautigam, MD, FACS

Scenario

A 25-year-old man was working on a tree 30 feet above the ground when he lost his footing and fell, striking his right upper quadrant on a branch that he had previously cut from the tree. On the arrival of the paramedics, the patient had difficulty with breathing, but was hemodynamically stable. He was intubated. A cervical collar and long backboard were applied and he was transferred to the trauma room. After primary and secondary surveys were completed, a CT scan of the abdomen and pelvis revealed an avascular head of the pancreas and a large hematoma surrounded the second part of the duodenum. He was taken directly to the operating room for an exploratory laparotomy.

Management

Combined injuries to the pancreas and duodenum carry a high mortality due to the involvement of the underlying vascular structures. High-grade injuries caused by blunt force or penetrating trauma to the pancreatic head and duodenum provide a challenge for the surgeon. Injuries to the pancreas and duodenum causing devascularization and significant tissue loss may warrant pancreaticoduodenectomy. After a thorough assessment of the pancreatic and duodenal injuries a staged approach to reconstruction may be optimal. Once the initial resection of the duodenum and head of the pancreas has been completed, the abdomen is washed thoroughly with normal saline. Large closed suction drainage tubes are placed at the gastric, transected pancreas and proximal jejunum staple lines to control any leakage. If possible, the abdomen is closed at completion of this first damage control procedure. The patient is then taken to the intensive care unit for continued resuscitation and issues of hemodynamic instability, hypothermia, acidosis and/or coagulopathy are corrected. After the patient's resuscitation is complete, which may take more than 24 hours, the patient will return to the operating room for definitive reconstruction. At this time, the abdomen is inspected for injuries and attention is focused at reconstruction. If the bowel and surrounding tissues remain significantly edematous, precluding a safe stapled and hand sewn anastomosis, it may be warranted to close the abdomen over closed suction drainage tubes at the completion of this second damage control procedure. Resuscitation of this critically injured patient in the intensive care unit will continue. At this time, the patient's fluid status should be assessed and if they are euvolemic, attempts at fluid restriction to decrease bowel wall and tissue edema should be a priority.

After 24 to 48 hours of fluid restrictive therapy, the patient should return to the operating room for the third exploration. At this time, significant bowel wall and tissue edema should have decreased secondary to restrictive management of intravenous fluids in the intensive care unit. In addition, limiting intravenous fluids and limiting bowel manipulation during the operative reconstruction will also limit tissue edema and provide optimal circumstances for stapled and hand sewn anastomosis.

- A staged reconstruction may be optimal

- Once the initial resection of the duodenum and the head of the pancreas are completed, large suction drains are placed

- The patient is taken to the intensive care unit for further resuscitation

- The patient is returned to the operating room when bowel and tissue edema has resolved

- This provides for optimal anastomosis

TECHNICAL OPERATIVE PROCEDURES:

HOW I DO IT

Partial Pancreatic Transection

Thomas M. Scalea, M.D., FACS, FCCM

Scenario

A 20-year-old female presents after a blunt trauma to the abdomen. After exploration she has a partial transection of the pancreas just distal to the portal vein. Pancreatic juice is leaking from the pancreatic duct.

Management

I generally approach the mid portion of the pancreas through the lesser sac. I completely divide the gastro-colic omentum and perform a full Kocher maneuver. This allows me to fully inspect the portal structures and perform a cholangiogram if necessary. This also allows for an exploration of the superior mesenteric vein and the portal vein at the juncture of the splenic and superior mesenteric veins.

Diagnosing pancreatic ductal injury can be difficult. A number of methods exist such as intraoperative cholangiography attempting to fill the pancreatic duct. Other options include amputating the tail of the pancreas and trying to perform a retrograde pancreatic ductal study. Finally, intraoperative ERCP can be an attractive option. I have not had good success with intraoperative cholangiography or retrograde studies. Intraoperative ERCP is generally not available on off hours when these patients often present. An experienced surgeon can generally make the diagnosis of ductal transection by simply carefully inspecting the pancreas. It may be necessary to mobilize the inferior margin of the pancreas to examine the back wall, in order to be certain. In this case, the diagnosis is obvious as pancreatic juice is leaking into the injured organ.

Procedure: *Managing a partial pancreatic transection*

A number of options exist and my decision would be based on the amount of pancreas present proximal and distal to the injury. This can be quite variable from patient to patient. It is necessary for the surgeon to completely mobilize the pancreas in order to make this judgment. If distal pancreatectomy would preserve adequate pancreatic function in the surgeon's opinion, that can be curative. A Whipple procedure is an option here, but I believe a bad choice. I reserve the Whipple procedure for patients with exsanguinating hemorrhage or complete destruction of the area

- It is necessary to completely mobilize the pancreas

- The distal pancreas is inserted into the roux-en-Y limb of the jejunum

- Two layer invagination

- Fibrin sealant to buttress the repair

around the ampulla. If in the surgeon's opinion distal pancreatectomy is not a good choice, two other options exist. The first is simply to drain the area. This will result in a well-controlled pancreatic fistula. Postoperative ERCP can then be employed to stent the duct, particularly if it is only partially transected. This is attractive as there is no pancreatic anastomosis necessary, and the chance of leak is minimal. The final option involves transecting the pancreas at the level of injury. One would then over-sew the proximal end allowing the head of the pancreas to drain normally into the duodenum. The distal pancreas can then be plugged into a roux-en-Y limb of jejunum. The roux-en-Y limb is constructed in a standard manner. If the size match is good, the pancreas can be dunked into the end of the roux limb. The pancreas is generally too large and then an end to side pancreatic jejunostomy can be used. As the size of the pancreatic duct is small, there is no role for a mucosal to mucosal anastomosis between the duct and the jejunum. Instead, I dunk the pancreas into the jejunum. I generally do this in two layers invaginating the cut end of the pancreas into the jejunum. I then place a second layer, between the pancreatic capsule and the seromuscular layer of the jejunum. The pancreas is generally soft and the capsule may not hold suture well. Thus, one must roll the jejunum onto the pancreas. When the anastomosis is completed, I use fibrin sealant to buttress the repair.

It is wise to widely drain the area. In addition, I believe that placement of a post-pyloric feeding tube is essential to provide early enteral nutrition. These patients virtually all have a protracted course and enteral nutrition can be life saving.

The choice of pancreatic jejunostomy versus simple drainage should be made based on the experience of the surgeon and comfort he or she has with this relatively complicated injury. If there is reason to believe that a skilled endoscopist may be able to stent even a completely transected duct, drainage will suffice. Even if that is not possible, a well-controlled pancreatic fistula should be well tolerated. If it does not close, one can return some months later and place a roux-en-Y loop of jejunum over the pancreatic fistula to internally control the fistula.

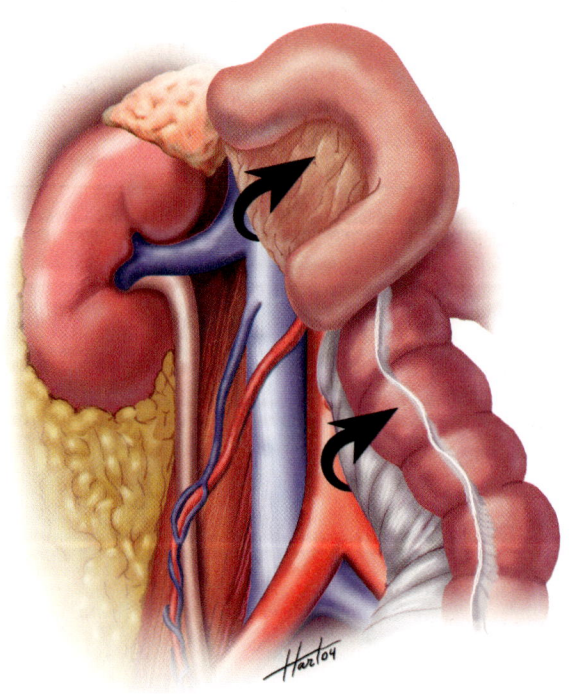

TECHNICAL OPERATIVE PROCEDURES:

HOW I DO IT

Operative Management of Combined Duodenum and Pancreas Injury

Patricia M. Byers, MD, FACS

Scenario

This is a 26-year-old gentleman who had sustained an abdominal gunshot wound 8 hours ago and was brought to the trauma center by helicopter. On arrival, he was alert and oriented in mild distress due to abdominal pain, with a blood pressure of 93/60, a heart rate of 120 in sinus tachycardia, a respiratory rate of 32, and a temperature of 38.2°C.

On physical exam his chest was clear and his abdomen had a single bullet hole in the right flank and was tender with peritoneal signs. The rectal exam was negative and the urine was clear. His extremities were normal. Plain radiographs demonstrated a bullet in the left flank, and a normal chest x-ray, except for free air under the diaphragm. The patient was taken to the operating room for exploratory laparotomy with a diagnosis of perforated viscus.

Management

After receiving antibiotics and anesthesia with endotracheal intubation, the patient was prepared and draped from the xiphoid to mid-thigh. A midline incision was made from the xiphoid to the pubis with a scalpel and cautery through the linea Alba. Approximately 750 mL of blood and bilious fluid was noted to be present primarily on the right side of the abdomen and all four quadrants of the abdomen were packed off. A Bookwalter retractor was used to provide exposure to the abdomen. The left-sided packs were removed first and no injury was noted there. The right lower quadrant had no injury and the liver was not injured, however there was bleeding and bile leaking in the right mid-abdomen with a hematoma over the duodenum. The duodenum was Kocherized and a 1.5 cm laceration was noted in the third portion of the duodenum along the antimesenteric border. Two intestinal clamps were used to control the contamination and the lesser sac was opened via the gastrocolic omentum to evaluate the pancreas.

There was noted to be significant inflammation and edema of the pancreas and the duodenum with surrounding saponification. A hematoma with active bleeding was noted to be coming from the pancreas, and this area was packed. The gastrocolic omentum was opened all the way to the gastrocolic venous trunk in order to gain exposure to the pancreas. A large Penrose drain was placed through the lesser omentum, around the body of the stomach, and retracted toward the head on the retractor's ring using a Kelly clamp. A laceration was noted along the inferior border of the pancreas to the left of the portal vein. There was no injury to the vein; however, the laceration itself was bleeding from tiny pancreatic vessels. The inferior border

> - A thin malleable retractor is placed through the laceration into the duodenum to inspect the Ampulla
>
> - Laceration closed with a running Cannel suture
>
> - A Hickman catheter was placed through the left upper quadrant into the stomach
>
> - The catheter was directed into the efferent limb of the gastrojejunostomy
>
> - An elemental low fat diet is started as soon as the base deficit is corrected

of the body of the pancreas was dissected free to examine the posterior surface, but there did not seem to be a major ductal or venous injury. To control the bleeding from the pancreatic laceration 4-0 silk sutures were used. The bullet tract was noted to have missed the aorta and penetrated the retroperitoneum.

Attention was then turned to the duodenal laceration. The edges of the wound were débrided to fresh tissue, creating a 2 cm transverse laceration. A thin malleable retractor was placed into the duodenum to palpate and examine the ampulla. The ampulla was intact, as was the medial wall of the duodenum. The laceration was then closed with a running Cannel suture of 3-0 Vicryl, followed by a layer of interrupted silk Lembert sutures. A final exploration was performed of the right peritoneal cavity and retroperitoneum, again noting the porta hepatis to be without injury as well as the inferior vena cava and right ureter. The left retroperitoneum was also explored and was noted to have an intact ureter. The lesser sac and posterior wall of the stomach were once again carefully inspected as was the small and large intestine.

When no further injury was noted, the area of injury was once again examined. Due to the combined pancreatic and duodenal injury, especially with the active pancreatitis and edema, the decision was made to perform a pyloric exclusion procedure. A 4 cm transverse incision is made over the anterior gastric body, placing a malleable retractor on either side and using long Allis clamps to deliver the pylorus closer to the incision. A 2-0 Prolene suture was selected to run the pylorus closed, rather than an absorbable suture or a closure by a row of exterior staples. I feel this technique is reliable in closure of the pylorus for several weeks, as it was possible that the pancreatitis would persist during the postoperative period. If necessary, the suture can be cut and the pylorus can be opened endoscopically at a later date. A gastrojejunostomy was performed to the gastric opening, again using a two-layer technique of Vicryl and silk as described above. After closing the posterior row, a 9.6 Fr. Hickman catheter was placed through the left upper quadrant. A purse string suture using 2-0 silk was made in the lateral border of the stomach at the greater curve. The Hickman catheter was trimmed to 70 cm and the 16 gauge introducer needle was placed through the middle of the purse string in an oblique manner. The guide wire was then placed through the needle and the needle was removed. A dilator and 10 Fr. introducer were carefully placed through the purse string, being careful not to injure the back wall of the stomach. The dilator was removed and the Hickman catheter placed through the introducer into the efferent limb of the gastrojejunostomy. The introducer was then removed and the purse string secured. Note that the decision to place feeding access was based on the significant pancreatitis and edema that might create a scenario of impaired gastric emptying. In addition, this patient was requiring fluids due to fluid sequestration and plans were made to place the patient in the intensive care unit for possible respiratory support. Using a predictive model, more than 80% of trauma patients with emergency surgery who were triaged to the intensive care unit will not tolerate a regular diet in five days, and thus early enteral support is indicated. A Hickman catheter was selected due to its flexible tubing, which would not put pressure or tension on the anastomosis. The anterior layer of the anastomosis was then closed with the feeding access in place. The area of the purse string was then brought up to the abdominal wall using four 2-0 silk sutures.

After the gastrojejunostomy was completed, a 10 mm flat Jackson-Pratt drain was placed posterior to the duodenal repair and taken out through the right upper quadrant. A second drain was placed adjacent to the body of the pancreas and taken out through the left upper quadrant. A tongue of omentum was created and placed over the pancreatic laceration to help to isolate it from the gastrojejunal anastomosis. After the abdomen was irrigated and once again checked for laparotomy pads, the fascia was closed with two strands of number 1 looped PDS suture. The drains were anchored with several 0 silk sutures, as was the Hickman catheter so they would not be accidentally removed. The cuff was left in place within the subcutaneous anterior fascia interface. The drains should remain in place until the patient is recovered and tolerating a regular diet. An elemental low fat feeding will be started at 20 mL/hr as soon as the base deficit is corrected, and increased by 20 mL/hr every 12 hours until a goal of 85 mL/hr is reached. If abdominal distention develops, the rate will be reduced by half until the distention resolves.

TECHNICAL OPERATIVE PROCEDURES:

HOW I DO IT

Laceration of the Second Portion of the Duodenum

David B. Hoyt, M.D., FACS

Scenario

An 18-year-old is stabbed in the right epigastrium and remains hemodynamically stable during transport. He has obvious peritonitis on physical exam.

Management

Immediately following identification of the stab wound and the determination that laparotomy is required, antibiotics should be given and the patient taken to the operating room.

Procedure

A midline incision is made and immediate exploration would identify blood and intestinal contents which would be distinctly characteristic because of bile staining.

The abdomen would be packed in all four quadrants and following control of hemostasis attention would be directed to the source of bilious leakage. The laceration would be identified in exploration of the sweep of the duodenum. This would be accomplished by a Kocher maneuver to mobilize the duodenum posteriorly all the way to the aorta so that the undersurface of the head of the pancreas, the anterior pancreas, and the entire duodenal sweep can be evaluated. When a 2 cm laceration is identified on the antimesenteric border the lumen should be inspected and if possible, the origin of the ampulla of Vater identified to assure that this is not part of the injury. In addition, one should look very carefully for an additional wound corresponding to the antimesenteric wound. One would then

- Mobilize the duodenum posteriorly to the aorta

- Evaluate the entire duodenum and the head of the pancreas

- Identify the ampulla of Vater to exclude an injury

- Primary two-layer closure of the duodenal injury

- Buttress with omental pedicle

- Lateral Jackson-Pratt closed suction drainage

evaluate the actual length of the wound and if it were judged to be less than 50% of the circumference of the duodenum, the wound would be closed primarily with one layer of 2-0 or 3-0 silk sutures. If there was any question regarding the adequacy of the repair, a pedicle of omentum would be placed over the wound and held in place with tacking sutures.

A Jackson-Pratt drain would be placed lateral to the wound and a nasogastric tube would be placed to provide decompression for several days postoperatively. It would not be necessary to protect the pylorus in this circumstance. Additional surgery other than débridement and repair would be considered excessive. The patient could be fed after about five days and the drain removed thereafter.

TECHNICAL OPERATIVE PROCEDURES:

HOW I DO IT

Laceration of the Third Portion of the Duodenum

Alasdair K.T. Conn, MD, FACS

Scenario

A young male with a stab wound was taken to the operating room. At laparotomy, a 2 cm laceration of the antimesenteric border of the third portion of the duodenum was discovered. There were no other injuries.

Management

Once a decision to take this patient to the operating room was made, preoperative antibiotics were administered. A generous midline incision allows for complete exploration of the abdominal cavity. The exact length of the injury to the duodenum may be difficult to determine; and as exploration is initiated, Kocherization of the second part of the duodenum, together with the head of the pancreas is required. Mobilization using this technique should be sufficient to identify the complete length of the injury. As this is on the antimesenteric border, primary repair may be performed.

The danger with duodenal injuries is excessive constriction of the duodenal lumen so I find that attempts to débride the wound edges are normally not required. Beginning at one end of the wound, I would start with a single layer closure of an absorbable suture and for the duodenum I would use Dexon or Vicryl. I would leave the tag long once the first knot has been tied and gently approximate the edges. Try to take full thickness bites of the duodenum. It is most important in duodenal, rather than other bowel injuries, to ensure that the edges are approximated sufficiently such that a leak does not occur but not so tight as to produce ischemia. Once the first layer has been performed, a decision needs to be made as to whether it is possible to perform a second layer of interrupted sutures. Although some surgeons state that it is preferable to place a second layer of interrupted, non-absorbable 3-0 silk sutures, I think that if there is compromise of the lumen then an omental

- Mobilization using a Kocher procedure is sufficient to identify the injury

- Take full-thickness bites of the duodenum

- An omental patch to buttress the repair

- Suction drainage is essential

patch can be applied to buttress the wound. A portion of omentum can be brought down and lightly secured in place to reinforce the single layer closure. It is especially important not to have the sutures produce ischemia to the omentum, but rather merely to tag it in place. The proximal and distal ends of the primary closure can be used to assist in tagging down this omental patch.

With a duodenal injury of this nature I usually leave a suction drain in place. I do not personally believe in Penrose drains. I would also ensure that the stomach is adequately drained and that the nasogastric tube is in place.

A feeding tube can be placed through the repair and fed into the proximal small bowel and may be used for feeding in the immediate postoperative period. I do not routinely provide feeding jejunostomies or feeding gastrostomies, preferring to keep the integrity of the rest of the bowel. After thorough irrigation, the wound should be closed in layers. I use a running suture for the fascia to speed up the closure.

TECHNICAL OPERATIVE PROCEDURES:
HOW I DO IT

Laceration of the Third Portion of the Duodenum

Rao Ivatury, MD, FACS

Scenario

A 40-year-old man presents with a stab wound to the abdomen. The knife has created a 50% laceration of the antimesenteric border in the third portion of the duodenum. The patient has been resuscitated and is in the operating room. There is no other injury.

Management: *Exposure of the duodenum*

I begin by mobilizing the duodenum by a Kocher maneuver, incising the peritoneum on the lateral border of the C-loop of the duodenum and bluntly mobilizing the duodenum and the pancreatic head off the retroperitoneum, exposing the vena cava. For further evaluation of the third portion of the duodenum, I do a Cattel Braasch maneuver by mobilizing the hepatic flexure of the colon, incising the root of the mesentery from the right lower quadrant to the duodenal jejunal junction and reflecting the small bowel towards the head of the patient. Now I have complete visualization of the second and third portions of the duodenum and the duodenal jejunal junction.

Repair

The type of surgical repair of the injury described depends upon whether the diagnosis is early or late. When operating early, simple techniques yield excellent results. I débride the edges of the duodenal laceration, ensure good vascularity and repair the duodenum transversely in two layers: inner absorbable and outer non-absorbable. I drain the area with a closed suction Jackson-Pratt drain. If the repair is deemed unsatisfactory because the laceration is too close to the mesenteric border, another easy technique is to do a side-to-side anastomosis between the duodenum and a loop of proximal jejunum. I avoid putting any intraluminal tubes in the duodenum. They are unnecessary and may cause complications.

If the operation is for a missed injury, the duodenal wall may be thick and inflamed and may not hold sutures well. In such instances, a variety of techniques have been proposed: duodenorrhaphy with pyloric

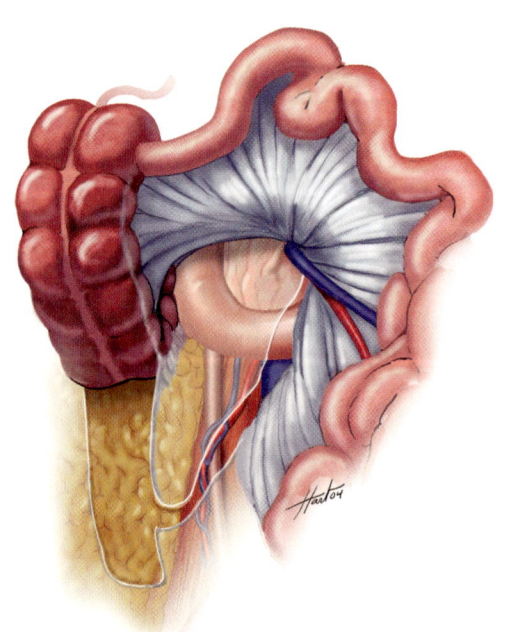

> - Repair the duodenum transversely in two layers
>
> - Consider a pyloric exclusion procedure
>
> - Drainage is essential

exclusion procedure which is generally reserved for pancreatoduodenal injuries; jejunal mucosal patch or pedicle graft; or division of duodenum and a roux-en-Y duodenojejunostomy.

If the duodenum can be débrided and closed reasonably well, I would consider adding a pyloric exclusion procedure. This is performed through a gastrostomy and the pylorus is sutured closed with 2-0 Prolene sutures. A gastrojejunostomy is constructed at the gastrostomy site.

If the duodenum is macerated and cannot be safely closed, I would resect that portion of the duodenum and perform a roux-en-Y duodenojejunostomy. In all instances, drainage of the area is essential.

TECHNICAL OPERATIVE PROCEDURES:

HOW I DO IT

Exposure and Repair of the Third and Fourth Portions of the Duodenum

Erwin F. Hirsch, MD, FACS

Scenario

Gunshot wound to the abdomen with a 1 cm lesion at the junction of the third and fourth portions of the duodenum.

Management

The scenario described mandates an exploratory laparotomy. Perioperative broad-spectrum antibiotics should be administered and an adequate amount of blood should be available depending on the hemodynamic status of the patient. A preoperative chest x-ray and KUB are desirable, however, a nasogastric tube in these patients is mandatory.

Procedure

A conventional midline laparotomy should be performed. Upon entering the abdomen, the initial thrust should be directed to the identification and control of hemorrhage while the anesthesiologist optimizes the patient's hemodynamic status. Following hemorrhage control and surgical exploration of the abdomen, the options as to how to manage the duodenal injury should begin.

A complete mobilization of the involved area should be carried out prior to repair. The possibility of injuries proximal or distal to the observed lesion mandates Kocherization of the duodenum to visualize the second and third portions as well as the pancreas. Equally important is the mobilization of the fourth portion and proximal jejunum by dividing the ligament of Treitz. Once the injuries have been thoroughly staged, identified, and non-viable areas débrided, repair options should be considered.

- Mobilize the fourth portion and proximal jejunum by dividing the ligament of Treitz

- Two layer closure

- May require a T-tube feeding jejunostomy

A 1 cm wound or even two 1 cm wounds (entrance and exit) in most instances will not significantly compromise the lumen of the duodenum. Therefore, a primary repair using a two-layer technique, 4-0 catgut or Vicryl and 4-0 silk sutures should solve the problem.

Postoperative nutritional support for these patients needs to be discussed during the surgical procedure. Associated injuries, the length of the operative procedure and the degree of resuscitation may require enteral access to be provided via a T-tube feeding jejunostomy.

TECHNICAL OPERATIVE PROCEDURES:

HOW I DO IT

Methylene Blue Pancreatography

Vicente Cortes, MD, FACS

Scenario

A 26-year-old female restrained driver of an automobile involved in a head on collision at moderate speed arrives to the trauma center with a Glasgow Coma Score of 15, a revised Trauma Score of 12, a systolic blood pressure of 131, and a respiratory rate of 20. She maintains normal cardiorespiratory function during the course of the trauma evaluation.

Management

She is found to have blunt torso trauma with a tender left chest wall, upper abdominal seat belt contusion and ecchymosis, left upper quadrant tenderness, a chest film with left seventh to tenth rib fractures, an equivocal FAST, no fracture on AP pelvis film, elevated amylase and lipase and macroscopic hematuria. Chest, abdomen and pelvis CT scan shows left lower lobe pulmonary contusion, hemoperitoneum, Grade I liver injury, Grade III to Grade IV splenic injury and Grade III left renal injury.

Procedure: *Methylene blue pancreatography*

She is taken for exploratory laparotomy. She is found to have approximately 1000 mL hemoperitoneum and all four quadrants are packed. No injuries are found in the small bowel, large bowel, mesentery and pelvic organs. Inspection of the liver shows partial avulsion of the gallbladder from the liver bed that is actively bleeding and this is temporarily packed. Inspection of the spleen shows multiple 1 cm to 3 cm deep lacerations not actively bleeding. The spleen and tail of the pancreas are completely mobilized with plans to perform a Dexon mesh splenic wrap. To complete the exploration, the lesser sac is opened to inspect the neck and body of the pancreas and upon doing so it becomes apparent that the splenic artery near its takeoff has been stretched and appears thrombosed. The artery is dissected free and ligated in continuity proximally and distally to the injury to avoid the formation of pseudoaneurysm and a splenectomy is performed dividing and ligating the splenic artery and vein at the hilum and the short gastric vessels on the fundus of the stomach. Inspection of the body and tail of the pancreas shows contusion and saponification at the site of the injury to the splenic artery but there is no clear-cut parenchymal laceration.

The attention is redirected to the partial gallbladder avulsion from the liver bed and a cholecystectomy is undertaken. However before dividing the cystic duct a cholangiogram catheter is inserted into the cystic duct and secured and using a C-arm fluoroscopic cholangiography is performed. The initial injection shows normal biliary tree and easy passage of contrast into the duodenum.

Methylene Blue Pancreatography

The anesthesiologist is then asked to inject intravenous fentanyl to achieve spasm of the sphincter of Oddi and a repeat cholangiography injection is performed hoping to fill the pancreatic duct. The injection shows extravasation from the pancreatic duct but it is not clear whether it is coming from the neck or from the tail of the pancreas. Therefore methylene blue stained normal saline is injected via the cholangiography catheter and the dye is easily seen extravasating at the site of contusion and saponification. It is therefore surmised that a major ductal injury is present at that location. After removing the cholangiography catheter and completing the cholecystectomy a distal pancreatectomy is done using a stapling device and PDS sutures to close the stump. Two Jackson-Pratt drains are left to drain the pancreatic stump.

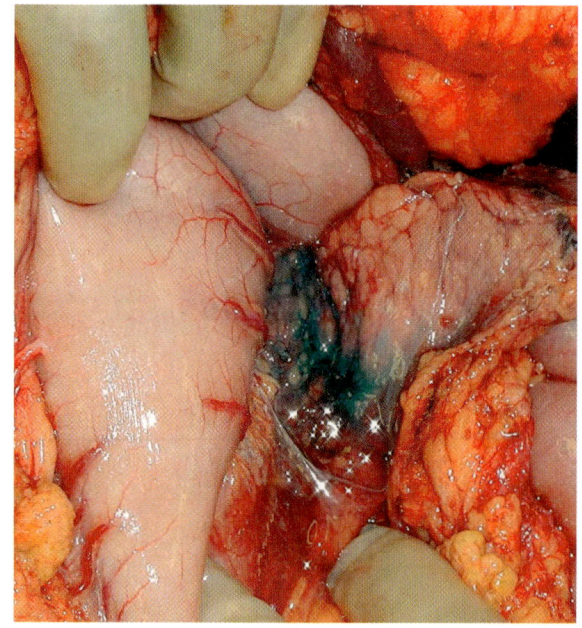

- Intravenous fentanyl causes spasm of the sphincter of Oddi

- Methylene blue cholangiography precisely identifies the site of the injury

TECHNICAL OPERATIVE PROCEDURES:

HOW I DO IT

Penetrating Duodenal Injury to the Second Portion of the Duodenum

Peter Rhee, MD, MPH, FACS

Scenario

A 30-year-old man was shot in the right upper quadrant with a 9 mm handgun. The defect is in the second portion of the duodenum along the antimesenteric border. The exit wound is through the back along the posterior axillary line. The patient was initially hypotensive in the field but now his heart rate is 100 and systolic blood pressure is 110 mmHg.

Management

The patient is talking and breathing normally. I roll the patient to identify all the injuries. I then ensure that two large bore intravenous lines are started but withhold fluids. Blood and fluids are started if mentation decreases or if the systolic blood pressure falls below 90 mmHg. The operating room and radiology are notified. A chest x-ray is obtained and, if possible, an abdominal KUB. The films are useful to locate the bullet or bullet fragments and obtain an idea of the possible injuries. If time is really crucial, the chest x-ray is the only essential film to obtain since it evaluates the structures in the chest and the diaphragm. This includes a hemopneumothorax. The patient is rapidly transported to the operating room. Antibiotics are initiated as soon as possible. I prefer Unasyn – ampicillin/sulbactam. The patient is prepped from the chin to mid thigh.

- Controlled hypotensive resuscitation until bleeding has been controlled

- Intubate the ampulla to ensure ductal patency

- Two layer closure

- Use the omentum to protect the suture line

- Closed suction drainage

A celiotomy incision is performed from the xiphoid to the pubis. Intraoperatively, the principles of management remain the same: hemorrhage control; identification of all injuries; and reconstruction. The third phase can be delayed with damage control surgery, but in general, reconstruction during the first operation is always better if possible. Although the vital signs are normal, the extent of bleeding is unknown and one has to always assume ongoing hemorrhage until proven otherwise. Controlled hypotensive resuscitation is performed attempting to use minimal fluids to obtain a systolic blood pressure of 90 mmHg. The anesthesiologist is instructed to transfuse fluids carefully until the bleeding has been controlled.

Once in the abdomen, I pack off the injury and ensure that there are no other injuries. For penetrating injuries to the abdomen, packing the four quadrants is not an effective method of gaining tamponade. I put pressure to the most likely site of injury and then pack laparotomy packs into the four quadrants and the pelvis. The injury is then isolated and identified. A concern in this situation is an injury to major vascular structures. If the injury is to the antimesenteric border of the duodenum, and the tract passes laterally, it is likely to miss the inferior vena cava. The other potential vascular structures in this region are the adrenal vessels and the right renal vessels. The ascending colon is identified and rotated to the midline to expose the kidney and the vena cava. The rest of the exploration is completed to make sure that there are no other injuries. The pancreas is carefully inspected. The anesthesiologist can now work towards resuscitation of the patient to correct the base deficit but avoid over resuscitation.

Procedure: *Repair of the duodenum*

I cauterize the mucosal edges of the duodenum laceration as it is well vascularized and can bleed significantly. A Kocher maneuver is performed to allow for complete inspection of the liver and posterior portion of the duodenum as well as the posterior surface of the pancreas. The patient has a 2 cm injury to the duodenum. In this case the ampulla of Vater has bile coming from it. A pediatric feeding tube is used to intubate the ampulla and obtain a pancreatogram to ensure there is no injury to the duct. The duodenum is the only injury. The edges of the duodenal laceration are débrided sharply. The duodenum is closed primarily in a transverse fashion using a continuous non-absorbable monofilament Maxon or PDS suture. The second layer is performed with interrupted Maxon or PDS sutures. Fibrin glue is then applied to the suture line and the omentum is sutured to the injury site.

A Jackson-Pratt drain is positioned in close proximity to the site. For an isolated injury to the second portion as described in this injury, I do not routinely perform pyloric exclusion, nor place a feeding jejunostomy. I pass a small nasogastric feeding tube into the stomach, through the pylorus and into the duodenum and guide it past the fourth portion of the duodenum into the jejunum. Enteral nutrition through the tube is started on the second to third day and increased very slowly. A duodenal leak can occur postoperatively. It is the complication to watch for.

TECHNICAL OPERATIVE PROCEDURES:

HOW I DO IT

Pyloric Exclusion for Tenuous Complex Duodenal Injury

Edward Cornwell, MD, FACS

Scenario

A 22-year-old male with multiple gunshot wounds to the abdomen. He has a burst injury of the second and third portion of the duodenum which necessitates a complex repair. It is necessary to protect the repair with pyloric exclusion.

Management

The pyloric exclusion procedure has replaced duodenal diverticulization. In addition to repair and external drainage of the duodenum, retrograde intraluminal decompression and enteral feeding via jejunostomy tubes, the pyloric exclusion procedure is performed to divert gastric flow from the duodenum.

Procedure: *Technique of pyloric exclusion for tenuous complex duodenal injury*

A 6 cm to 8 cm incision is made across the anterior wall of the distal antrum approximately 5 cm proximal to, and parallel to the pylorus. Two Allis clamps are used to grasp the pyloric ring from the inside and evert it towards the gastrotomy incision. The pylorus is then sutured closed with two running layers created by taking large bites with 0 Prolene sutures. Alternatively a TA stapler can be fired just distal to the pylorus, but care must be taken not to allow the stapler to slip proximally. This would create antral G cells distal to the staple line and produce an ulcerogenic situation secondary to retained antrum. Once the pylorus is sutured closed the gastrotomy is closed in two layers with a continuous Vicryl suture and a 3-0 seromuscular silk suture. A separate incision across the greater curve of the stomach is made in a dependent position to facilitate gastrojejunostomy. A loop of jejunum approximately 40 cm distal to the ligament of Treitz is positioned parallel to the greater curve and the anastomosis is performed in a two-layer closure using 3-0 seromuscular interrupted silk sutures for the outer layer and a running 3-0 Vicryl suture full thickness for the inner layers. Alternatively a stapled GIA anastomosis with one arm each fired through the stomach and jejunum may be utilized to complete the gastrojejunostomy.

- Two Allis clamps are used to grasp the pylorus

- The pylorus is closed with two layers of continuous 0 Prolene

- A separate incision is made for a dependent gastrojejunostomy

TECHNICAL OPERATIVE PROCEDURES:

HOW I DO IT

Pyloric Exclusion

Michael Rhodes, MD, FACS

Scenario

A 45-year-old moderately obese female after blunt abdominal trauma is found to have a blow-out laceration at the second portion of the duodenum. The wound is irregular with devitalized edges. There appears to be a contusion of the head of the pancreas without evidence of ductal injury.

Management

Most simple duodenal injuries require only simple repair and drainage. In cases requiring resectional débridement, or large lacerations greater than 50% of the circumference, pyloric exclusion can be considered to protect the repair.

The duodenum is fully mobilized. After resecting the devitalized edges, a 5 cm oblique rent on the anterolateral surface of the duodenum is repaired with a single layer of interrupted 3-0 silk sutures. A decision is made to protect the repair with a pyloric exclusion.

Procedure: *Pyloric exclusion*

A 2 cm transverse gastrostomy is made with the electrosurgical unit in the anterior surface of the antrum approximately 2 cm superior to the greater curvature and 5 cm to 7 cm proximal to the pylorus. It is usually not necessary to remove the omentum from this area of the stomach.

The index finger of the left hand invaginates the wall of the first portion of the duodenum from lateral to medial so as to advance the pylorus toward the stomach. Using the finger as a guide, a large Babcock clamp is placed through the gastrostomy toward the pylorus. Both the anterior and posterior pyloric rings are grasped with the Babcock, and it is pulled toward the gastrostomy while simultaneously pushing the gastrostomy toward the end of the clamp. Sometimes a second Babcock is required. This allows enough visualization of the pylorus to place a running 2-0 PDS suture from posterior to anterior to close the pylorus. Usually only 3 or 4 bites are required. Deep pyloric bites are advised, but the closure should be done under minimal tension so as not to crush the tissue.

Next, a loop of jejunum approximately 20 cm to 25 cm from the ligament of Treitz is positioned in an antecolic, isoperistaltic position adjacent to the gastrostomy. The arms of a GIA stapler are then placed in the gastrostomy and an adjacent jejunal opening directed away from the pylorus toward the body of the stomach, but parallel to the greater curvature. The stapler is fired and the staple line inspected for hemostasis. The gastrostomy and jejunostomy opening is then closed with either a TA stapler or interrupted 3-0 silk sutures.

A closed suction drain is placed lateral to the duodenal repair and over the pancreatic contusion.

Depending on the extent of associated injuries, a nasogastric tube may be positioned proximal to the gastroenterostomy prior to closing the gastrostomy. As an alternative for patients with multiple associated injuries, a gastrojejunostomy tube is placed in the proximal stomach with the jejunal portion positioned in the efferent limb of the jejunum for enteral access. An acceptable alternative is to place a needle catheter jejunostomy beyond the gastroenterostomy and decompress the stomach with a nasogastric or gastrostomy tube. I recommend postoperative somatostatin for the first five days and an H2 blocker for the first two weeks, or until the patient is tolerating a full diet.

It is anticipated that the pyloric closure is temporary and will eventually open with preferential transport of stomach contents through the pylorus rather than the gastroenterostomy. Therefore, the gastroenterostomy is not a long-term risk for ulceration and a vagotomy is not indicated. Also, since the gastroenterostomy is a short-term conduit, it is acceptable for expeditious placement on the anterior antrum rather than the classic posterior-inferior surface of the lesser curvature of antral-fundic junction.

A contrast study as an outpatient at six weeks postoperatively is useful to demonstrate pyloric patency. If not patent, endoscopic dilation may be considered.

- Anterior transverse gastrostomy

- Pylorus grasped with a Babcock

- Continuous PDS suture to close the pylorus

- Antecolic isoperistaltic gastrojejunostomy

- Temporary pyloric closure

- No need for a vagotomy

TECHNICAL OPERATIVE PROCEDURES:

HOW I DO IT

Stapled Pyloric Exclusion

Orlando Kirton, MD, FACS

Scenario

A 32-year-old male sustains a gunshot wound to the second portion of the duodenum. There is a 3 cm blast injury with devitalization to the antimesenteric border. It is essential to protect the repair with a pyloric exclusion procedure.

Management

The diagnosis of duodenal injury is based primarily on a high degree of suspicion on the part of the surgeon since signs of retroperitoneal injury are often difficult to elicit and the diagnostic modalities currently available are notoriously deficient. The majority of duodenal injuries are the result of penetrating trauma.

Findings that directly affect the morbidity and mortality of these patients with duodenal injuries include the type of agent, the size and location of the injury, the interval to repair, and associated adjacent injuries. Corresponding large injuries to the first and second portion of the duodenum, long elapsed time from injury to repair, and associated injuries to the bile duct or pancreas are all associated with increased morbidity and mortality.

- Pyloric exclusion is accomplished by stapling across the distal edge of the pylorus

- A retrocolic gastrojejunostomy is then performed

Procedure : *Pyloric exclusion*

The majority of duodenal injuries which include stab wounds, injury of less than 50% of the wall, injury of the third or fourth portion of the duodenum, injury interval of less than 24 hours, and no associated biliary or pancreatic injuries can be repaired primarily with periduodenal drainage. For more complex injuries, a procedure which effectively diverts the gastric contents away from the duodenal repair is recommended. Pyloric exclusion is a technique that is less disruptive and less time consuming than a true duodenal diverticulization.

A self-retaining device, a Balfour retractor, is employed for wide exposure of the upper abdomen. I mobilize the duodenum by performing a generous Kocher maneuver encompassing and mobilizing the ligament of Treitz. Pyloric exclusion is accomplished by firing a staple line across the distal edge of the pylorus using a TA-55 device with extra-length staples. A 2 cm to 3 cm gastrostomy is made in the body of the stomach along the greater curvature after suture ligation of an appropriate distance of the right gastroepiploic vessels. A retro-colic gastrojejunostomy is constructed either by a stapled, i.e. triangulated with TA 55 or combined GIA/TA stapler technique or hand sewn anastomosis with two layers. An alternative approach involves closure of the pylorus from within the lumen of the stomach via the gastrostomy using a running or interrupted suture line of absorbable 0 PDS or Vicryl sutures. Intraluminal pyloric closure is followed with construction of the gastrojejunostomy. The pylorus usually reopens after two to three weeks and the gastric jejunostomy functionally closes. The primary duodenal injury is closed in either two layers with running 3-0 Vicryl and 3-0 silk Lembert or a single layer inverting mattress Gambee stitch of 3-0 Prolene.

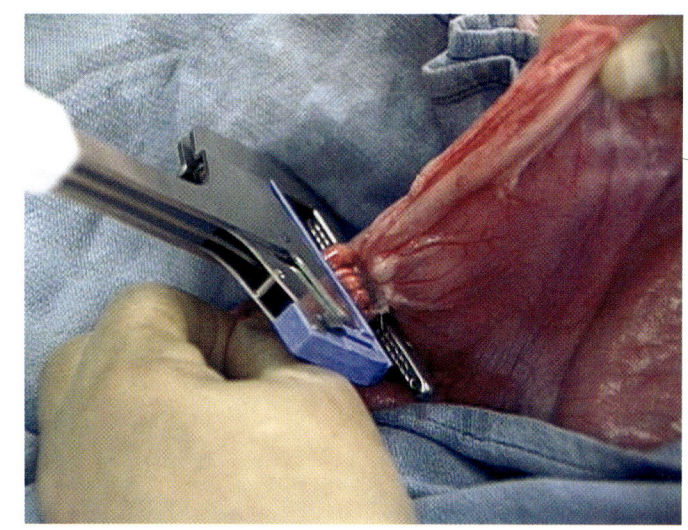

References

1) Cogbill T, Moore EE, Feliciano DV, et al:
Conservative management of
duodenal trauma: A multi-center
perspective.
J Trauma 1990;30:1469.

2) Vaugham G, Grazier O, Graham D, et al:
The use of pyloric exclusion
in the management of severe duodenal
injuries.
Am J Surg 1977;134:785.

TECHNICAL OPERATIVE PROCEDURES:

HOW I DO IT

Management of Injury to the Common Bile Duct

Jameel Ali, MD, FACS

In the setting of blunt and penetrating abdominal trauma, bile duct injuries are very uncommon unless there is a direct penetrating injury such as a stab wound. Generally, common bile duct injuries occur in the setting of severe associated injuries which usually take priority. The timing and type of ductal repair depend on the hemodynamic status of the patient, the ability to control other injuries as well as the location and extent of the injury to the common bile duct.

In the patient who is hemodynamically compromised from associated major injuries, attention is first directed at control of hemorrhage by appropriate means through a generous midline abdominal incision and adequate exposure. Damage control techniques and placement of drains with return of the patient to the intensive care unit take priority over any bile duct injury. Under these circumstances the bile duct injury is either left alone or if it is easily identified, a 7 Fr. red rubber tube may be placed in a transected duct which may be combined with a quickly placed cholecystostomy tube with the intention of following with cholecystectomy at the time of the definitive laparotomy.

I very seldom employ ERCP in this setting or for that matter in general, in assessing or managing common bile duct injuries. One situation where ERCP may be of benefit is where there is bile staining and the injury is not clearly evident. An intra-operative ERCP to assist with the location of the injury may be of use and, indeed, if the spillage is very minimal this could be combined with a papillotomy and stent placement with conservative management of the small laceration. In general, however, I prefer direct repair of the duct.

Procedure: *Common bile duct repair*

At surgery, care is taken to visualize the extrahepatic biliary tract but undue manipulation and dissection should be avoided in order to preserve the blood supply.

If the injury to the common bile duct consists of a laceration involving 50% or less of the circumference of the duct and there is no associated devitalization of the wall then direct suture repair is conducted.

The repair is conducted in meticulous fashion using absorbable interrupted 5-0 PDS, sutures with accurate mucosa-to-mucosa approximation.

Placement of a T-tube is not mandatory in this type of injury but it has the theoretical advantage of postoperative decompression of the biliary tree in the presence of edema which may limit internal drainage. If a T-tube is placed it should be silastic rather than the traditional rubber T-tube and it should not be brought out through the suture line but through a separate small choledochotomy, the size being just large enough to allow introduction of the tube. One of the arms of the intra-luminal portion of the tube should traverse the suture line. If a T-tube is used in these injuries I recommend that it be left in for at least 4 weeks to allow formation of a mature tract so that on removal of the T-tube, spillage of bile into the general peritoneal cavity is avoided. I employ a Jackson-Pratt drain brought out through a separate stab wound for control of fluid collections in the subhepatic space. I always combine repair of the common bile duct injury with a cholecystectomy which is conducted in the usual fashion.

If there is a laceration involving greater than 50% of the circumference of the duct or if there is a large area of ischemia precluding a tension free anastomosis after débridement of devitalized tissue then I employ a biliary enteric reconstruction.

Procedure: *roux-en-Y choledochojejunostomy*

My preferred procedure is a roux-en-Y choledochojejunostomy. This procedure is also combined with a cholecystectomy.

If there is uncertainty regarding the blood supply, reconstruction should be done more proximally. The distal end of the common bile duct is ligated with a 2-0 silk ligature.

The jejunum is transected with a GIA stapler at an appropriate distance from the ligament of Treitz that would ensure a tension free anastomosis to the side of the ascending jejunal segment. The distance between the jejuno-jejunal anastomosis and the end of the ascending jejunal limb should be at least 40 cm to allow a tension free anastomosis to the common bile duct.

The ascending jejunal limb is brought up to the proximal end of the transected common bile duct through a small opening in the transverse mesocolon, the opening being just large enough to allow jejunum access. Two or three interrupted 3-0 Vicryl sutures are placed to attach the jejunum to the edge of the mesocolon to prevent future herniation.

- Undue manipulation and dissection should be avoided to preserve the blood supply of the common bile duct

- If a T-tube is used in the common bile duct, it should remain in place for at least 4 weeks

The biliary enteric anastomosis is conducted between the end of the common bile duct and the side of the jejunum. This is conducted as a single interrupted closure using absorbable suture (e.g. 4-0 PDS). Meticulous technique is necessary to ensure mucosa-to-mucosa approximation and to avoid ischemia of the anastomotic ends. The size of the opening in the jejunum should be just enough to accommodate the end of the common bile duct. I use 3-0 silk sutures to secure the jejunum to surrounding peritoneal attachments.

I do not routinely use a T-tube for this biliary enteric anastomosis but, again, if a T-tube is used it should be inserted at a site separate from the anastomotic suture line and one limb of the T-tube should traverse the suture line and be placed in the jejunum.

The jejuno-jejunal anastomosis is conducted by placing interrupted posterior seromuscular 3-0 silk sutures between the end of the proximal jejunum and the side of the ascending jejunal limb. The staple line is then excised and a continuous 3-0 Vicryl suture is placed in the mucosal layer approximating the ascending and transverse limb after incising the ascending limb to create an opening of the same size as the end of the proximal jejunum. After completion of the inner mucosal layer the anterior seromuscular layer is completed with interrupted 3-0 silk sutures. I also employ a Jackson-Pratt drain with these procedures in the trauma situation.

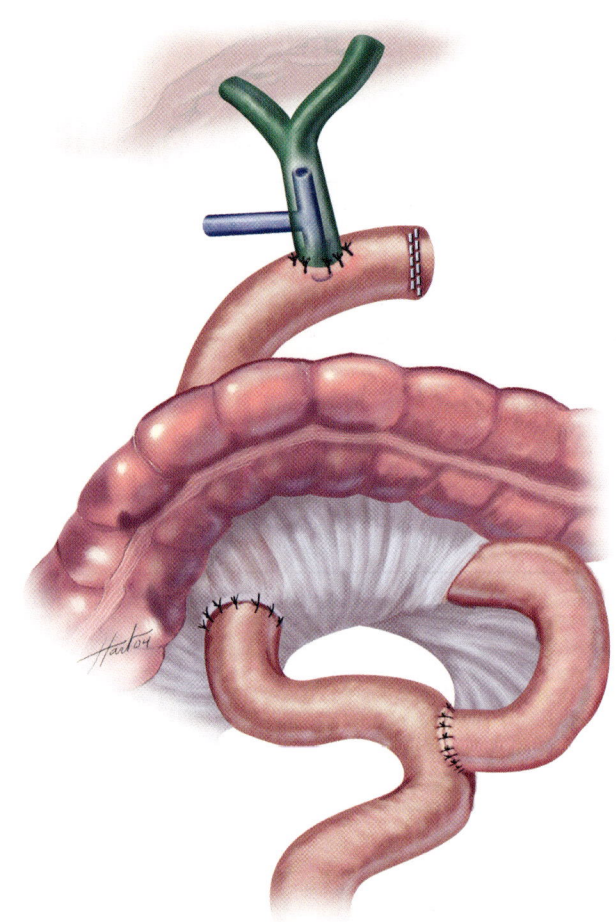

TECHNICAL OPERATIVE PROCEDURES:
HOW I DO IT

Stab Wound to the Pancreas with Ductal Injury

Margaret Knudson, MD, FACS

Scenario

The patient was a 30-year-old man who was stabbed once in the epigastrium just to the right of midline. His blood pressure on arrival was 130/90 and his pulse rate was 120. He was somewhat intoxicated but answered questions appropriately. He had no significant medical history and his only previous surgery was orthopedic in nature. On physical examination, he had a deep wound measuring 3 cm in length in the epigastrium with obvious deep penetration. He was tender in the upper abdomen only without peritoneal signs. A chest x-ray was unremarkable. The patient was given tetanus prophylaxis and a dose of a second-generation cephalosporin with anaerobic coverage and signed a consent form for exploratory laparotomy. Blood was sent to the blood bank for type and cross matching.

Operative Report

The patient was given general anesthesia and a Foley catheter was inserted. Intravenous access was assured with two large-bore catheters. Because he was presumed to have a full stomach, a nasogastric tube was also inserted. The patient was then prepped widely including the chest, abdomen and one groin for potential vein harvest and draped in a sterile fashion. After achievement of adequate anesthesia, a generous midline incision was created (from the xiphoid to below the umbilicus) with a knife and carried down into the peritoneum sharply. There was no free blood or intestinal contents noted on entering the peritoneum. A thorough inspection of the abdomen was then accomplished. The liver and right hemidiaphragm were free of injury. Inspection of the spleen and left hemidiaphragm were also normal. Next, the stomach was inspected and was normal. The ligament of Trietz was identified and the small and large bowel run in their entirety. There was no injury to the intestines or to the mesentery.

Attention was then directed toward the

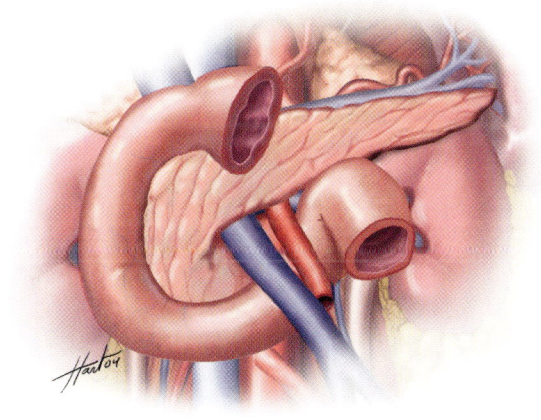

retroperitoneum. The wound appeared to enter the retroperitoneum just below the stomach. In order to inspect this area thoroughly, an extended Kocher maneuver was conducted. To do this, the right colon was mobilized at the hepatic flexure and retracted medially. The right lateral duodenal attachments were taken down sharply with the electrocautery and the head of the pancreas palpated and inspected. It appeared to be uninjured. In order to inspect the body of the pancreas, the lesser sac was entered through the gastrocolic ligament. Several small vessels were clamped and tied in order to get a wide window into the lesser sac through the greater omentum. The stomach was retracted superiorly with a wide retractor and the body of the pancreas was fully inspected. A hematoma in the area of the superior mesenteric vessels was noted with no active hemorrhage. The rest of the body appeared uninjured.

Gently, the hematoma was unroofed to reveal the source of the bleeding, which was venous and originated from venous tributaries to the splenic vein. These vessels were controlled with small clips. The avascular plane at the base of the pancreas was entered sharply and the body of the pancreas mobilized in order to inspect the posterior aspect. It appeared that the injury was very central and extended through the back. This was consistent with an injury to the main pancreatic duct. At this point, it was felt that a distal pancreatectomy was indicated. To accomplish this, we continued to mobilize the area of injury, both from the bottom and from the top, taking down attachment to the splenic vein in the area just proximal to the injury until we could safely slide a finger under the pancreas from bottom to top. Taking the TA-55 stapler with wide staples, we divided the pancreas in this area, taking care not to injure the superior mesenteric vessels. Using the distal, transected end of the pancreas as a handle, we worked our way from medial to lateral, taking down all arterial and venous attachments carefully from the pancreas to the splenic vessels with clips or suture ligatures as needed. During this procedure, the spleen was left intact. We were successful in mobilizing the tail without injuring the splenic vessels and the distal pancreas was then handed off the field.

- Area of injury to pancreatic body is mobilized from superiorly and inferiorly proximal to the injury until a finger could slide under the pancreas

- Pancreas to be resected is mobilized from midline laterally using the distal transected end of the pancreas as a handle

- All arterial and venous attachments from the pancreas to splenic vessels are taken down using clips or suture ligatures

- Nasojejunal tube feeds are initiated on postoperative day two with high protein, low fat diet

- Peripancreatic drains are left in place for two weeks

The staple line on the pancreas was inspected. There was minimal bleeding and the area where the main pancreatic duct had been transected was suture ligated with a figure-of-eight suture of 3-0 Prolene. The staple line was then oversewn with interrupted suture of 3-0 PDS on a tapered needle. Two large Jackson-Pratt drains were placed, one below and one above the pancreatic remnant and brought out through separate stab incisions. The nasogastric tube was removed and a nasojejunal feeding tube placed and directed into the proximal jejunum for post-operative nutritional support. After irrigation and inspection for hemostasis, the abdomen was closed, including the skin.

Postoperative Care

The patient was extubated and taken to the ICU for close observation. His glucoses were monitored carefully. On his second post-operative day, nasojejunal feeds were initiated with a high-protein, low-fat diet and advanced to goal as tolerated. No octreotide was used. When the patient's ileus resolved, he was given a liquid diet and gently advanced to a low-fat diet. The drains were observed to any increase in drainage with the resumption of an oral diet. Noting none, the drains were left in place for 2 weeks and an outpatient CT scan was performed to assess for pseudocyst formation before removal of the drains.

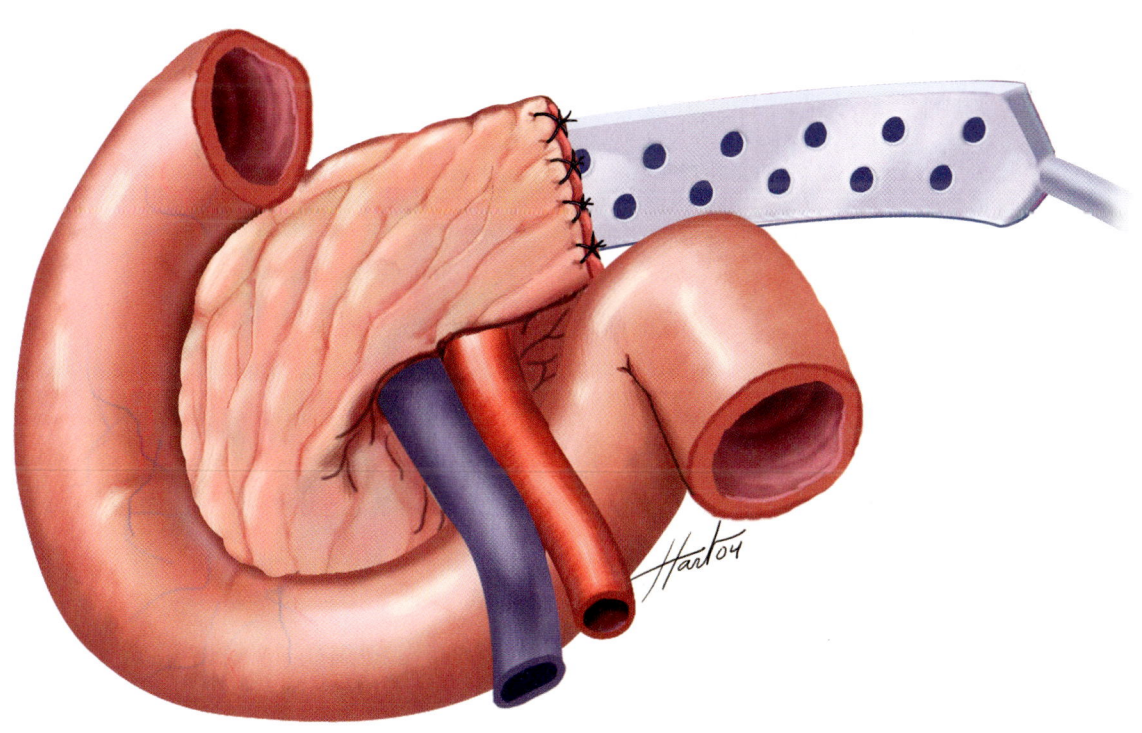

TECHNICAL OPERATIVE PROCEDURES:
HOW I DO IT

Stab Wound to the Pancreas with Ductal Injury Splenic Preserving Distal Pancreatectomy

Aurelio Rodriguez, MD, FACS

Scenario

The patient is a 30-year-old man who was stabbed once in the epigastrium just to the right of midline. His blood pressure on arrival is 130/90 and his pulse rate is 120. He is somewhat intoxicated but answers questions appropriately. On physical examination, he has a deep wound measuring 3 cm in length in the epigastrium with obvious deep penetration. He is tender in the upper abdomen only without peritoneal signs. A chest x-ray is unremarkable. The patient is given tetanus prophylaxis and a dose of a second-generation cephalosporin with anaerobic coverage. Blood is sent to the blood bank for type and cross matching.

Management

The patient is given general anesthesia and a Foley catheter is inserted. Intravenous access is assured with two large-bore catheters. A nasogastric tube is also inserted. The patient is then prepped widely including the chest, abdomen and one groin for potential vein harvest and draped in a sterile fashion. A generous midline incision is created. There is no free blood or intestinal contents noted on entering the peritoneum. A thorough inspection of the abdomen is then accomplished. The liver and right hemidiaphragm are free of injury.

Inspection of the spleen and left hemi-diaphragm are also normal. Next, the stomach is inspected and is normal. The ligament of Treitz is identified and the small and large bowel run in their entirety. There is no injury to the intestines or to the mesentery.

The wound appears to have entered the retroperitoneum just below the stomach. In order to inspect this area thoroughly, an extended Kocher maneuver is conducted. The right colon is mobilized at the hepatic flexure and retracted medially. The right lateral duodenal attachments are taken down sharply with electrocautery and the head of the pancreas palpated and inspected. It appears to be uninjured. In order to inspect the body of the pancreas, the lesser sac is entered through the gastrocolic ligament. Several small vessels are clamped and tied in order to get a wide window into the lesser sac through the greater omentum. The stomach is retracted superiorly with a wide retractor and the body of the pancreas is fully inspected. A hematoma in the area of the superior mesenteric vessels is noted with no active hemorrhage. The rest of the body appeared uninjured.

Procedure: *Spleen saving pancreatectomy*

The avascular plane at the base of the pancreas is entered sharply and the body of the pancreas mobilized in order to inspect the posterior aspect. It appears that the injury is very central and extended through the back. This is consistent with an injury to the main pancreatic duct. At this point it is felt that a distal pancreatectomy is indicated. The splenic vein in the area just proximal to the injury is mobilized until a finger can be passed under the pancreas from bottom to top. Taking the TA-55 stapler with wide staples, the pancreas is divided in this area, taking care not to injure the superior mesenteric vessels. Using the distal, transected end of the pancreas as a handle, all arterial and venous attachments are carefully dissected and controlled from the pancreas to the splenic vessels with clips or suture ligatures. During this procedure, the spleen is left intact.

The staple line on the pancreas is inspected. There is minimal bleeding and the area where the main pancreatic duct has been transected is suture ligated with a figure-of-eight suture of 3-0 Prolene. The staple line is then oversewn with interrupted suture of 3-0 PDS on a tapered needle. Two large Jackson-Pratt drains are placed one below and one above the pancreatic remnant and brought out through separate stab incisions. The nasogastric tube is removed and a nasojejunal feeding tube placed and directed into the proximal jejunum for postoperative nutritional support. After irrigation and inspection for hemostasis, the abdomen is closed.

- Open the avascular plane at the base of the pancreas

- Pass a finger under the pancreas

- Divide the pancreas with a stapler

- Oversew the staple line with interrupted sutures

- Suture ligate the pancreatic duct

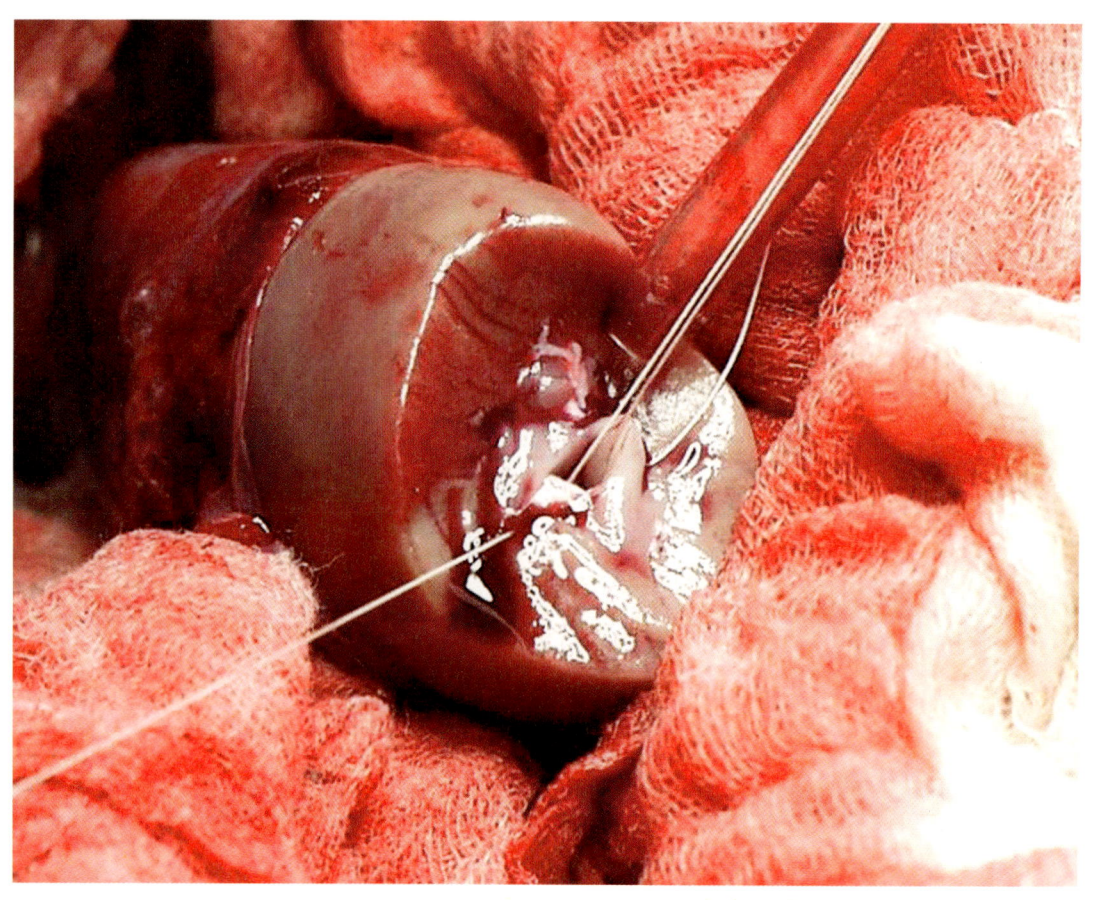

The Genitourinary System

5

Urologic Injuries

Injuries to the genitourinary tract are seen in less than 5% of all trauma patients and in 10% of patients who have sustained penetrating injury. About 80% of all urological injuries involve the kidneys, and almost 90% of these are due to blunt trauma. Conservative nonoperative management is successful in treating the vast majority of genitourinary injuries.

Urologic Injuries

- Occur in less than 5% of trauma patients
- 80% of these are renal injuries
- Mechanism is predominantly blunt
- Majority of these injuries do not require operative intervention

Hematuria

Hematuria is the hallmark for injury to the genitourinary system. However, the amount of hematuria does not correspond to injury severity. Although gross hematuria always requires a work-up for genitourinary injury, the presence of microscopic hematuria does not need to be immediately addressed in the absence of shock. On the other hand, persistence of microscopic hematuria should always be worked-up.

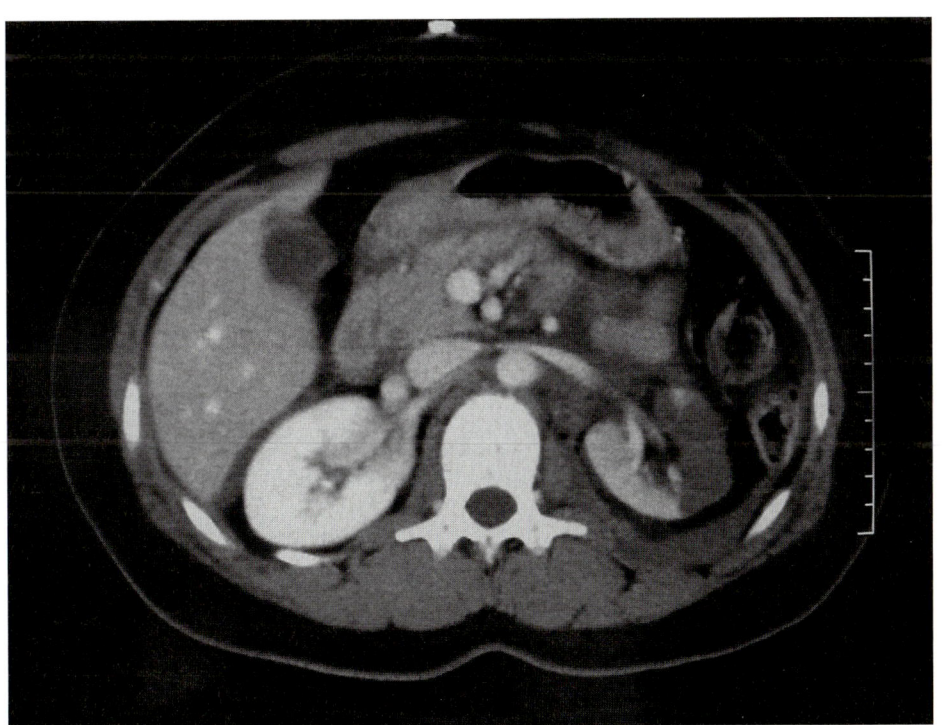

Diagnostic Studies

- **Intravenous pyelogram (IVP):**
  - one shot in trauma room or operating room
  - 2 mL/kg of contrast
  - radiograph after 10 minutes

- **Cystogram**
  - use at least 300 cc to fully distend bladder
  - two views required – distension and post drainage

- CT
  - able to evaluate the entire system with one study

Diagnostic Studies

In the past, the intravenous pyelogram (IVP) was the traditional radiographic diagnostic study used to evaluate the genitourinary system. This time-consuming radiographic examination has been abbreviated for use in trauma. The shorter procedure consists of a one-shot IVP performed in either the trauma bay or the operating room. A nonionic intravenous contrast (2 cc/kg) is administered, and an x-ray is taken after 10 minutes. Although the one-shot IVP is useful in establishing the presence and functionality of both kidneys and ureters, it is not useful for evaluation of the bladder or the urethra.

Examination of the bladder requires a cystogram or a CT scan cystogram (CT cystogram). Adequate evaluation of the urethra requires a retrograde urethrogram (RUG). When performing a cystogram using conventional x-ray, it is important to remember that a minimum of 300 cc of contrast must be instilled into the bladder. The preferred volume of contrast is 450 cc. Two x-rays are then required: one immediately following distention of the bladder and another immediately after complete drainage of the bladder. The postdrainage film is used to fully examine the perivesical space for extravasation that might have been obscured by the full bladder.

The introduction of multislice CT scanning has made CT evaluation of the genitourinary tract the diagnostic gold standard. With the addition of a CT cystogram, the entire genitourinary tract can be examined in one study. Not only does this study provide information with respect to the anatomy and function of the entire genitourinary tract, it can also be used to evaluate the renovascular system in a time-efficient manner.

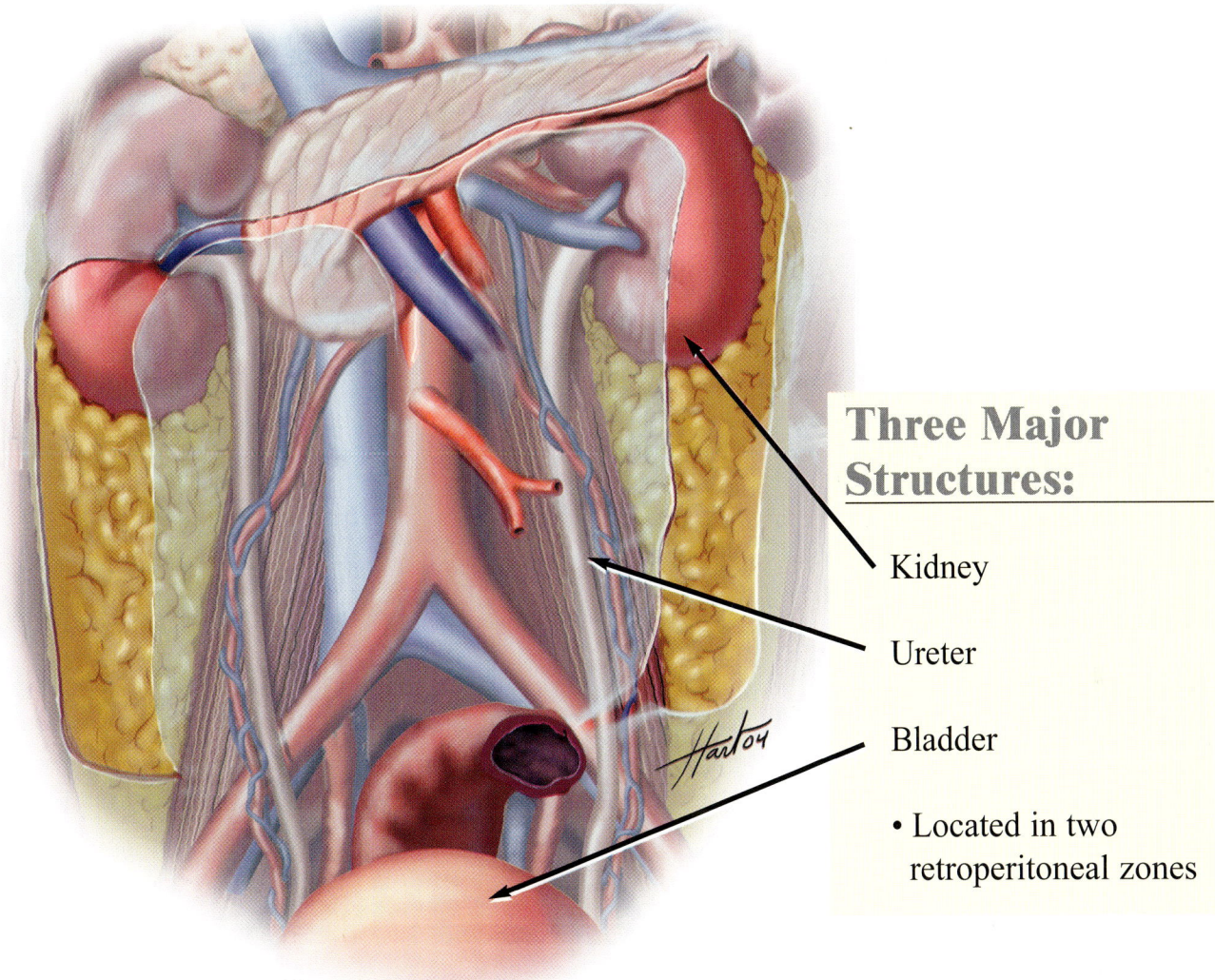

Three Major Structures:

- Kidney
- Ureter
- Bladder

• Located in two retroperitoneal zones

Anatomy

The major anatomic structures to be considered when evaluating the genitourinary system are the kidneys, ureter, bladder, and, to a lesser extent, the urethra. These major structures can be located in two retroperitoneal zones; the lateral structures are located in Zone II and the caudal structures in Zone III. However, the renovascular structures are located in Zone I. The genitourinary system is at risk for injury with any injury to the retroperitoneum, regardless of location.

AAST Grading System

The Organ Injury Scale of the American Association for the Surgery of Trauma (AAST-OIS) is used to grade injuries to most of the organ systems, including the kidney. Injury grading is based on the appearance of the kidney on CT scan.

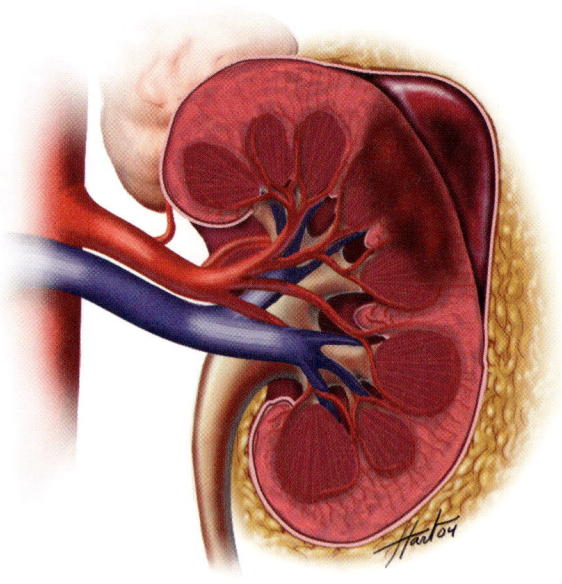

AAST Grading System

- Grade I:
  - contusion: hematuria without x-ray abnormalities

  - subcapsular hematoma: no parenchymal laceration

Grade I

Grade I injuries to the kidney are characterized as a contusion presenting as hematuria without any x-ray abnormalities, or a subcapsular hematoma with no parenchymal laceration visualized. There is no disruption of the cortex, and the calyceal system is intact.

Grade II

A Grade II renal injury presents as a perinephric hematoma that is confined to the retroperitoneum, or a laceration that involves the cortex but is less than 1 cm in depth. The calyceal system remains intact in Grade II injuries, as it does with Grade I injuries.

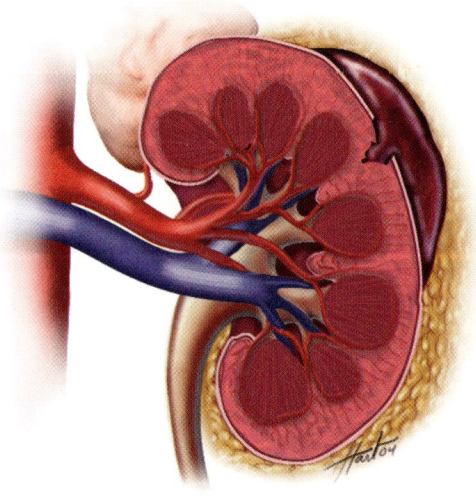

AAST Grading System

- Grade II:
  - perinephric hematoma confined to retroperitoneum

  - Laceration < 1 cm in depth of renal cortex

Grade III

Grade III and Grade IV injuries to the kidney are the first levels of injury that might require operative intervention. A Grade III injury is an injury to the renal cortex that is greater than 1 cm in depth. A Grade IV injury is a kidney laceration that involves the collecting system. Both grades of injuries will often have an associated perinephric hematoma.

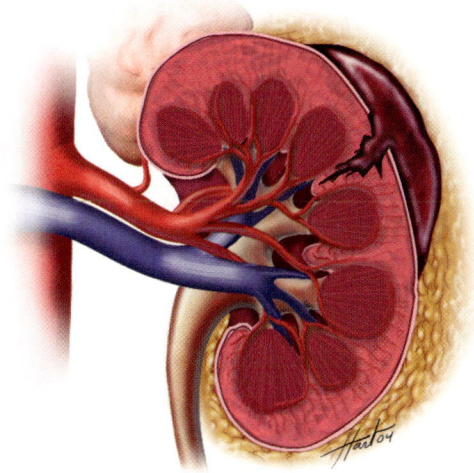

AAST Grading System

- Grade III:
  - laceration > 1 cm in depth

- Grade IV:
  - laceration through collecting system

Grade IV

In addition to cortical and calyceal injuries, Grade IV injuries can also be characterized by the presence of a vascular injury with contained hemorrhage.

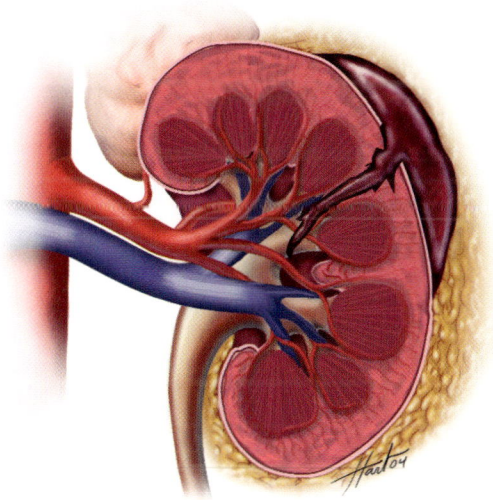

AAST Grading System

- Grade IV:
  - vascular injury with contained hemorrhage

- Grade V:
  - vascular avulsion
  - shattered kidney

Grade V

Grade V injuries to the kidney are the worst injuries sustainable. They involve disruption of the vascular supply to the kidney, or a shattered kidney. Grade V injuries almost always result in loss of function of the injured kidney.

Three Scenarios for Renal Injury

- Penetrating trauma
- Blunt trauma for renal injury
- Blunt trauma with other indications for celiotomy

Three Operative Scenarios for Renal Injury

As previously discussed, 80% of all urogenital injuries involve the kidney, and most of these are managed nonoperatively. However, penetrating truncal trauma that involves Zone II of the retroperitoneum and results in ongoing hemorrhage, with or without shock, requires operative intervention for renal trauma. Similarly, blunt trauma resulting in renal injury with subsequent ongoing bleeding and shock also necessitates operative intervention. Patients who have sustained blunt truncal trauma, and have other indications for celiotomy, may require operative intervention for an injured kidney, that might have otherwise initially been managed nonoperatively.

Exposure

Optimal exposure is one of the most important factors that influence the outcome for renal injuries requiring operative intervention. As mentioned earlier, the kidneys are retroperitoneal structures located in Zone II. The right kidney is located more inferior than the left. The superior pole of the right kidney is located at the level of the twelfth rib, and the superior pole of the left kidney is located at the level of the eleventh rib.

Exposure of either kidney will involve medial visceral rotation. This can be accomplished by using a Mattox maneuver on the left kidney or by reflecting the hepatic flexure of the colon on the right. The addition of a Kocher maneuver will improve visualization of the right renal vascular pedicle.

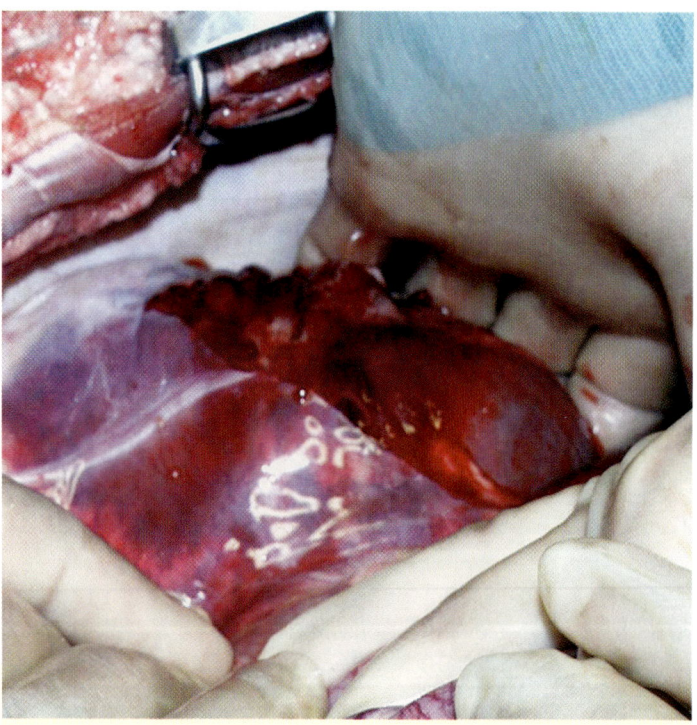

Exposure

- Medial rotation of intestinal structures
- Vascular control either by isolating the hilar vessels first or by medially rotating the kidney

Control of the vascular pedicle is imperative once the injured kidney has been adequately exposed. In the absence of significant retroperitoneal bleeding, the renal hilum can be dissected out sharply, and vascular clamps can be applied directly to the renal artery and vein. However, this approach may be impossible in the face of massive hemorrhage or a large retroperitoneal hematoma. In these cases, the kidney can be carefully mobilized using digital dissection. The kidney is elevated out of its retroperitoneal bed, and manual compression is used to obtain control of the hilar vessels. Application of a vascular clamp can follow.

With either approach, the time that vascular occlusion occurred must be recorded. Total occlusion time must be carefully followed. In general, warm ischemic time exceeding four hours cannot maintain an optimally functioning kidney.

Treatment: Grade I

The AAST-OIS grade assigned to the injury and the patient's clinical status will determine the initial management of the renal injury. Grade I injuries to the kidney, the least severe of all injuries, are managed conservatively. Grade I injuries are not operated on unless any unforeseen changes develop in the patient's status, or the injury progresses to require reclassification.

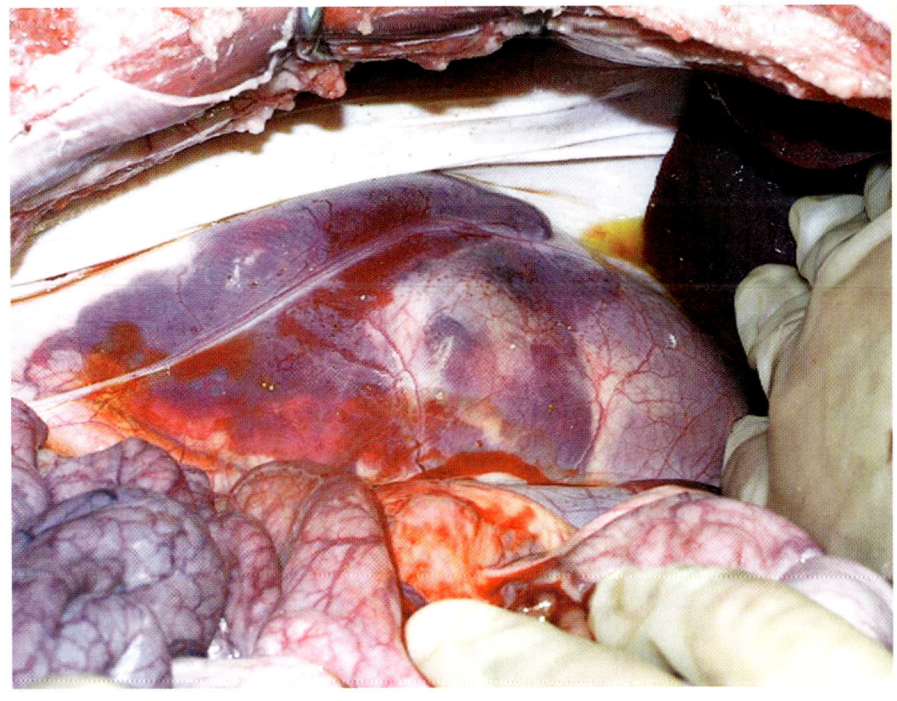

Grade I

- Observation

Treatment: Grade II and Grade III

As with Grade I injuries, Grade II and Grade III injuries that have resulted from blunt trauma in hemodynamically stable patients with no other reason for celiotomy are managed nonoperatively. Surgical intervention may be indicated if celiotomy is required for other injuries and the observed retroperitoneal injury appears to be expanding during the course of the celiotomy.

Grade II and Grade III

- Observe in stable blunt injury patients

- Renorraphy with capsular approximation

- Pledgeted sutures or mesh wrap

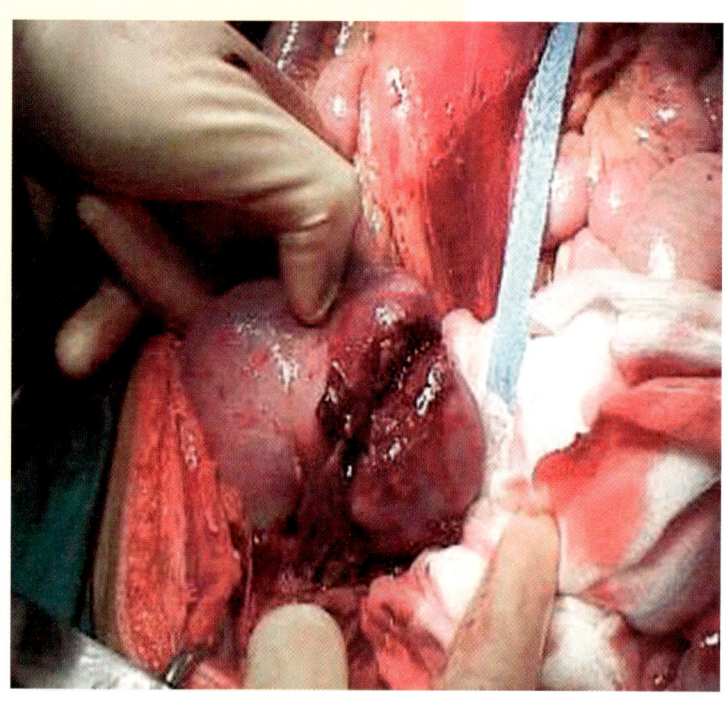

Renorrhaphy may be indicated for Grade III injuries with either cortical or calyceal disruption. In these cases, the calyceal system should be closed with absorbable sutures in a hemostatic and hydrostatic fashion, and the renal parenchyma approximated with pledgeted sutures. The primary goals of this repair are to achieve and maintain hemostasis of the renal parenchyma and prevent the formation of a urinoma due to urine leaking from the injured calyceal system. Although some surgeons advocate the use of a mesh wrap of the injured kidney, the pledgeted repair is more commonly performed.

Treatment

- Closure of calyces during repair or partial nephrectomy

- Absorbable interrupted suture

- Prevents urinoma

- Perinephric drain

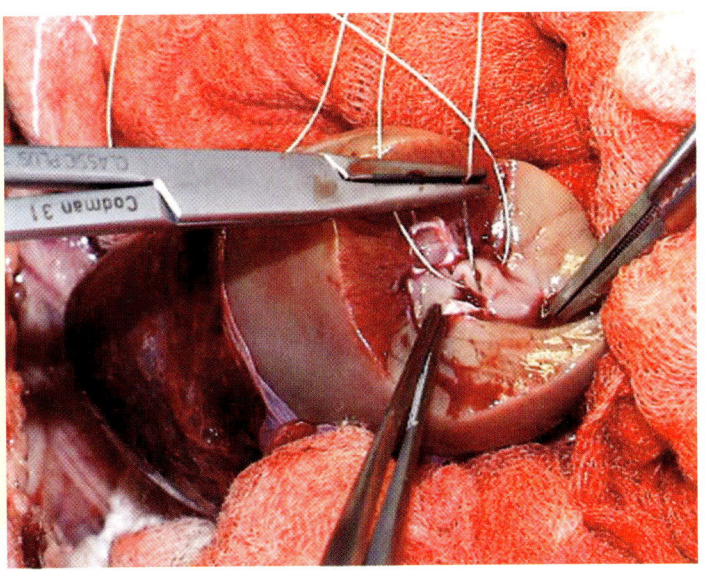

Treatment: Grade IV and Grade V

The vast majority of Grade IV and Grade V renal injuries require surgical intervention. In the stable patient, the ideal treatment would be repair of the injured kidney, with or without partial nephrectomy. However, this may not always be possible, and nephrectomy may be necessary.

An open calyceal system resulting from either the initial trauma or subsequent partial nephrectomy requires a watertight closure in order to prevent the formation of a urinoma. A fine absorbable suture should be used for closure of the calyceal system. Nonabsorbable sutures should not be used because of their tendency to promote calculus formation. The retroperitoneal perinephric space must be drained with closed-suction drains after renal salvage and repair have been accomplished.

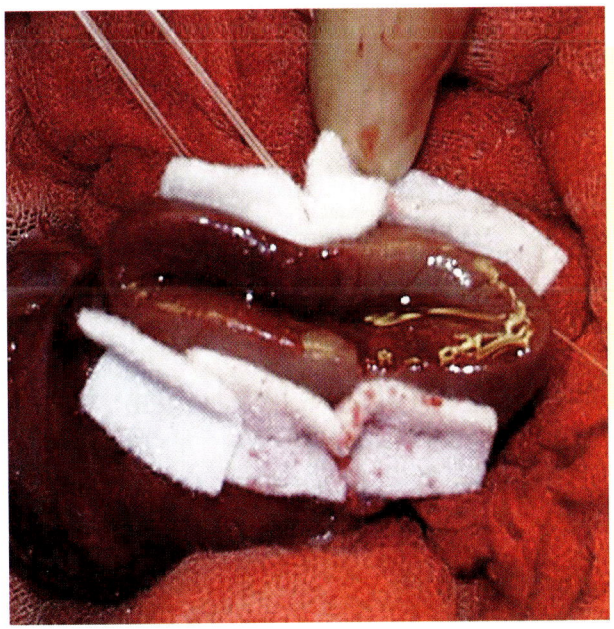

Grade IV and Grade V

- Stable Patient:
    - repair
    - partial nephrectomy
    - nephrectomy

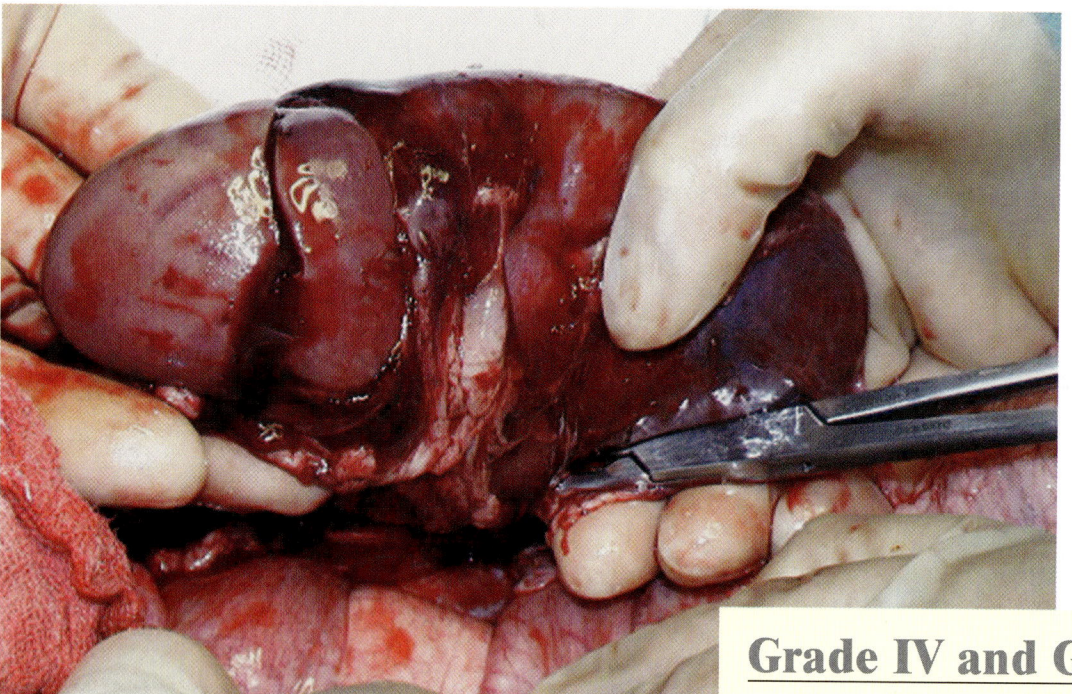

Grade IV and Grade V

- Unstable Patient:
  - nephrectomy
  - ureterectomy

Trauma patients who have sustained Grade IV or Grade V renal injuries and are hemodynamically unstable as a result of their renal injury require nephrectomy and ureterectomy. It is ideal to be able to document a functioning contralateral kidney. However, nephrectomy may be the only option if the patient is hemodynamically unstable or if renal salvage fails.

A ureterectomy is obviously necessary when performing a total nephrectomy. However, the patient's clinical status will determine the extent of the procedure. Ureterectomy should involve removal of the entire ureter down to the ureterovesical junction. Although it should be the goal when performing a nephrectomy, the patient's clinical status (i.e., hemodynamic instability, a large retroperitoneal hematoma, and/or significant coagulopathy) may preclude performance of this procedure. Simple ligation of the ureter distal to the renal pelvis is indicated in these patients. Dissection through the retroperitoneum down to the bladder is discouraged.

Ureterectomy

It has been shown that resection of the ureter at the ureterovesical junction decreases the subsequent risk for developing transitional cell carcinoma and ureteral calculi in the stable patient requiring a nephrectomy. It also decreases the risk for developing hydroureter, stasis within the remaining ureter, and subsequent infections. However, ureterectomy in the unstable, cold, and coagulopathic patient increases operative time and causes further bleeding by requiring dissection in an area of the retroperitoneum that could have otherwise been left untouched.

Contralateral Kidney

It is extremely important to determine the presence and functionality of a contralateral kidney in any patient who has sustained renal injury, regardless of whether or not surgical intervention is necessary. The presence and size of a contralateral kidney can be established with a plain abdominal x-ray, one-shot IVP, abdominal CT scan, or FAST exam. In the hands of an experienced sonographer, the FAST exam is a very quick and reliable tool for determining the presence of a kidney and demonstrating normal architectural anatomy. A one-shot IVP or an abdominal CT with contrast can also be used to demonstrate renal function on the uninjured side.

Ureterectomy

Pros
- Transitional cell carcinoma
- Calculi
- Hydroureter
- Infection

Cons
- Time consuming

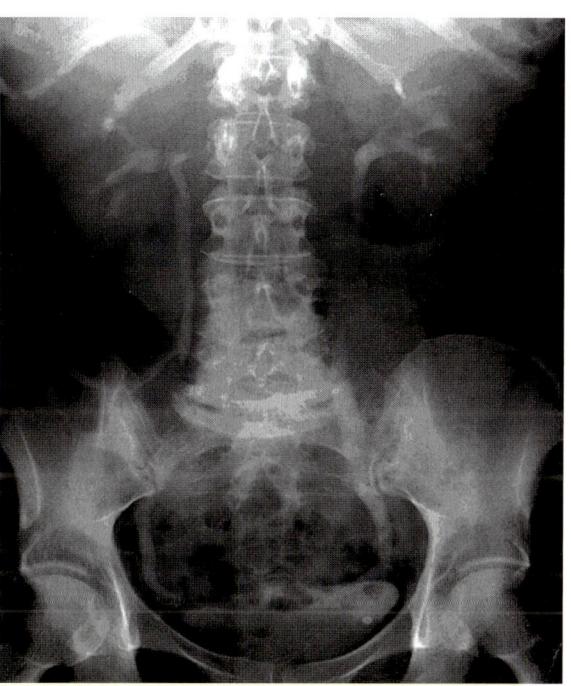

Assessment of Contralateral Kidney

- Presence
- Size
- Injury
- IVP
- Methylene blue
- FAST

Intravenous methylene blue can be administered if there is a questionable injury to the kidney and the patient is already in the operating room for a celiotomy for other injuries. Methylene blue will be quickly seen in the perinephric or periureteral tissues if there has been an injury to the collecting system of that kidney.

Reimplantation

- Bench top repair

- Preservation of vascular pedicle and ureter

- Four hour warm ischemic time limit to allow for meaningful function

Reimplantation

Reimplantation is occasionally discussed for Grade V renal injuries, characterized by vascular disruption of the renal pedicle. The procedure requires removal of the injured kidney, with subsequent débridement of the proximal and distal ends of the injured vessels and ureter. The kidney is then returned to its normal anatomic position with the anastomosis of the renal pedicle. This is possible only in patients who have remained hemodynamically stable, have no other significant traumatic injuries, and have had preservation of the vascular pedicle and the ureter. Careful attention must be paid to the total warm ischemic time. It is widely accepted that a maximum of four hours warm ischemic time will allow for meaningful postreimplantation renal function, but some physicians argue that this is a very generous time frame and that the reconstruction and reimplantation should be accomplished in less than four hours.

Renovascular Injury

Renovascular disruption is one form of a Grade V renal injury, but a more common form of vascular disruption is renal artery thrombosis. These thromboses result from marked blunt trauma, where the kidney itself moves within Gerota's fascia and stretches the arterial supply. The resultant injury is not a disruption of the renal artery but, rather, thrombosis within the artery caused by an intimal injury. These renal artery thromboses are not indications for operative intervention. The potential role for interventional radiology and endoluminal stenting has not been well studied to date. Although acute surgical intervention is not indicated, these injuries may eventually require operative intervention for the complications of a nonfunctional kidney. Postinjury hypertension (the Goldblatt kidney phenomenon), postinjury infection, and chronic pain are established complications that require nephrectomy.

Renal Artery Thrombosis

- Thrombosis from stretch injury
- Blunt trauma
- Not an indication for operative intervention
- Delayed intervention for complications:
  - hypertension
  - infection
  - chronic pain

Ureteral Injury: Exposure

The ureters extend from Zone II of the retroperitoneum into Zone III. Under elective surgical conditions, the ureter is usually fairly easy to identify anywhere along its course in the retroperitoneum. However, the ureter can be difficult to identify when it is injured or when a significant retroperitoneal hematoma is present. The easiest way to identify the ureter in the trauma patient with a retroperitoneal hematoma is at the bifurcation of the iliac vessels, where the ureter passes directly anterior to the common iliac artery. Once identified at this level, the ureter can be traced proximally and distally with relative ease.

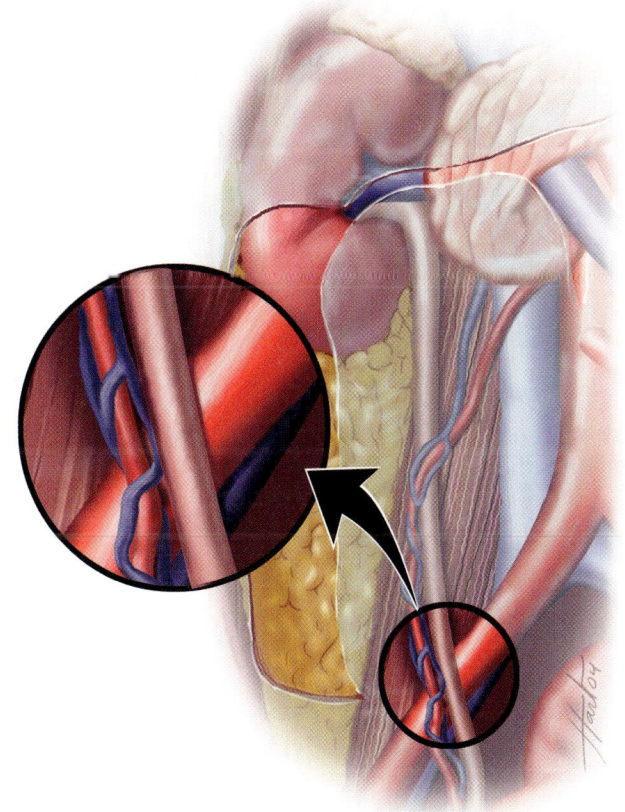

Locate ureter at the level of the iliac bifurcation then trace proximally and distally

Ureteral Injury: Treatment

It is always best to repair the injured ureter primarily whenever possible. In order to minimize the risk of stenosis or stricture at the repair site, any devitalized tissue should be débrided once the ureteral injury has been identified, and the ureter should be spatulated. Once a double J stent has been appropriately placed within the ureter, absorbable sutures are used to repair the ureteral injury. Stay sutures should be placed on either side of the ureteral injury and used as guides. The interrupted absorbable sutures are then placed at regular intervals in order to completely close the defect and minimize the possibility of urinary leakage.

All ureteral repairs must be drained with closed-suction drains. A 10 mm Jackson-Pratt drain is most commonly used. It is placed adjacent to, but not contiguous with, the repair. When the degree of hemodynamic instability is profound, ureteral injuries can be ligated and repaired during subsequent surgical intervention.

Treatment

- Repair with interrupted absorbable suture over double J stent

- Drain adjacent to repair

- IVP prior to removal of stent

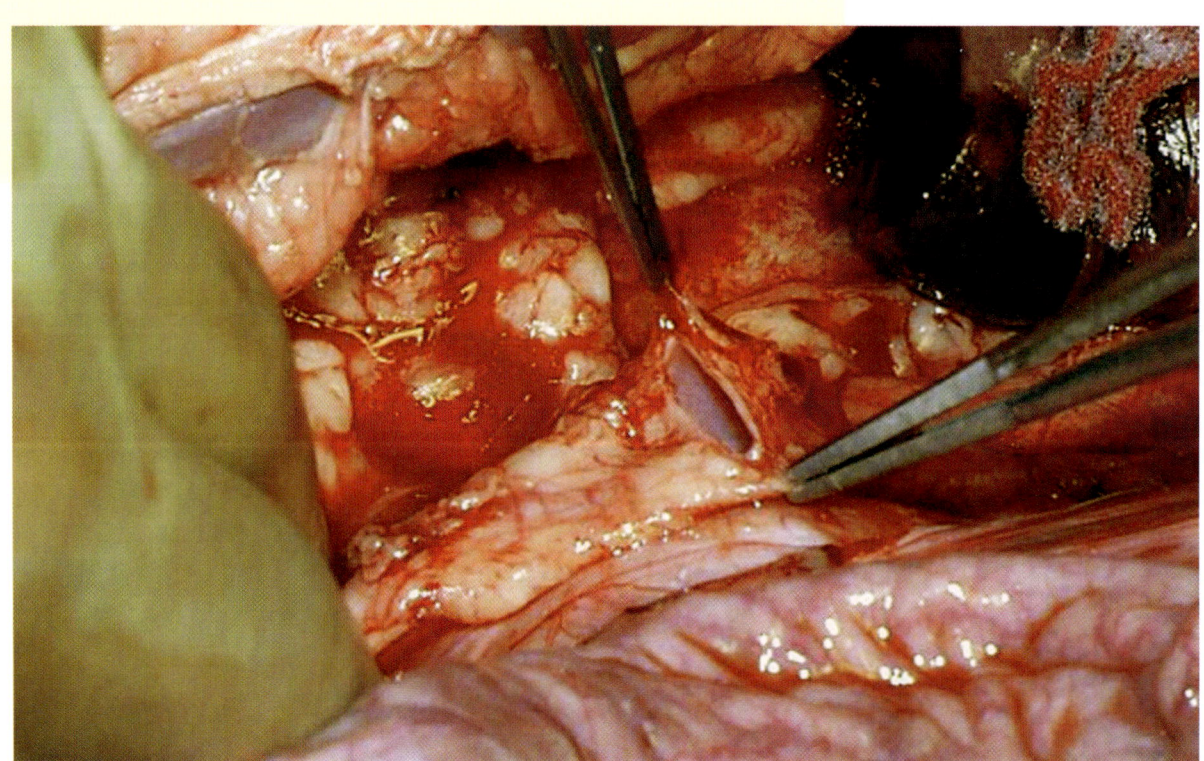

Complete Transection

- Débride to viable tissue
- Primary repair with spatulation over stent
- Interrupted absorbable suture

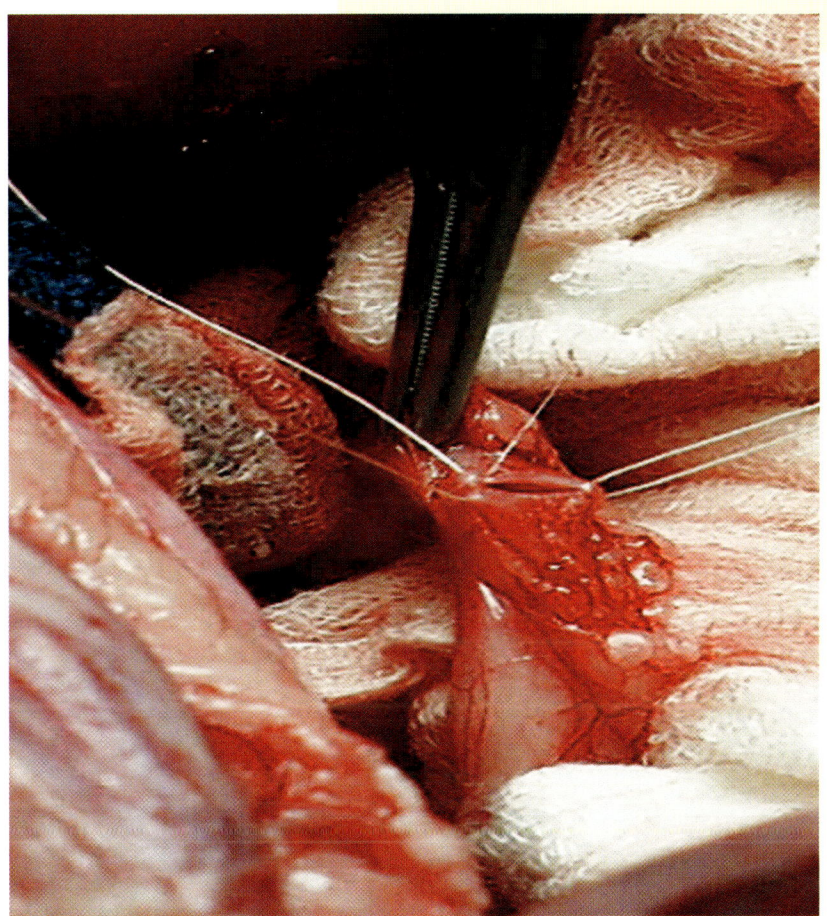

Ureteral Injury: Complete Transection

Ureteral injuries require débridement of all damaged tissue. Viable tissue is used for the anastomosis. Repairs must be tension free, as is the case for any other anastomosis. The two ends of the injured ureter are spatulated to avoid stricture or postoperative stenosis. The use of absorbable suture material avoids presenting a permanent foreign body within the lumen of the ureter. Foreign bodies are known to act as a nidus for stone formation and should be avoided.

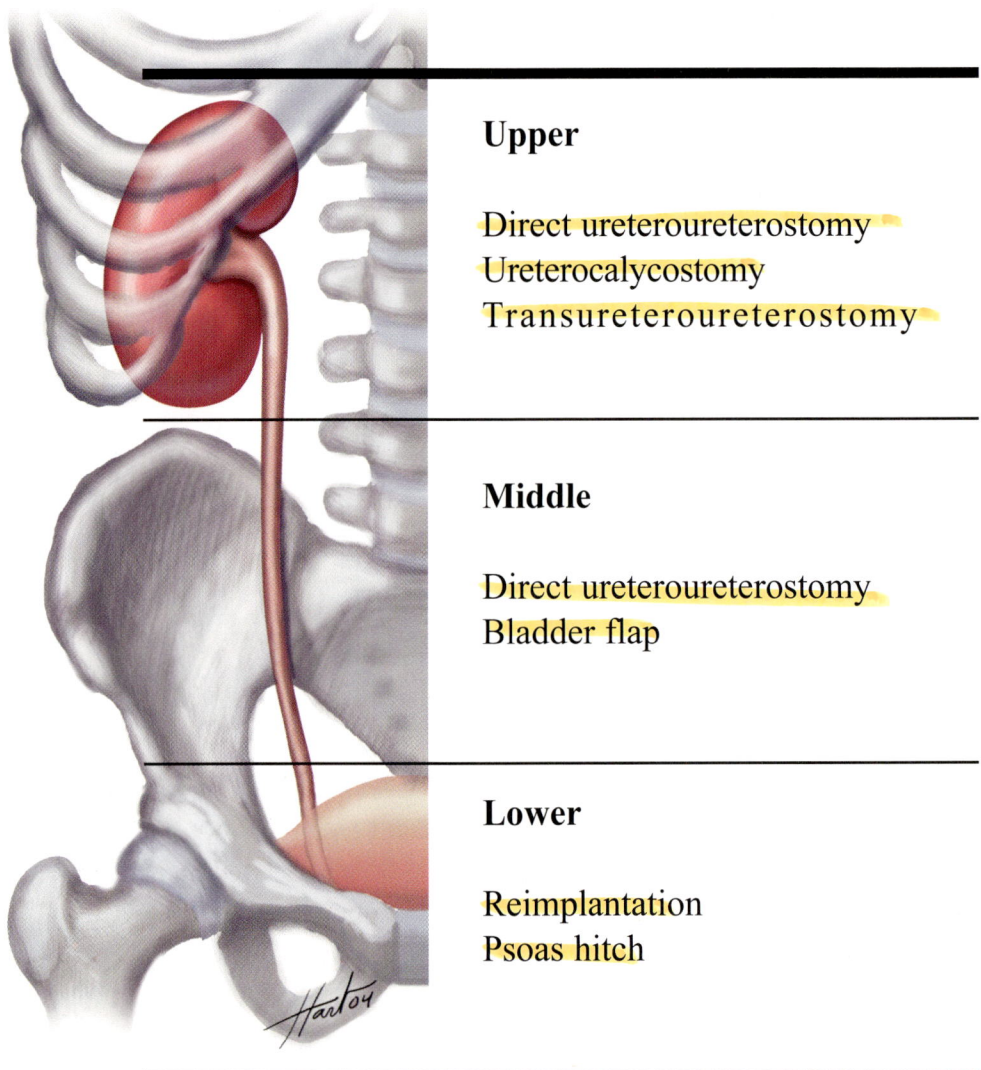

Ureteral Injury: Treatment Options

The ureter has traditionally been divided into three segments, each of which has a different blood supply. The upper, middle, and lower ureter segments are dealt with differently if a primary repair of the injured ureter is not possible due to tissue loss or devitalization.

The repair of choice for the upper and middle ureter would be a direct ureterostomy. However, injury to the upper third of the ureter can be treated with a ureterocalycostomy or a transureteroureterostomy. If a tension free ureteroureterostomy is not possible in the lower two thirds of the ureter, a bladder flap with implantation of the ureter can be performed. This involves implanting the ureter into a Boari flap. A Psoas hitch can be performed if there appears to be any tension on the flap and tunneled ureter. This technique will be described in more detail later.

Proximal Ureter: Transureteroureterostomy

Transureteroureterostomy is not recommended as the primary method of ureteral repair. Implantation of one ureter into the contralateral ureter puts the contralateral kidney at risk.

Transureteroureterostomy

- Puts the uninjured kidney at risk
- NOT recommended

A nephrectomy with ureterectomy should be considered if a ureteral injury is accompanied by concomitant ipsilateral renal injury, and the contralateral kidney and ureter are normal. As with any other decision-making process in the trauma patient, hemodynamic stability will affect the procedure chosen. Damage control procedures must be used if the patient is not stable.

Middle Ureter: Boari Bladder Flap

Injury to the middle third of the ureter poses a challenge because the proximal and distal thirds of the ureter remain intact, while the middle portion cannot be used. The best treatment approach for these cases is a distal ureteral resection down to the ureterovesical juncture, and the formation of a Boari bladder flap. This can be accomplished by creating a rectangular-shaped flap of bladder tissue, with primary closure of the defect caused on the bladder. The resulting bladder appendage is closed in a tubular fashion with implantation of the proximal end of the ureter well down into the flap. Once the construction of the tube is completed and the ureter is implanted, recreating continuity of the urinary stream from the kidney into the bladder, constriction of the bladder musculature should minimize reflux into the implanted ureter.

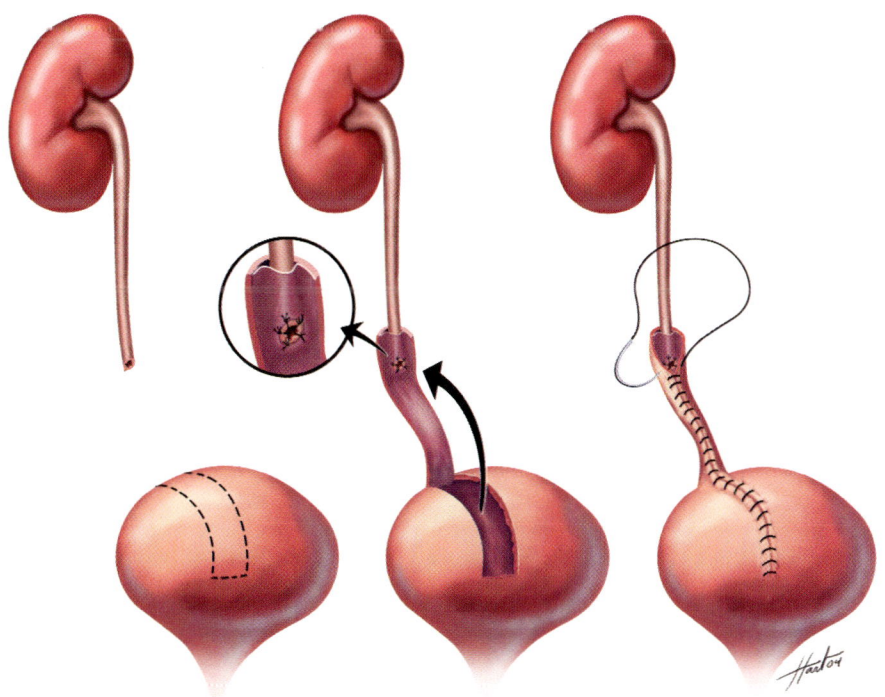

Distal Ureter: Psoas Hitch

A Psoas hitch can be performed if any tension is noted once the repair has been completed. The bladder is mobilized cephalad and to the side of injury, and it is sutured to the psoas muscle with a 2-0 Vicryl stitch. Care must be taken to avoid incorporating any neurovascular structures within this suture. Resection of the distal ureter minimizes stasis and should decrease the risk of stone formation and infection.

Destruction of the distal ureter presents a significant challenge but can be handled by mobilizing the bladder and performing a Psoas hitch. The distal ureteral remnant must be débrided and the ureterovesical junction suture ligated and closed. This closure must be watertight in order to prevent urinary leakage from the bladder. After the Psoas hitch is performed, the distal end of the ureter is implanted into the bladder. As with all other ureteral repairs, the area is drained widely.

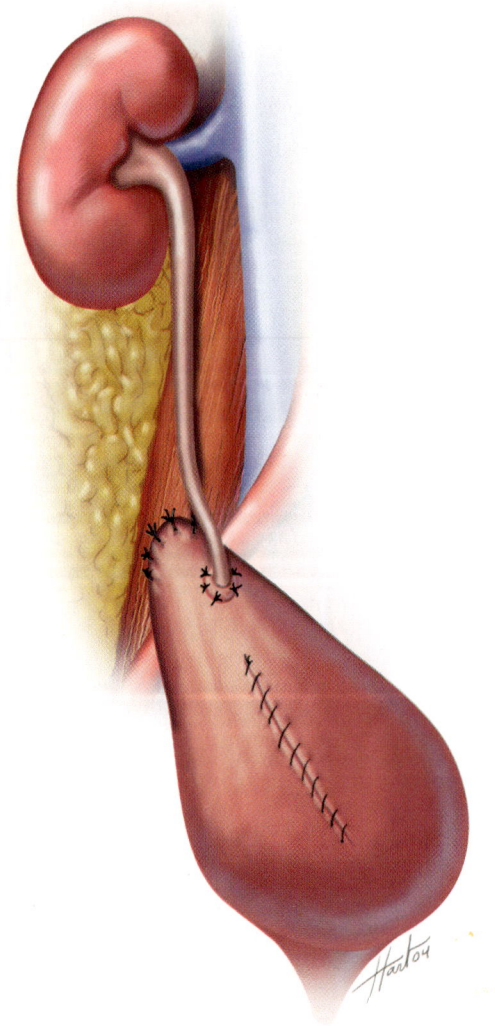

CYSTOGRAM OR CT CYSTOGRAM

- Requires retrograde filling of bladder with at least 300cc

- Standard cystogram requires x-ray with bladder full and after drainage

Diagnosis: CT or Cystogram

Although intraperitoneal and extraperitoneal bladder injuries are managed differently, the diagnoses are arrived at similarly. Diagnosis of bladder injuries requires a cystogram or a CT cystogram. The CT cystogram, which tends to be the method of choice with multislice CT scans, requires retrograde filling of the bladder with contrast material through a Foley catheter. The Foley is clamped once the bladder has been filled with at least 300 cc preferably with as much as 450 cc of contrast. As with a regular cystogram, the CT scan must be performed with a full bladder. The bladder region must be rescanned once the Foley is unclamped and the bladder is drained.

As mentioned earlier, the standard cystogram requires two x-rays; the first when the bladder has been filled as it is for the CT cystogram and the second image a postdrainage view.

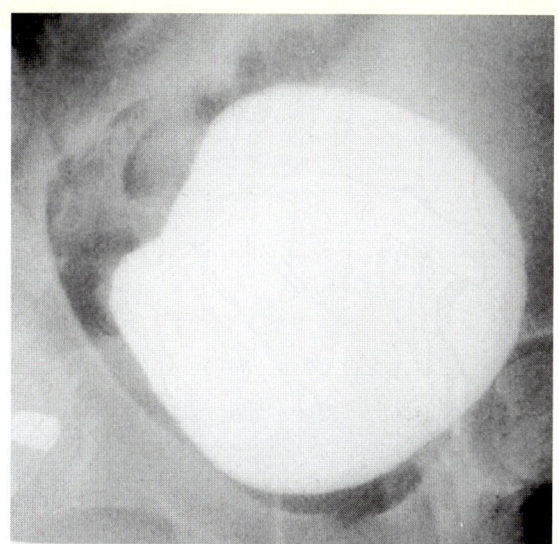

Extraperitoneal Injury

The vast majority of extraperitoneal bladder injuries result from puncture of the bladder by bony fragments of a pelvic fracture. The diagnosis is made by extravasation of contrast material from the bladder that remains within the extraperitoneal tissues. These injuries do not require operative intervention and are best treated by Foley catheter drainage. If there is significant bleeding, a three-way catheter can be

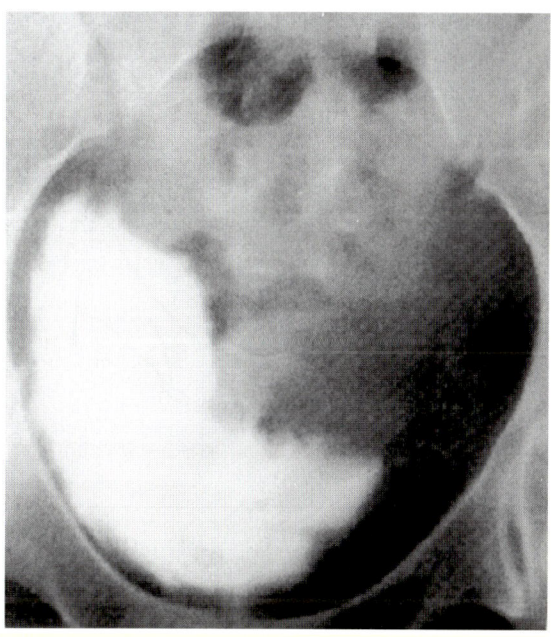

Extraperitoneal Injury

- Usually secondary to tear by bone fragments

- Majority of bladder injuries are associated with pelvic fractures

- Foley catheter drainage

inserted and the bladder irrigated free of clots. Catheter drainage is maintained for at least seven days. Prior to removal of the Foley catheter, a cystogram is performed to ensure complete healing and the absence of any further extravasation.

Intraperitoneal Injury
- Blunt force to distended bladder
- Penetrating trauma
- Requires operative intervention

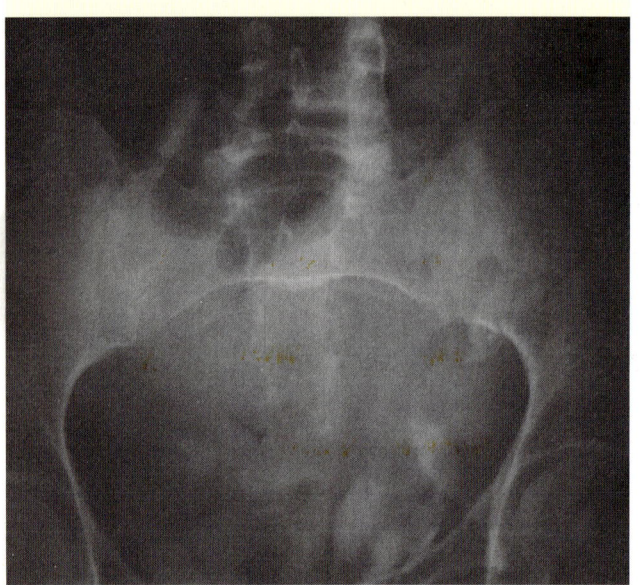

Intraperitoneal Injury

Unlike extraperitoneal bladder disruption, an intraperitoneal bladder injury requires operative intervention. Intraperitoneal bladder injury most often results from blunt abdominal trauma in the presence of a markedly distended bladder, or as a result of penetrating abdominal trauma.

Treatment

Intraperitoneal bladder disruption requires surgical repair. Exploration of the inside of the bladder is imperative once the bladder injury has been identified. The trigone is identified in order to ensure the integrity of the urethral and both ureteral orifices. The repair is then performed in two layers, using absorbable sutures to eliminate the presence of a permanent intraluminal foreign body, which can act as a nidus for stone formation. Although the first layer of absorbable sutures can be a simple running suture, a running locking suture will be more hemostatic and hydrostatic. The second layer is performed using Lembert sutures to imbricate the first layer.

Once the repair has been completed, 300 cc to 400 cc of saline must be instilled into the bladder to distend the bladder and ensure that the repair is hydrostatic. Putting methylene blue into the saline will make it easier to determine if there is any leakage through the repair. A Foley catheter is left in place.

The use of a suprapubic drain after repair of a bladder has always been recommended in the past. However, this is now only done in selective cases, for example, in

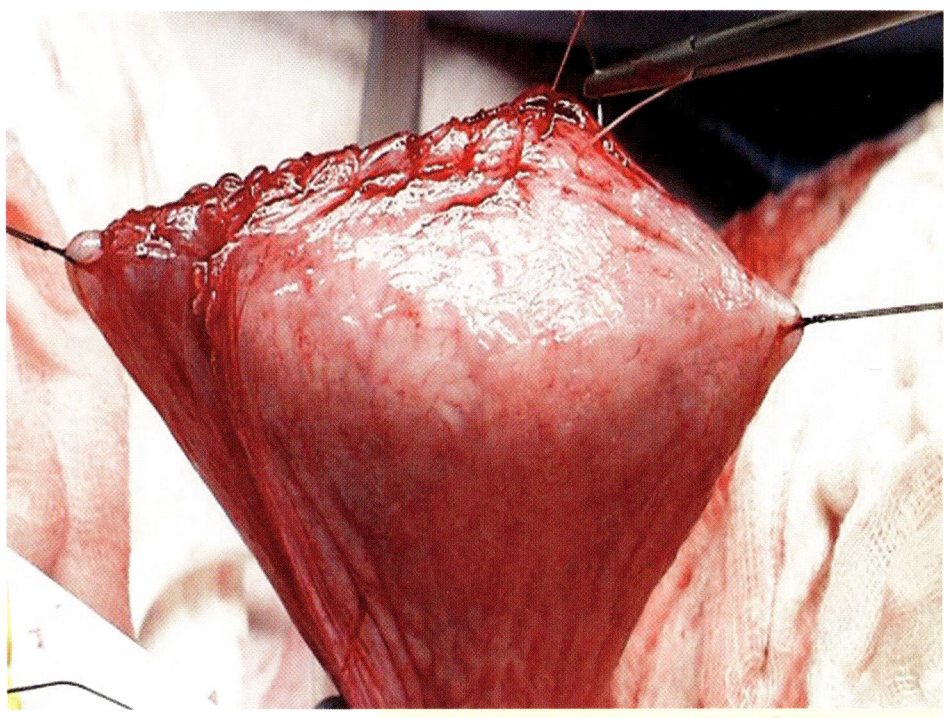

patients with a high likelihood of intravesicular clots, in cases where long-term bladder drainage is anticipated, and in patients where the long-term presence of a Foley might increase the risk for urethral stricture. Perivesical drainage is no longer routinely recommended.

Postoperative Management

Postoperative management of bladder injuries is fairly straightforward. A Foley catheter should be left in place for at least seven to ten days, and a formal cystogram should be performed before removing the Foley. If there is no extravasation of contrast material, the Foley catheter can be safely removed. The bladder should be assessed for postvoid residual using a bladder ultrasound to assess the postvoid residual volume.

Intraperitoneal Injury

- Two layer absorbable closure
- Identify ureteral orifices
- Identify uretheral orifice
- Foley catheter

Optional

- Perivesical drain
- Suprapubic drain

Postoperative Management

- Foley drainage 7 to 10 days
- Cystogram prior to Foley removal

ADVANCED TRAUMA OPERATIVE MANAGEMENT
Selected Readings
Chapter 5 - Genitourinary System

Holcroft JW et al. Renal trauma and retroperitoneal haematomas: indications for exploration. J Trauma 1975;15:1045-1052.

Wessels H et al. Criteria for non-operative treatment of significant penetrating renal lacerations. J Urol. 1997;157:24-27.

Velmahos GC et al. Selective management of renal gunshot wounds. Br J Surg. 1998;85:1121-1124.

Gonzalez RP et al. Surgical management of renal trauma: Is vascular control necessary? J Trauma 1999;47:1039-1044.

Wessells H et al. Renal injury and operative management in the United States: Results of a population-based study. J Trauma 2003;54:423-430.

Parry NG et al. Traumatic rupture of the urinary bladder: Is the suprapubic tube necessary? J Trauma 2003;54:431-436.

Tips From the Masters

There are a number of safe methods to manage blunt and penetrating trauma in the operating suite. The following technical surgical tips have been successfully used by the authors to deal with difficult or challenging operating situations.

Chapter 5: Genitourinary

TABLE OF CONTENTS

Exposure and Management of a 3 cm Burst Laceration of the Bladder 251
L. D. Britt, MD

Exposure and Management of Grade V Renal Injury 252
Michael F. Rotondo, MD, FACS

Penetrating Injury to the Bladder 254
Peter Rhee, MD

Intraperitoneal Bladder Laceration Involving Trigone 256
Kimball I. Maull, MD

Penetrating Injury to the Bladder Including the Trigone 258
Thomas E. Knuth, MD

Repair of Intraperitoneal Bladder Laceration 261
Kimball I. Maull, MD

Repair of Laceration of the Bladder 262
Glen Tinkoff, MD

Nephrectomy with Laceration of the Renal Artery and Vein 264
Stephen S. Luk, MD

Renal Laceration Involving the Collecting System 266
Erwin F. Hirsch, MD

The Management of a 3 cm Deep Laceration to the Lower Pole of the Left Kidney in Which There is Active Extravasation of Urine 267
L.D. Britt, MD

Management of a Kidney Laceration Involving the Collecting System 269
David B. Hoyt, MD

Ureteral Repair 271
Michael Rhodes, MD

Ureteral Repair 273
Thomas Scalea, MD

TECHNICAL OPERATIVE PROCEDURES:
HOW I DO IT

Exposure and Management of a 3 cm Burst Laceration of the Bladder

L.D. Britt, MD, MPH, FACS

Scenario

A 36-year-old woman was involved in a motor vehicle crash. She was the restrained driver of a vehicle which struck a telephone pole. The patient was alert and hemodynamically stable but complaining of severe pelvic and lower abdominal pain.

Management

Upon the patient's arrival to the emergency department, ATLS protocol was initiated, including the insertion of a large bore catheter in each antecubital fossa. Although there was no evidence of an unstable pelvic fracture, the patient has tenderness with palpation of the symphysis pubis. Foley catheter insertion demonstrates a scant amount of gross blood. The FAST exam demonstrates a large amount of free fluid in the pelvis. The patient is taken to the operative theater for an exploratory celiotomy.

Procedure: *Exposure and management of a 3 cm burst laceration of the bladder*

A midline incision is made from the xiphoid to the pubis, being careful not to enter a possible pelvic hematoma. Upon entering the peritoneal cavity, approximately 1 liter of straw-colored fluid was suctioned from the pelvis. A rupture of the dome of the bladder was found. Prior to definitive repair of this injury, the abdominal cavity is thoroughly explored for associated injuries. With the exception of a small, non-expanding pelvic hematoma, there is no other injury. The bladder is inspected internally through the laceration to determine if there are any other associated vesical injuries. The edges of the bladder wound require minimal débridement. Closure of the laceration is performed with a two-layer closure, using a thick absorbable suture, e.g. Vicryl or chromic catgut. The inner layer of the bladder wall is closed with an interrupted 1-0 chromic suture and the outer layer is closed with the same suture in a continuous fashion.

> • The bladder is inspected internally through the laceration

> • Two layer closure with heavy absorbable sutures
>
> • First layer interrupted; second layer continuous

A large bore transurethral catheter is used for bladder drainage. The entire abdominal cavity is copiously irrigated and the abdominal wall is subsequently closed primarily.

TECHNICAL OPERATIVE PROCEDURES:

HOW I DO IT

Exposure and Management of Grade V Renal Injury

Michael F. Rotondo, MD, FACS

Scenario

The patient is a 30-year-old male who presents with a stab wound to the right flank and hypotension. The laceration is located in the mid-axillary line and the costal margin on the right.

Management

The need for operation is immediately recognized upon discovery of the right flank stab wound in the presence of hypotension. After obtaining large bore peripheral intravenous access, blood is obtained for type and crossmatch, an abbreviated neurologic examination is performed, and the patient undergoes rapid sequence induction and intubation for immediate airway control. Resuscitation is initiated with warm crystalloids and universal type O blood. The patient is fully exposed and examined for additional penetrations and no other injuries are identified. A rectal examination is completed, which reveals no gross blood. A Foley catheter is placed, which reveals gross blood. A nasogastric tube is placed, which reveals no gross blood. The initial temperature is 37°C and the patient's blood pressure improves to 110 systolic.

The patient's total resuscitation time is 12 minutes, and he is taken to the operating room for exploratory laparotomy.

Procedure: *Exposure and management of right renal artery laceration*

The patient is brought to the operating room and placed on the table in a supine position. Patient is prepped and draped from chin to knees and two suction devices are placed on the operative field, including a device for blood scavenging and auto transfusion. A midline incision is made through the skin, subcutaneous tissue, and fascia from xiphoid to the pubic symphysis. The peritoneum is identified and a small opening is created and a cell saver suction inserted. 1.5 liters of gross blood are evacuated and the peritoneum is further opened throughout the extent of the incision. Four quadrant and central retroperitoneal packing is performed. The Bookwalter retractor is set up for general exposure. Resuscitation is ongoing.

At this point, the packs should be systematically removed and it is my practice to remove the packs that are least likely to be involved with hemorrhage first. This creates more room in the abdomen for exposure of the bleeding area. Systematic trace of the trajectory of the stab wound should then take place starting in the right upper quadrant. Examination of the right upper quadrant begins with gentle traction of the hepatic flexure inferiorly and medially, identifying a large right pericolic gutter hematoma and free blood oozing through a rent in the posterior parietal tissues. It is also noted that there is a large contained central retroperitoneal hematoma. Given the presumed trajectory of this injury, a Cattel Braasch maneuver is immediately performed. This is done by retracting the hepatic flexure medially and inferiorly and bluntly incising the posterior parietal attachments of the colon. A right medial visceral rotation is then performed bluntly, encompassing both the hepatic flexure and the duodenum using digital and blunt dissection. The surgeon on the left side of the patient most easily accomplishes this. The dissection should be carried posterior-medially to include the head of the pancreas, but should be carried anteriorly to Gerota's fascia of the right kidney. In this circumstance, with a patient who is hypotensive from a stab wound to the perinephric region, it is not my practice to obtain central vascular control. From my experience, this is a difficult and time-consuming dissection, contributes to ongoing blood loss and shock perfusion injury, and does not increase the likelihood of renal salvage. Upon placement of packs in the right upper quadrant, the exposure is reset again with the Bookwalter retractor to include medial retraction of the right colon and the duodenum and the perinephric hematoma is entered using a combination of sharp and blunt dissection. Again, the surgeon on the left side of the table most easily accomplishes this. Upon entering the renal capsule, the thumb and forefinger of the surgeon's left hand should be used for hilar control. The kidney should be inspected with proximal digital control for salvage. In this case, the kidney is lacerated down to the hilum and all hilar structures are damaged. Nephrectomy is indicated. After proximal digital control, a more proximal curved vascular clamp should be applied en masse to the pedicle. The pedicle should then be transected using the Metzenbaum scissors and the area assessed for control of hemorrhage and immediately repacked. This sort of nephrectomy should take no longer than two to four minutes.

At this point, it is my practice to perform mass suture ligation of the hilum. This is done using a 0 silk suture on a large needle in standard fashion, flashing the clamp, and further securing the hilum with the second 0 silk suture ligature. The clamp is then removed and the area is inspected for hemostasis. It is customary that the renal capsule will have some persistent bleeding, and this should be controlled using electrocautery. Additional bleeding of the posterior parietal tissues should be controlled with cautery as well. If the patient is physiologically unstable, I do not hesitate to use a damage control approach, pack this area and return within 36 hours for pack removal and definitive closure. If hemostasis is adequate and the patient is physiologically stable, the rest of the abdomen is carefully inspected and finding no other abnormalities, the fascia is closed using a running #1 monofilament suture and the skin is closed using skin staples.

- The kidney is lacerated at the hilum. Central vascular control is difficult and time consuming

- The thumb and forefinger are used for digital hilar control

- A curved vascular clamp is applied to the pedicle

- Suture ligation of the pedicle

TECHNICAL OPERATIVE PROCEDURES:

HOW I DO IT

Penetrating Injury to the Bladder

Peter Rhee, MD, MPH, FACS

Scenario

A 25-year-old man presents with a single stab wound to the suprapubic region. He has a 7 cm full thickness laceration to the dome of the bladder. His vital signs are normal and he has abdominal pain and tenderness to the lower abdomen. There are no other injuries.

Management

A second-generation cephalosporin is given and a Foley catheter inserted preoperatively. The urine should be evaluated to determine if there is hematuria. A careful secondary survey must be performed and any additional injuries should be identified preoperatively. The incision should be large enough to provide complete exploration of all abdominal and retroperitoneal viscera and should extend from the xiphoid to the symphysis pubis. Controlled hypotensive resuscitation allows for the use of minimal fluid volumes while maintaining adequate mentation or a systolic blood pressure of 90 mmHg. Once in the abdomen, I pack off the injury and ensure that there are no injuries to the rectum and ureters. I try to envision and recreate the stab wound tract to ensure identification of any possible associated injuries. Once it has been proven that the bladder is the only organ injured, I inspect the interior of the bladder. For a knife to have created such a large wound to the bladder, a "juug" maneuver was probably performed with the stabbing instrument. This motion is a lateral ripping motion with the fulcrum pivot point at the skin, and the skin usually has a hockey stick appearance.

Procedure: *Repair of the bladder*

If the bladder was full during the assault, it is possible to only lacerate one wall of the bladder without causing a second through-and-through injury that would be expected from a gunshot wound. However, it must be assumed that a second injury may have occurred. To evaluate the bladder, if the opening is not large enough to visualize the entire interior of the bladder, I enlarge it with electrocautery using the cutting function. Efforts to control bleeding using cautery should be minimized because this can adversely affect healing. Once the dome of the bladder has been opened, I insert one radiopaque sponge and use

- Two malleable retractors are used to inspect the entire mucosa of the bladder

- The dome is closed in two layers

- Closed suction perivesical drains are placed

two small malleable retractors bent in the middle to inspect the entire mucosa of the bladder. The assistant uses the suction device during the exploration inside the bladder to facilitate complete inspection. Once it has been verified that the opposite wall does not have an additional injury and that the ureter and the ureteral orifices are not injured, the retractors and the sponge are removed. The dome of the bladder is closed in two layers with 3-0 chromic continuous suture. A generous portion of muscularis and minimal accurate bites of mucosa facilitate meticulous mucosal approximation. This procedure enhances healing and minimizes the risk of a urinary leak. The second layer inverts the first suture line using a continuous absorbable Maxon or PDS suture. The bladder is a distensile organ. Use of non-absorbable sutures will make the suture line relatively non-expansile. Non-absorbable sutures can form a nidus for stone formation. For this reason they should not be used. A Jackson-Pratt drain is then placed over the injury and minimal suction applied. The drain should be brought out through a separate stab wound lateral to the midline incision. The Jackson-Pratt drain should be connected to low suction to decrease the potential for creation of a fistula. The subcutaneous tissue is irrigated with saline prior to closing the skin. The abdominal cavity is irrigated and the abdominal incision is closed. The drain can be removed in two to three days. I do not routinely keep the drain in for seven days nor do I perform a cystogram before the removal of the drain. A suprapubic drainage catheter is not necessary in this case and will only increase morbidity and length of stay. Perioperative antibiotics are given for 24 hours. The patient can be discharged with the Foley in place with instructions on drain care.

TECHNICAL OPERATIVE PROCEDURES:

HOW I DO IT

Intraperitoneal Bladder Laceration Involving Trigone

Kimball I. Maull MD, FACS

Scenario

A 24-year-old woman was injured when a tree fell on her vehicle during a storm. She sustained a direct crushing injury to her pelvis but otherwise escaped unhurt.

Management

Initial assessment confirmed suprapubic contusions and an inability to void. Bloody urine returned via the urethral catheter and fractures of both superior and inferior pubic rami were confirmed on plain films. On CT, there was minimal intrapelvic hematoma but easy egress of contrast was detected near the bladder neck. No intraperitoneal injuries were identified.

Procedure: *Repair of bladder laceration involving trigone*

A midline incision is made extending from superior to the umbilicus to approximately 6 cm above the pubis. Scant serous fluid is present in the peritoneal cavity. Using body wall retractors, the upper abdomen is visualized and explored thoroughly. No injuries are found. The remainder of the peritoneal cavity is inspected. Initially the bladder is not palpable. At this point, an assistant instills saline per urethral catheter to distend the bladder. The bladder is identified and grasped with Babcock clamps. Using a #11 blade, the lumen is entered, followed by the egress of blood-tinged fluid. Using sharp tissue scissors, the dome of the bladder is opened between the Babcock clamps and the bladder is suctioned. Using the Babcock clamps as countertraction, a pediatric sweetheart retractor is placed in the bladder demonstrating a posterior laceration just to the right of the midline extending inferiorly to involve the trigone. The ureteral orifices are sought. The left orifice is located but uncertainty exists about the right orifice.

At this point, the anesthesiologist is requested to inject one ampule of indigo carmine. Within four minutes, discolored urine is seen to emanate from the previously identified left ureter and from its mate on the other side. Because of the proximity of the ureters to the laceration, 5 Fr. whistle-tipped catheters are inserted up both ureters for a distance of approximately 15 cm and temporarily secured by an assistant. The extent of the laceration is inspected. Using two 2-0 chromic catgut sutures, each one is placed through the muscular wall of the bladder at the superior and inferior ends of the laceration from the inside of the bladder. Using the index finger and thumb of one hand, the course of each ureter is determined by palpating the ureteral catheters through the wall of the bladder. Beginning with the inferiorly placed suture, the muscular wall of the bladder is closed with a running locking mattress suture, being careful to avoid the ureters. Once the ureters are no longer in danger, several stitches are taken in like fashion with the superior suture until they meet and are tied together. The repair is carefully inspected to assure completeness of closure and hemostasis. The mucosal layer is anatomically re-approximated using 3-0 chromic catgut sutures, again being careful to avoid injuring the ureters. This intraluminal suture line may be completed by either interrupted individually placed sutures or by a running technique or a combination of the two. The ureteral catheters are removed.

Because the injury lies close to the bladder neck, it is best to remove the urethral catheter to avoid irritation or erosion of the repair. This requires the placement of a cystostomy. With the bladder still open, a pointed hemostat is passed through the anterior wall of the bladder from the outside to the inside and a 20 Fr Malécot catheter is pulled back through by the proximal end. Two circumferential purse string sutures of 2-0 chromic are placed around the catheter in the anterior bladder wall. At a site inferior to the midline incision, a 1 cm incision is made and the pointed hemostat is passed through the abdominal wall into the suprapubic space. The catheter is grasped and pulled through the abdominal wall where it is secured to the skin by a 2-0 nylon suture.

The site of entry into the bladder is closed as previously described. Adequacy of closure of both the cystostomy and the entry site is confirmed by irrigation and distention via the cystostomy. If there is lingering concern about any of the closures, closed suction drains can be placed in proximity to, but not in contact with any suture lines.

- The dome of the bladder is grasped with Babcock clamps and opened

- Indigo carmine facilitates identification of the ureteric orifices

- Catheters are inserted into both ureters

- The trigone is repaired avoiding the ureters and the urethra

TECHNICAL OPERATIVE PROCEDURES:
HOW I DO IT

Penetrating Injury To The Bladder Including The Trigone

Thomas E. Knuth, MD, MPH, FACS

Scenario

A 22-year-old male presents with a stab wound to the anterior left lower quadrant of the abdomen. There is a large laceration with evisceration and obvious bowel injury. He is taken directly to the operating room for a laparotomy. Upon insertion of the Foley, gross hematuria is discovered, and a urinary tract injury is suspected. A rectal exam is negative for blood. Gastric contents from the nasogastric tube are also negative for blood. The patient is placed in the supine position.

Management

Broad-spectrum antibiotics are started preoperatively. A long midline incision is made from mid-abdomen to the pubis. The abdomen is eviscerated and quickly explored. Multiple small bowel injuries and an anterior bladder injury are noted. No other injuries are noted; specifically, there is no colon, vascular, kidney, nor ureter injury. The liver, stomach, spleen and retroperitoneum Zones I and II are normal. Small bowel containing several injuries < 3 cm apart is resected between GIA staplers. The small bowel mesentery is transected between Kelly clamps and ligated with 3-0 Vicryl. A functional end-to-end anastomosis is performed using a GIA stapler and the mesenteric defect is repaired using 3-0 Vicryl. Several other small bowel injuries are closed in a horizontal manner using a single layer of running 3-0 Vicryl.

Procedure

Attention is then directed toward the bladder injury. 2-0 stay sutures are placed at both ends of the bladder laceration and two thin Deaver retractors are inserted to allow visualization of the inside of the bladder. A 4 cm laceration involving the posterior wall, including the left inferior aspect of the trigone just above the Foley balloon is discovered. The laceration is within a half centimeter of the left ureteral orifice. A double J stent is inserted into the left ureter to protect it from the repair or subsequent stricture. Although the preoperative rectal exam was negative for blood, the high potential for associated rectal injury warrants proctoscopic confirmation, which is planned prior to leaving the operating room.

Because the retrovesical space will need to be drained, the peritoneal reflection along the posterior aspect of the pubis is incised and the bladder is bluntly dissected off the posterior wall until the neck and injury are clearly visualized. The ureters are clearly identified and found to be uninjured. The anterior rectal wall appears intact. Stay sutures of 2-0 chromic are placed on both sides of the laceration and a single layer full-thickness closure using a running 2-0 chromic suture is performed. Care is taken to include mucosa with each throw. The inside of the bladder is then inspected. The trigone is again inspected to ensure patency of both ureters; the double J stent is left in place. Attention is then directed to repairing the anterior bladder wound. Stay sutures are placed on both ends of the wound and it is repaired in two layers using running 2-0 chromic catgut sutures. The first layer includes the mucosa, submucosa, and muscular layers; the second layer closes the serosa.

A 10 mm closed suction drain is placed in the retrovesical space and is brought out through a separate stab incision in the abdominal wall. The anterior abdominal wall defect is closed from the inside using 0 PDS in a running fashion. The position of the sigmoid colon is identified and placed in a position where it can be easily located.

The abdomen is irrigated with copious quantities of sterile saline. The midline fascia is closed with #1 PDS in a running fashion, the skin is closed using staples, and a sterile dressing is applied. The estimated blood loss was minimal. The operative time was about two hours. The patient received about two liters of warmed intravenous crystalloid, and his postoperative temperature was 35°C.

The patient is then placed in the lithotomy position. A repeat rectal exam is again negative for blood and no anterior wall defect is palpable. A gentle soapsuds enema is performed. The proctoscope is introduced and the rectum insufflated. The rectum is visualized and confirmed to be uninjured. If it had been injured, a single layer trans-anal repair using 3-0 Vicryl would be indicated. The patient would be re-prepped and draped and a loop sigmoid diverting colostomy performed through a left lower quadrant incision.

Post-Op Management

A cystogram is performed at 10 to 14 days. If there is no leak from the bladder, the Foley is removed. If the patient is able to void, the Jackson-Pratt drain is removed.

A single dose of pre-operative broad-spectrum antibiotics is all that is necessary, however I continue them for 24 hours.

This is considered a contaminated case, which carries a 15% to 40% risk of wound infection. If the patient remains afebrile, with a normal WBC, I leave the sterile dressing alone for 72 hours then remove it. Depending on how the wound looks, the patient can generally shower at this time. If the patient has a fever or leukocytosis, the wound should be looked at twice daily. A low threshold is maintained for removing staples if there is any drainage or periwound erythema.

- A Double J stent is inserted into the ureter to identify and protect it

- The bladder is closed with two layers of continuous absorbable sutures

- A closed suction drain is left in the retrovesical space

The risk of a urinary tract infection is 20-30%. Any fever or leukocytosis warrants a urinalysis. The ureteral stent is removed after 30 days. The patient is kept on Macrodantin during this period.

Teaching Point

A single dose of broad-spectrum antibiotics is probably all that is necessary but the risk of opportunistic infection does not increase with 24 hour dosing so I use antibiotics for 24 hours. After this, PO Bactrim or Macrodantin is indicated for prophylaxis of infection from the ureteral stent.

Conventional repair of urinary bladder injuries includes débridement of devitalized tissue, identification of ureteral and urethra orifices, watertight closure, and drainage.

Urethral and ureteral orifices should be stented to prevent them from being inadvertently included in the repair and also to protect them from unpredictable scarring and stricture formation. When in doubt, use a stent. The bladder is reevaluated with cystoscopy 30 days following the repair.

The number of layers used in closing the bladder is controversial. Some surgeons close the bladder in three layers while others routinely use a single layer. The point is that a watertight closure is desired. The posterior base of the bladder is difficult to access so a good single-layer closure is sufficient.

External drainage is also controversial. If there is a concern that the closure may not be watertight either because the injury is difficult to access or because contused tissue may not readily heal, drainage is always indicated.

Suprapubic drainage versus transurethral drainage versus using both drains simultaneously is controversial. The rationale for using two drains has been to facilitate bladder irrigation in case the Foley becomes blocked with clot. With the use of irrigating catheters, this is no longer an issue. Long-term transurethral catheters carry a very small risk of urethral stricture and epididymitis and may be uncomfortable for the patient. Other complications, including urinary tract infection, appear to be equal.

Internal repairs of the bladder using cystoscopy have been reported. This injury might have been adequately repaired with lifting the bladder and without disturbing the retrovesical planes, however, the risk of a missed rectal injury and the need for drainage may outweigh the benefit of a less invasive procedure in this case.

TECHNICAL OPERATIVE PROCEDURES:
HOW I DO IT

Repair of Intraperitoneal Bladder Laceration

Kimball I. Maull MD, FACS

Scenario
A 20-year-old man was thrown from his motorcycle at 35 miles per hour after leaving a local beer hall.

Management
He initially appeared uninjured but began to complain of abdominal pain and he could not void voluntarily. FAST demonstrates intraperitoneal fluid, an absent bladder shadow, and placement of a urethral catheter returns gross hematuria. Cystography performed by gravity in the emergency unit shows intraperitoneal extravasation. No pelvic fractures are evident by examination or plain films.

Procedure: *Repair of intraperitoneal bladder laceration*

A standard midline celiotomy is performed and the peritoneal cavity is suctioned free of copious serosanguineous fluid. The pelvis is packed with laparotomy pads and a systematic exploration of the remainder of the peritoneal cavity is accomplished. No injury is detected. The pelvic packs are removed, demonstrating a 6 cm full thickness laceration of the dome of the urinary bladder. Bleeding is moderate from the cut edges but is readily controlled with gently applied Babcock clamps. With the aid of a pediatric sweetheart retractor, the interior of the bladder is inspected and no additional injury is found.

Allis clamps are placed at the lateral-most extents of the laceration and the Babcock clamps are removed. Using a running locking hemostatic suture of 2-0 chromic catgut, the bladder wall is closed in one full thickness layer. Two sutures are used, each placed lateral to the Allis clamp, thereby assuring no gap between the lateral extent of the laceration and the placement of the anchoring suture. The sutures are run medially and tied to each other. A second row of sutures is placed incorporating both the peritoneum and bladder wall. A single continuous non-locking "baseball" suture of 2-0 chromic is utilized for this layer. The peritoneal cavity is again irrigated and suctioned free of fluid.

Using the previously placed urethral catheter, the bladder is distended by an assistant with saline to assure a watertight closure. The bladder is irrigated to confirm hemostasis. For simple intraperitoneal bladder rupture, no drains or cystotomy tube are required.

- The dome of the bladder is repaired with a running locking hemostatic absorbable suture
- A second layer of sutures incorporates the peritoneum and the bladder wall
- No drains are required

TECHNICAL OPERATIVE PROCEDURES:

HOW I DO IT

Repair of Laceration of the Bladder

Glen Tinkoff MD, FACS

Scenario

A 6 cm laceration to the dome of the bladder is encountered during exploratory laparotomy for a stab wound to the left lower quadrant of the abdomen. The laceration extends from the dome to the area of the trigone and there is free extravasation of urine into the peritoneal cavity.

Technical Aspects of Repair

A urinary drainage catheter of appropriate size is placed prior to the procedure. Placing an appropriate retractor, such as a Balfour with bladder blade, attains adequate exposure of the pelvis. The patient should be placed in 30° of Trendelenburg. The small bowel and cecum, which have previously been thoroughly inspected from ligament of Treitz to the ileocecal valve, is covered with saline moistened lap pads and packed cephalad. The pelvic cavity is aspirated dry and inspected for any additional injuries to adjacent organs. A lap pad is placed in the pouch of Douglas as a sentinel sponge.

Procedure: *Repair of bladder laceration*

The remaining peritoneum adjacent to the laceration is dissected free of the dome of the bladder. The laceration is inspected and hemostasis attained with electrocautery or suture ligature. Occasionally, the edges of the laceration will need débridement if devitalized tissue is present. The edges of the laceration are separated using narrow retractors and a suction catheter to trifurcate the opening. The bladder lumen is thoroughly inspected and the bladder neck and ureteral orifices identified. If this area is involved in the laceration further assessment of the ureters should be undertaken and a ureteral stent should be considered.

- A retractor with bladder blade provides exposure

- The patient should be in 30° of Trendelenburg

- Laceration repair in two layers

- Perivesical closed suction drain

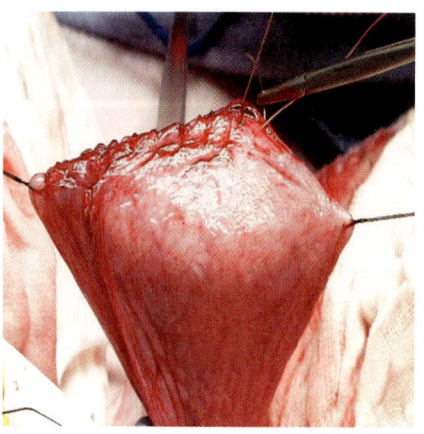

After inspection of the bladder lumen, the laceration is repaired in two layers. The mucosa and muscularis are closed using a running 3-0 absorbable suture, followed by a seromuscular closure utilizing 3-0 or 2-0 absorbable suture in continuous fashion. After completion of the repair, the perivesical space is drained using closed suction drainage placed through a separate stab wound and secured at skin level. The pelvis is copiously irrigated. The sentinel sponge in the pouch of Douglas is inspected for soilage. In most instances, suprapubic catheter drainage is not necessary.

TECHNICAL OPERATIVE PROCEDURES:

HOW I DO IT

Nephrectomy with Laceration of the Renal Artery and Vein

Stephen S. Luk, MD, FACS, FCCP

Scenario

A young female patient presents six hours after an assault with multiple stab wounds to the back and flank. She is hemodynamically stable and has no peritoneal signs.

Management

A triple contrast CT scan of the abdomen reveals no contrast flow to the left kidney with a large perinephric hematoma. There is a small amount of arterial extravasation from the renal artery. The right kidney appears normal. There is also a splenic laceration with intraperitoneal blood. The patient becomes hypotensive in the CT suite and responds to intravenous fluids. The decision is made to take the patient to the operating suite.

Procedure

Headlights are used to provide supplementary illumination, a self-retaining retractor is used, and a cell saver is available to recover blood from the patient. A standard trauma laparotomy prep is performed from nipple to knees. A midline laparotomy is performed from xiphoid to pubis symphysis and all four quadrants are packed. Exploration reveals the injury to the spleen and a large Zone II left retroperitoneal hematoma. The retroperitoneal hematoma is packed and the splenic injury does not respond to packing or splenorrhaphy. A splenectomy is performed.

Reevaluation of the retroperitoneal hematoma reveals that it has increased in size. A decision is made to explore an expanding retroperitoneal Zone II hematoma. If no assessment of the contralateral kidney has been performed, it is important to assess for its presence by palpation and, if time permits, assess its function by an IVP.

- Reevaluation of the retroperitoneal hematoma reveals that it has increased in size

- The renal artery is controlled with a vascular loop

- The kidney is mobilized

- Thrombosis of the renal vein

- An eight-hour delay in presentation indicated the need for a nephrectomy

In light of the expansion of the retroperitoneal hematoma control of the renal vessels is essential prior to exploration of the kidney. The small bowel is retracted upwards and to the right and placed into a plastic bowel bag and the bag loosely closed. A self-retaining retractor is utilized to free the surgeon and first assistant's hands. The posterior peritoneum is inspected for hematoma location and character. If there is no Zone I hematoma, the posterior peritoneum is incised lateral to the aorta and medial to the inferior mesenteric vein. The incision should extend cephalad through the ligament of Treitz to allow for proximal aortic control if necessary. The vena cava is identified and the left renal vein is identified and dissected free as it crosses over the aorta. A double looped vessel loop is loosely placed around the renal vein as it leaves the vena cava. The aorta is exposed and the left and right renal arteries can be identified as they exit the aorta. The left renal artery is dissected free and a vessel loop is passed twice around the vessel. The vessel loops are tightened and any bleeding from the kidney or renal vessel injuries should cease. The time should be noted when the vessel loops are tightened.

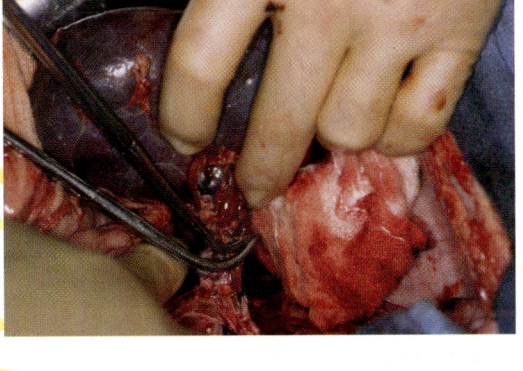

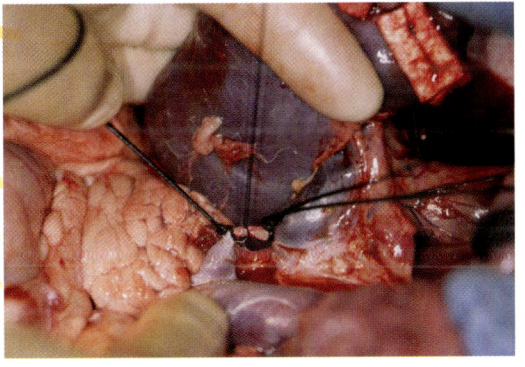

Next the kidney can be safely mobilized. The colon and mesocolon on the injured side are mobilized and rotated medially after incising the lateral peritoneal reflection. Wide exposure of Gerota's fascia is performed and the anterior surface of the fascia is incised vertically. The kidney is then mobilized utilizing sharp and blunt dissection techniques. Complete mobilization of the kidney is performed. This allows the kidney to be lifted anteriorly and medially, and allows for evaluation of the kidney and the hilar vessels.

This patient had complete transection of the renal vein that had thrombosed and was not actively bleeding. The renal transection bled significantly when proximal control was released. The patient presented in a delayed fashion and over eight hours passed since the time of injury to laparotomy. A nephrectomy was performed.

The ureter was dissected free by mobilizing the kidney and following it down to the pelvic brim. It was then ligated and transected. The renal bed was then inspected and irrigated with saline. Hemostasis was ensured. The abdomen was then closed.

TECHNICAL OPERATIVE PROCEDURES:
HOW I DO IT

Renal Laceration Involving the Collecting System

Erwin F. Hirsch, MD, FACS

Scenario

A 37-year-old man sustains a stab wound to the left flank. An enhanced CT scan shows a 4 cm laceration to the lower pole of the left kidney which involves the collecting system. There is free extravasation of urine and a significant hematoma.

Management

The overall approach to renal trauma is nonoperative management. Early intervention may result in nephrectomy while nonoperative management in most instances has a favorable outcome.

In the scenario described, the decision was made to proceed surgically because of the extravasation of urine and a significant expanding hematoma.

Renal salvage should be the overriding emphasis in this case. Control of the renal artery and vein by means of vessel loops should allow the surgeon to stage the magnitude of the injury and decide what procedure is indicated. The laceration is in the lower pole and measures 4 cm. Nearly 60% of the lower pole is involved. Furthermore, the presence of free extravasation indicates that the wound probably involves half the depth of the organ.

In this scenario, I would complete the partial lower nephrectomy by ligating the polar arteries and vein with Vicryl stitches. The collecting system is exposed. I approximate the free renal cut edges with Vicryl mattress stitches. The use of biological sealants, such as fibrin glue, may help to further control hemostasis. A Jackson-Pratt drain should be left in place and the wound closed.

- Control of the renal artery and vein allows the surgeon to stage the magnitude of the injury

- The collecting system is repaired with mattress sutures

- Closed suction drainage is essential

TECHNICAL OPERATIVE PROCEDURES:
HOW I DO IT

The Management of a 3 cm Deep Laceration to the Lower Pole of the Left Kidney in Which There is Active Extravasation of Urine

L.D. Britt, MD, MPH, FACS

Scenario

A 24-year-old man sustains a stab wound to the left flank. He is brought to the emergency department where he is assessed to be alert and hemodynamically stable but has grossly bloody urine.

Management

Crystalloid resuscitation is initiated and the patient is taken to the operative theater for an emergency celiotomy. The chest x-ray obtained demonstrates bilateral expanded lungs with no pneumothorax or hemothorax. The patient is taken to the operative theater for an emergency celiotomy.

Procedure

The abdomen is widely prepped and draped. A midline vertical transabdominal incision is made. Abdominal exploration demonstrates a large left perinephric hematoma which does not appear to cross the midline. With the small intestine lifted out of the abdominal cavity, the inferior mesenteric vein is identified. An incision is made just medial to the vein and over the aorta. The incision is extended superiorly to the ligament of Treitz. Dissection is performed on the anterior aspect of the aorta. The left renal vein is found superiorly. A soft silicone vessel loop is applied for vascular control. The left renal artery is found just superior and lateral to the renal vein. Vascular control of this vessel is also performed in the same manner. With the appropriate vascular isolation and control, an incision is made lateral to the left colon to facilitate medial mobilization and obtain better exposure of the perinephric hematoma. With

- Proximal control of the renal pedicle vessels

- The kidney is exposed

- The collecting system is repaired with a continuous suture

- The repair is buttressed with omentum

- Closed suction drains are placed in the retroperitoneal space

Gerota's fascia being distorted by the hematoma, dissection is done directly through the hematoma in order to expose the entire kidney. A 3 cm deep laceration is found in the lower pole of the left kidney with active extravasation of urine. There was no major bleeding or substantial nonviable tissue. A linear laceration in the collecting system is closed primarily with a running 4-0 Vicryl suture. The oozing from the lacerated renal parenchyma is controlled with the application of Gelfoam and the capsule is closed with interrupted 3-0 Vicryl, along with an omental buttress. A closed-suction drain is placed in the retroperitoneal space. The abdominal cavity is, again, thoroughly inspected prior to closure of the abdominal wound.

TECHNICAL OPERATIVE PROCEDURES:

HOW I DO IT

Management of a Kidney Laceration Involving the Collecting System

David B. Hoyt, M.D., FACS

Scenario

A 24-year-old is stabbed in the right flank and presents with hematuria, peritoneal tenderness, and has gross extravasation of contrast on preoperative IVP.

Management

This patient should be taken to the operating room and undergo exploration. The presence of a retroperitoneal hematoma in the area of the kidney on the right side would indicate the source of the injury. After adequate exploration of the rest of the abdomen the focus would be turned to this injury.

Procedure

A judgment would be made regarding the likelihood of repair versus the need for nephrectomy. Vascular isolation would be rapidly obtained after mobilizing the right colon and duodenum so that potential for repair is optimized. This would be done by careful dissection of the renal artery and vein just lateral to the great vessels and looped with vascular loops. Gerota's fascia would then be opened, usually easiest to identify in the area of the laceration, and the incision then continued in a curvilinear fashion around the kidney and the kidney is mobilized. A laceration would be identified in the inferior pole and while using manual compression to control bleeding, the kidney would be mobilized into the surgical field and inspected carefully. The wound would be evaluated for its depth and association with injury to the collecting system.

Parenchymal bleeders would be identified and ligated and the parenchyma exposed to reveal the laceration in the collecting system. With the collecting system well exposed, this would be closed using a running absorbable suture. The parenchyma would be inspected further for bleeding and then the parenchyma and renal capsule would be closed primarily with horizontal mattress sutures tied over an omental pedicle. Prior to tying the sutures, the pedicle would be mobilized and placed underneath the sutures to allow reinforcement of the suture line and provide further hemostasis. A suction drain would then be placed and monitored for urinary leak

- Parenchymal bleeders would be identified and ligated

- Two layer closure

- Omentum is placed over the repair

- Closed suction perirepair drainage

postoperatively for about seven days. An IVP would be obtained in 10 to 14 days to assure healing. The drain would be removed after approximately one week, if there was no urinary leak. In the event of a persistent urinary leak, cystoscopy and placement of a double J stent to decompress the collecting system would be done. The drain would be left in place until there was no further urinary drainage.

TECHNICAL OPERATIVE PROCEDURES:

HOW I DO IT

Ureteral Repair

Michael Rhodes MD, FACS

Scenario

A 19-year-old male suffers a stab wound to the right flank. His abdomen is tender prompting an exploratory laparotomy. He has a small laceration of the posterior medial cecum with minimal spillage which is repaired primarily. In reflecting the cecum medially, it is noted that he has an 80% laceration of the mid ureter.

Management

Injuries to the mid-ureter are usually repaired primarily over a stent. It is my practice to consult my urologic colleague either intraoperatively or postoperatively since the most difficult part of the case is finding and placing an appropriate stent. The urologist is also well suited to aid in dealing with postoperative care, including stent removal.

In this case, it may be tempting to leave the 20% bridge and repair the 80% rent. I recommend completing the laceration so that the edges can be sharply débrided. It is usually necessary to mobilize both ends of the ureter to avoid tension. It is an error in technique to skeletonize the ureter. Instead, the adventitial tissue around the ureter is kept intact when mobilizing. Only obviously non-viable edges should be excised so that as much ureter is spared as possible.

To avoid stricture, I spatulate the anterior wall of the superior segment and the posterior wall of the inferior segment. This is done by making a 3 mm vertical incision in the edge of the ureter. Prior to repair, a double J stent is placed proximally into the renal pelvis and distally into the bladder.

Ask for a 6 or 7 Fr., 22 to 30 cm double J ureteral stent with a Glidewire. The guidewire is placed through one of the stent side holes and advanced beyond the tip and then into the renal pelvis after which the stent is advanced over the guidewire. The guidewire is removed and redirected through a side hole distally into the bladder over which the distal portion of the stent is advanced. The guidewire is then removed from the side hole and the proximal and distal ends of the stents will curl into the renal pelvis and bladder.

I then repair the ureter using 4-0 Vicryl or 4-0 PDS interrupted sutures beginning with the

- It is an error to skeletonize the ureter

- The repair is performed over a stent

- A closed suction drain is brought out laterally

lateral sutures. The suture is tied with minimum tension, but the bites are no more than 2 mm apart to gain a good seal. Many surgeons recommend a continuous suture to gain a watertight repair. I think the same security can be gained with the interrupted technique with less narrowing of the lumen. Non-absorbable sutures should be avoided since they may become a nidus for stone formation.

The ureteral repair should have tissue placed between it and any other anastomosis of bowel or vessels. The ureter is drained laterally using a closed suction flat drain.

TECHNICAL OPERATIVE PROCEDURES:
HOW I DO IT

Ureteral Repair

Thomas M. Scalea, MD, FACS, FCCM

Scenario

A 20-year-old man presents with a gunshot wound through the ureter at the pelvic brim from a .32 caliber gun. There is a 1 cm defect in the ureter.

Management

Operative exploration for gunshot wounds to the ureter follows the same principles as exploratory laparotomy for all penetrating trauma. In general, these patients have evidence of retroperitoneal trajectory and usually have a retroperitoneal hematoma adjacent to the right colon. Depending on the presence or absence of vascular injury, this may be very large or relatively small. Injuries to the ureter are not life-threatening. Therefore, vascular injuries and other hollow visceral injuries take precedent. Once these are addressed, the ureter should be explored.

- Vascular injuries and other hollow visceral injuries take precedent

- It is important not to mistake the ureter for the gonadal vessels

Complete mobilization of the right colon allows for direct exploration of the retroperitoneum and identification of the ureter. I incise the peritoneum at the white line of Toldt. I generally fully mobilize the right colon around the hepatic flexure to the mid transverse colon. I also fully mobilize the cecum and the terminal ileum by doing a complete medial visceral rotation. Thus, I am able to trace the ureter in its entirety.

The ureter can be identified in the retroperitoneum as it courses along the psoas muscle. It is important to not mistake the ureter for the gonadal vessels. Some believe that gently pinching the ureter with a pair of pickups will promote peristalsis. While this can be helpful, it is not absolute. I generally identify the ureter by feel. Its wall is thicker than that of the adjacent vasculature.

If it is difficult to identify the ureter in the retroperitoneum, one is almost always able to identify it as it courses over the iliac vessels at the bifurcation of the common iliac artery. This anatomic relationship is surprisingly constant and varies very little from patient to patient. The ureter can then be traced retrograde. It is important to investigate the ureter throughout the area of potential injury. One should take care not to devascularize the ureter by stripping the adjacent tissue for long distances. This is counterbalanced by the need to circumferentially investigate the possibility of injury. I have found using methylene blue to be of very little help. The amount of time it takes for the urine to turn blue often exceeds the desired time in the operating room. Instead, I carefully examine the ureter throughout its course. A skilled surgeon should be able to identify ureteral injury.

Procedure: *Ureteral repair*

In this case, there is a 1cm defect in the ureter. As injuries at the pelvic brim are still a good distance from the bladder, I believe that end to end anastomosis is the best idea. Devitalized ureter should be débrided back to normal tissue. Mobilizing the ureter carefully should allow one to get sufficient length on the ureter to do an end-to-end anastomosis. To avoid ureteral stricture, I spatulate the ends of the ureter and assure adequate mobilization to obtain a tension free anastomosis. I generally use magnifying loupes to do the ureteral repair, so that I can place the suture with meticulous technique.

Ureteral repairs should be performed over a double J stent. The stent allows the ureter to heal with less likelihood of later stricture. The appropriate size stents should be selected and guidewire placed into the stent. And for this injury, I would thread the stent cephalad first. It is important to ensure that the stent is placed all the way into the renal pelvis. The guidewire can then be removed. The distal portion of the stent for an injury in this location often can be placed into the distal ureteral into the bladder without using a guide wire. If this is impossible, the guidewire can be again used. If it is difficult to pass the stent, one trick is to perform a cystotomy and then pass the stent in one motion up through the ureteral orifice through the injury and up to the kidney. The cystotomy can then be closed in two layers. Before I perform the ureteral repair, I obtain an x-ray to make sure the stent is positioned.

I generally repair the ureter using 4-0 Vicryl sutures. I tend to use interrupted sutures as I think that the chance of stricture is probably less. Even well-constructed repairs are not water tight. Therefore, I leave a Jackson-Pratt drain adjacent to the repair. This usually drains urine for a few days and then volume dries up.

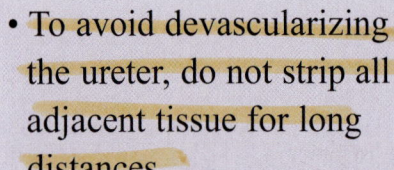

- To avoid devascularizing the ureter, do not strip all adjacent tissue for long distances

- Spatulate the ureteral ends and assure adequate mobilization to obtain a tension free anastomosis

- Leave a Jackson-Pratt drain adjacent to the repair

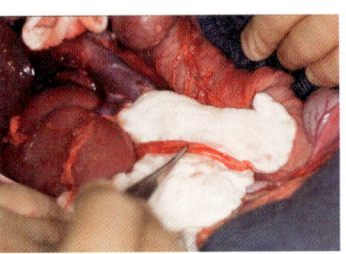
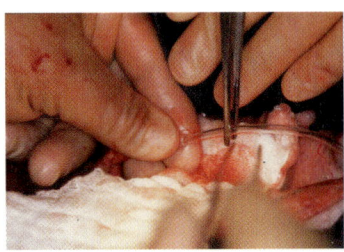
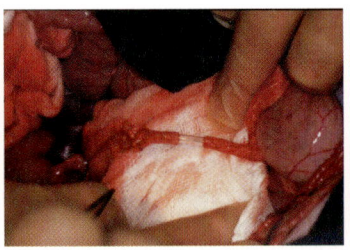
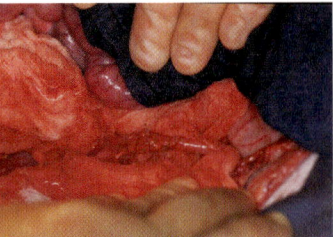

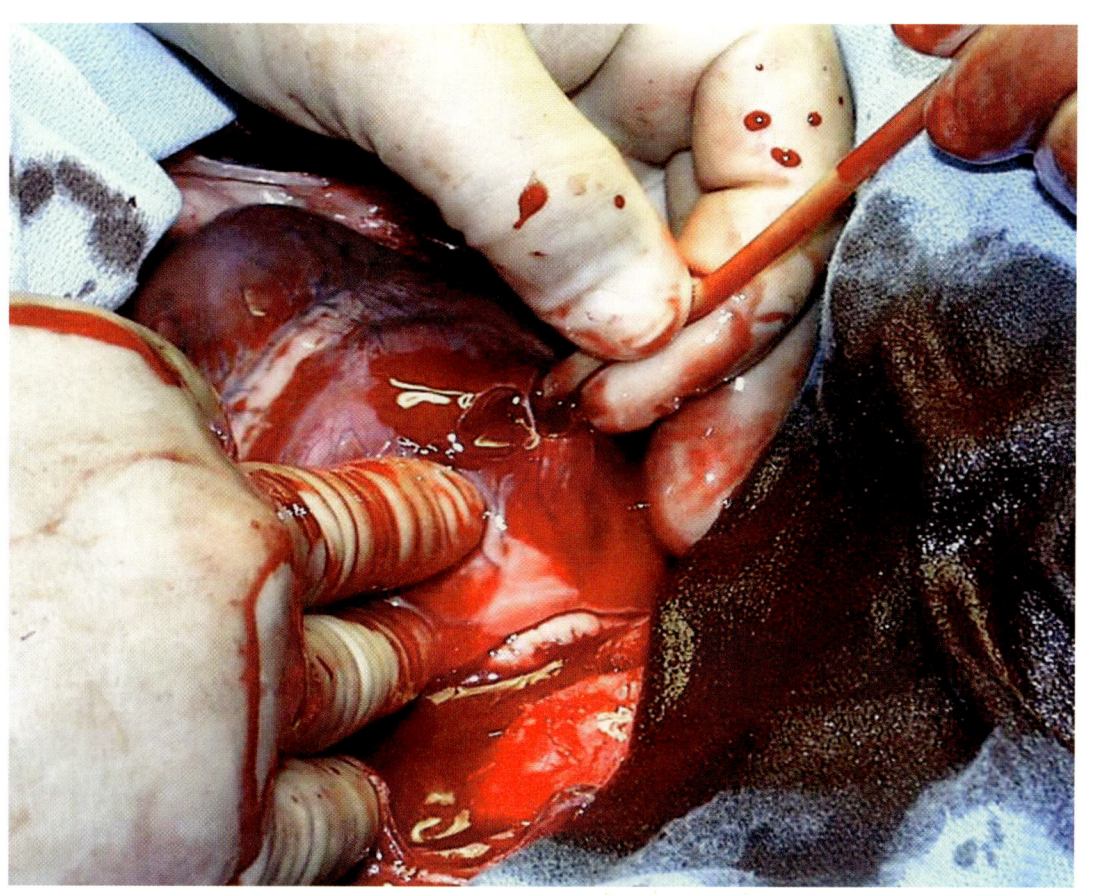

The Cardiac and Vascular System

6

Overview

- Penetrating cardiac injuries
- Emergency department thoracotomy
- Aortic injuries
- Inferior vena cava injuries
- Exposure of iliac vein injuries

Penetrating Cardiac Injuries

Immediate thoracotomy is indicated in only 5% of patients with penetrating thoracic injuries. Patients requiring immediate thoracotomy present to the emergency department with cardiac tamponade and massive hemorrhage.

Up to 15% of patients with penetrating thoracic injury require delayed thoracotomy. These patients' wounds consist of compensated cardiac tamponade, ongoing bleeding, and specific organ injury that includes the esophagus and great vessels, and delayed hemothorax.

About 80% of patients who present with penetrating injuries to the thorax require tube thoracostomy and evaluation. These patients' injuries include hemothorax and pneumothorax.

Penetrating Thoracic Injury
Types of Treatment Required

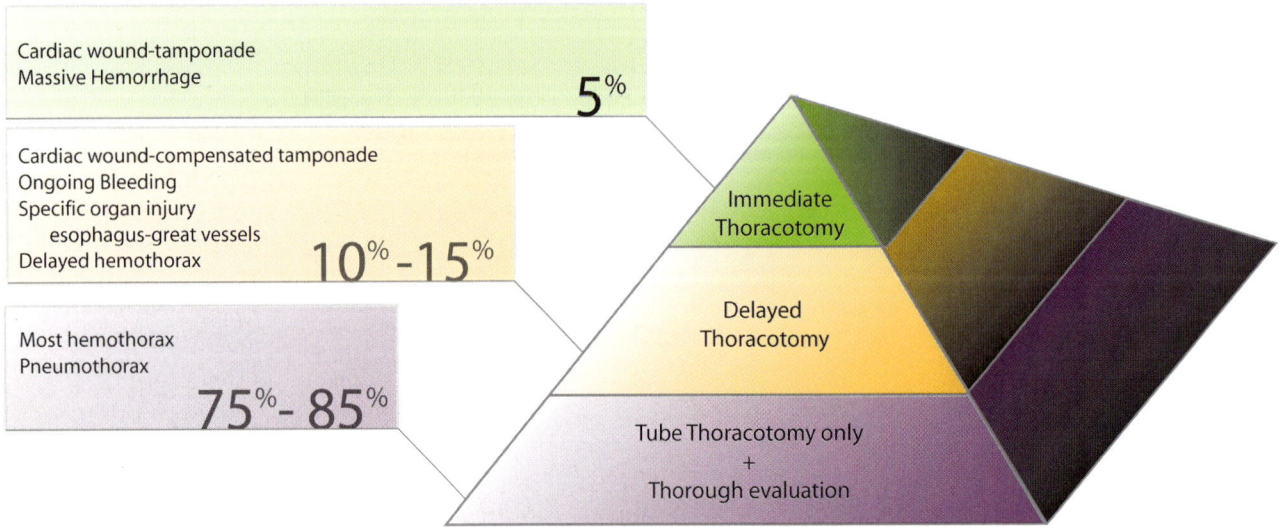

Ivatury et. al., The Textbook of Penetrating Trauma, 1996

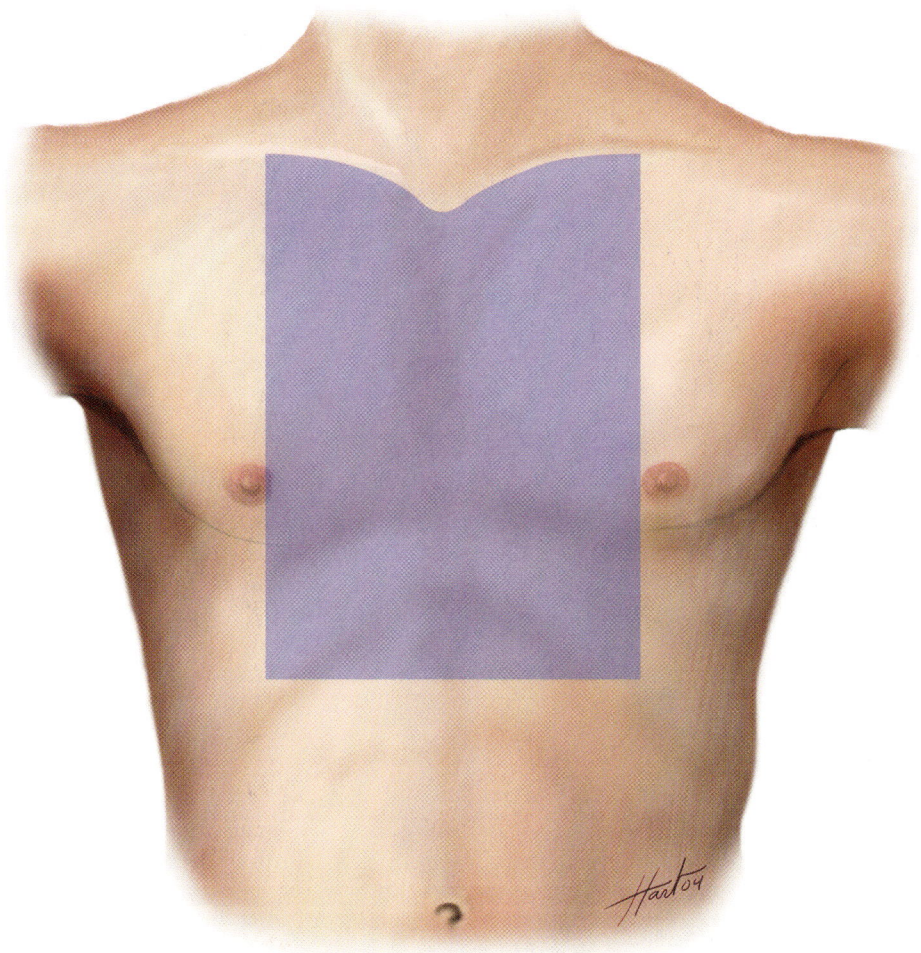

High Incidence of Cardiac Injury

The physician should maintain a high index of suspicion in order to diagnose potential cardiac injuries. A diagnosis can be made using echocardiography, chest x-ray, or intraoperative exploration. Patients at high risk for cardiac injuries include those with penetrating wounds to the anterior thorax between the nipple lines, clavicles, and costal margins.

INJURIES TO THE BOX

- Mid clavicular line bilaterally
- Suprasternal notch
- Xiphoid

Management of Cardiac Injuries
ABC's of Resuscitation

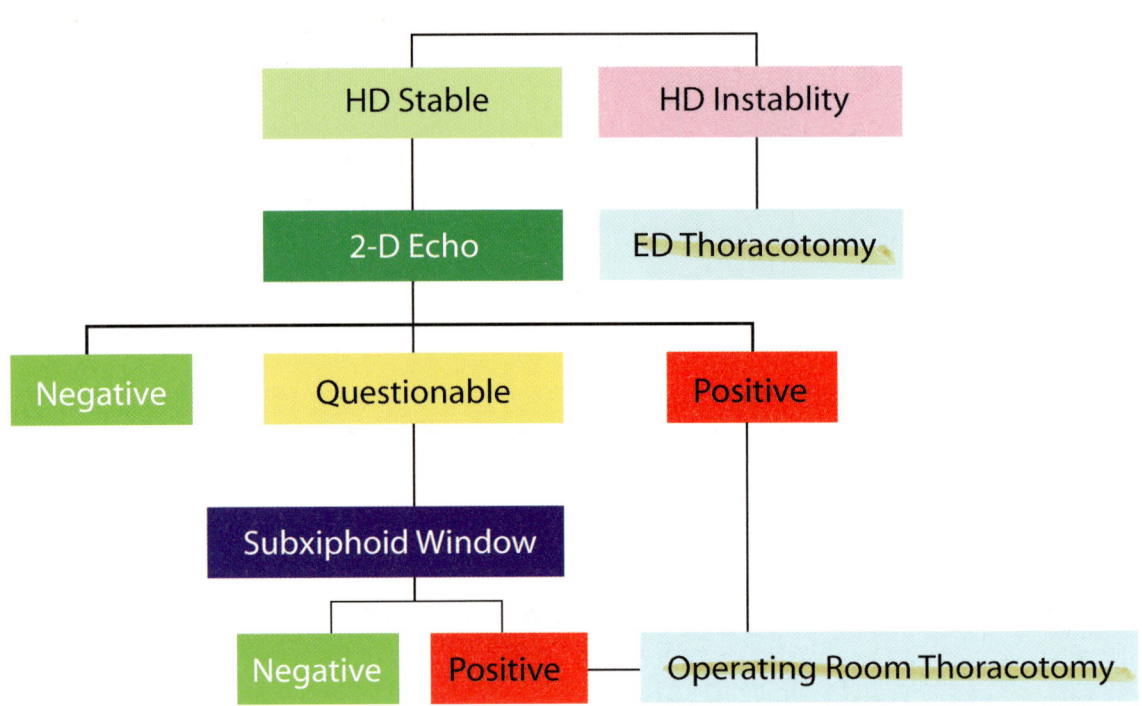

Mattox et. al., Trauma 4th Ed., 2000

Management of Cardiac Injuries

Hemodynamically stable patients presenting to the emergency department for evaluation of cardiac injuries should undergo echocardiography. No further work-up is needed if the results are negative. If the results are questionable, the patient should have a repeat echocardiogram. Some patients may instead require a diagnostic subxiphoid window in the operating room. No additional surgical intervention is needed if the results of this are negative. However, a thoracotomy will be required to repair cardiac injury if results are positive.

An emergency department thoracotomy may be indicated for hemodynamically unstable patients who arrive in the emergency department. The procedure should be followed by intraoperative exploration and repair of identified cardiac injuries.

Cardiac Injury

Cardiac injuries are most commonly caused by stab or gunshot wounds. Injuries associated with the ribs or sternum can also cause cardiac injuries, but this very rarely occurs. The cardiac structures likely to be injured, in order of decreasing frequency, include the right ventricle, left ventricle, right atrium, left atrium, and great vessels.

Symptoms

Symptoms of cardiac tamponade may not be present on the initial evaluation. Serial physical examinations should be done during the diagnostic evaluation. There should be a high suspicion for cardiac effusion developing into cardiac tamponade in patients with penetrating anterior thoracic injury.

Beck's triad, which consists of increased venous pressure, decreased blood pressure, and muffled heart sounds, may be difficult to assess in an injured patient secondary to a hypovolemic state and the noise level in the trauma resuscitation room. Pulsus paradoxus may also be difficult to assess in this environment.

CARDIAC INJURY

- Stab wounds or gunshot wounds

- Rarely, ribs or sternum

- Structures injured:

    - right ventricle: bleed more
    - left ventricle: bleed less, thick muscular wall
    - right atrium
    - left atrium
    - great vessels

SIGNS AND SYMPTOMS

- Asymptomatic

- Cardiac tamponade

- Beck's triad
    - increased central venous pressure
    - decreased systolic blood pressure
    - muffled heart sounds

- Pulsus paradoxus

- Hemothorax

DIAGNOSIS

- Clinically
- Echo

Cardiac Tamponade: Diagnosis

Clinical examination can be the basis for the diagnosis of cardiac tamponade, but echocardiography in the trauma room provides a more specific diagnosis.

Cardiac Tamponade: Treatment

A patient who has cardiac effusion and the subsequent development of tamponade should be treated with additional intravenous fluids to increase the preload to overcome the effects of fluid accumulation in the pericardial sac, which compresses the myocardium.

Once the diagnosis of cardiac tamponade or symptomatic effusion has been made, decompression in the operating room must occur immediately. The surgical approach may be either through a median sternotomy or left anterolateral thoracotomy, depending on the surgeon's operative approach and the pattern of injury.

Control of the bleeding is essential once the tamponade has been decompressed. Direct digital control of the injury stops the pulsatile hemorrhage and allows for an assessment of the injury and planned repair of the myocardium.

TREATMENT

- Increase preload
  - volume

- Decompression once identified
  - open in the operating room

- Repair myocardium

- Repair myocardial vascular injuries

Surgical Approaches

As stated earlier, surgical approaches to repair of cardiac injuries and decompression of tamponade may include a median sternotomy (A), or left anterolateral thoracotomy (C & D). Extension of the thoracotomy across the sternum to the contralateral chest (E) also provides exposure of the heart and great vessels. A trapdoor incision (B) gives complete exposure of the great vessels at the superior aspect of the heart.

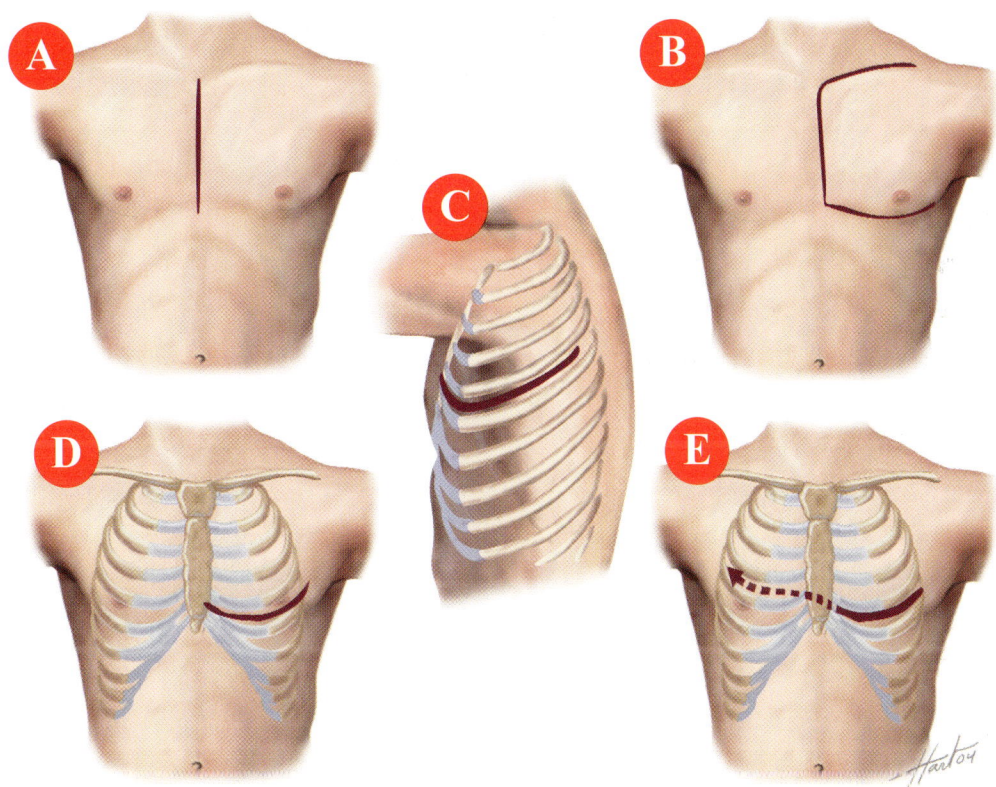

Emergency Department Thoracotomy

If an emergency department thoracotomy is indicated, the patient must be emergently intubated and have an orogastric or nasogastric tube inserted. Adequate intravenous access is needed for continued resuscitation and administration of anesthetics.

The patient must be supine for optimal exposure of the anterolateral left thorax. Extending the patient's left arm parallel to the head and neck facilitates positioning. A wide prep with Betadine and draping of the sterile field should follow.

Once the fifth intercostal space or inframammary fold has been identified, an incision is carried from the lateral edge of the sternum to the latissimus dorsi with a #10 scalpel blade. The intercostal muscles must be opened carefully to prevent an iatrogenic injury to the lung or heart.

APPROACH

- Intubated

- Orogastric tube

- IV access

- Supine

- Left arm above the head with wide prep

- 5th intercostal space

- Inframammary fold

- Sternum to latissimus dorsi

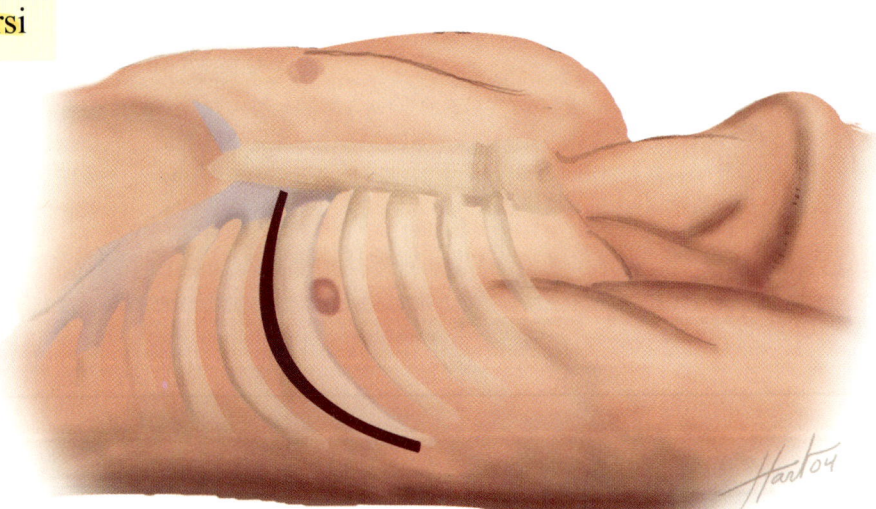

A Finochietto rib spreader is inserted into the incision between the ribs with the retraction arm parallel with the table and overlying the latissimus dorsi muscle. Next, the pericardium is identified and opened longitudinally, taking great care to avoid transecting the phrenic nerve. The tamponade is then decompressed.

The bleeding site is identified and digitally controlled. At this time, bleeding may be more effectively controlled with skin staples placed parallel and adjacent to each other. The heart and great vessels are then inspected for other injuries. Pledgeted sutures are used to reinforce the staple line once the heart has been inspected and all wounds have been controlled with digital control and/or staples.

The use of a vascular clamp on the descending aorta above the diaphragm has not been shown to improve survival. If a cross clamp is applied, an orogastric or nasogastric tube must be inserted to differentiate the esophagus from a volume depleted aorta. Making this differentiation can be difficult in the severely hypotensive patient. The inferior pulmonary ligament must be taken down to provide adequate access to the descending aorta above the diaphragm.

TECHNIQUE

- Place rib spreader

- Open cardiac massage

- Open pericardium longitudinally
  -avoid phrenic nerve

- Open cardiac massage

After the myocardium has been repaired, the vascular clamp on the aorta should be removed slowly to prevent a drop in blood pressure. The need for additional volume and pressors should be assessed at this time.

A left anterolateral thoracotomy with extension through the sternum to the right thorax provides excellent exposure of the heart, great vessels, and the structures of the right thorax.

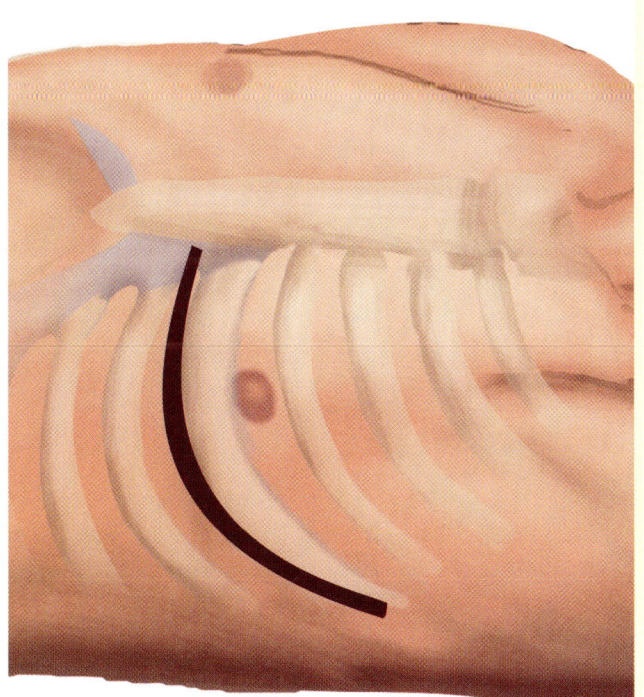

PROCEDURE

- Control hemorrhage

- Assess for coronary air emboli

- Perform:
  - cardiorrhaphy
  - vascular repair

- Examine posterior surface

- Intermittent cardiac massage

POST-REPAIR

- Defibrillate
- Assess for pressors
- Assure hemostasis
- Control mammary arteries
- Definitive care in the operating room

Penetrating Cardiac Injury

Emergency Department Thoracotomy: Maneuvers

Opening the pericardium longitudinally, while avoiding the phrenic nerve, completely exposes the heart and the tamponade is evacuated. In this case, the inferior pulmonary ligament is transected. A vascular clamp was placed on the hilum of the lung to prevent air emboli secondary to severe lung injury.

Digital Control

The use of digital control followed by the placement of multiple staples close to each other will control initial bleeding from the myocardium and allow for effective resuscitation. Pledgets can be used to reinforce a staple line.

Foley Control

A Foley catheter can also be used to control larger injuries to the heart, which require more extensive repair.

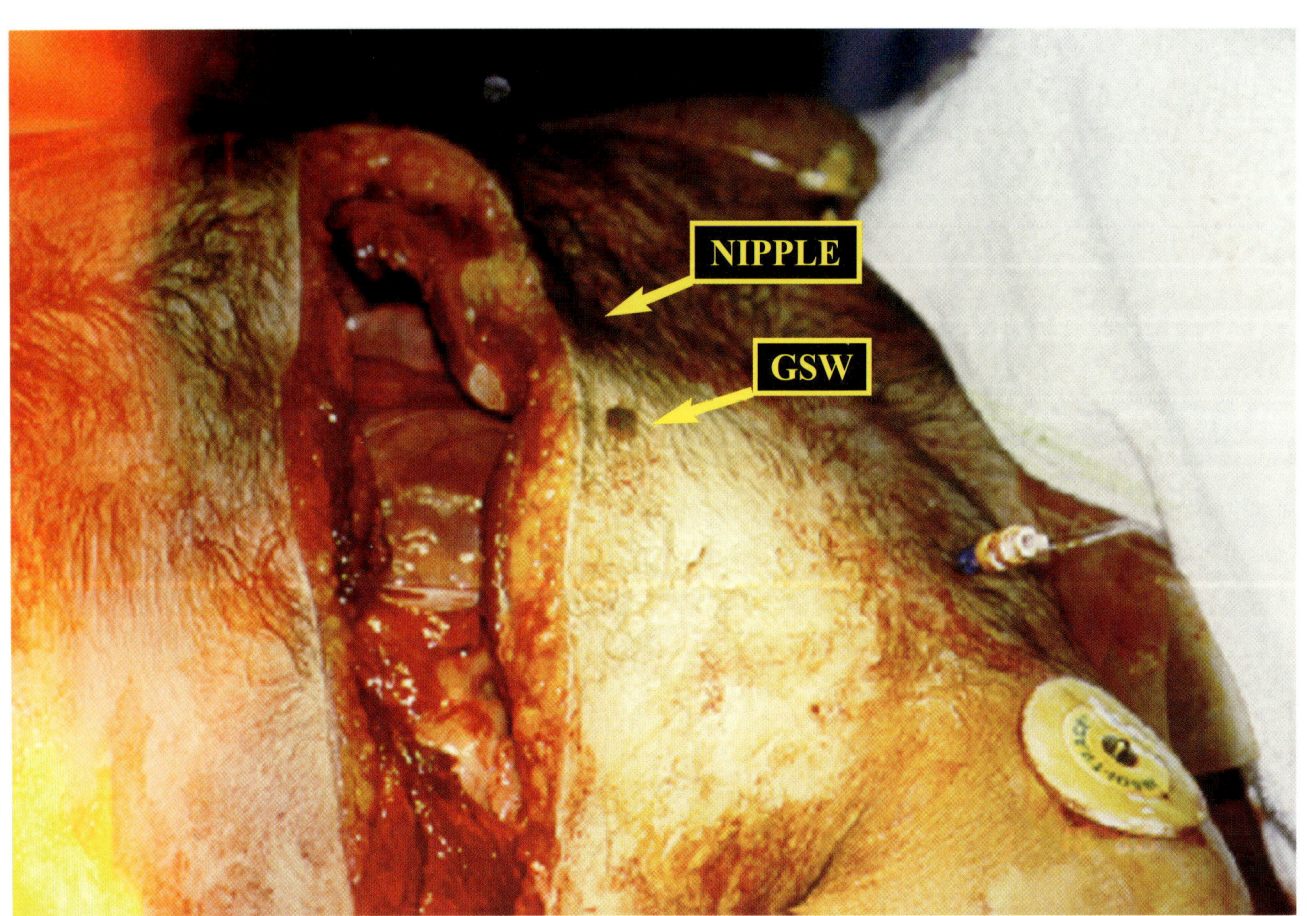

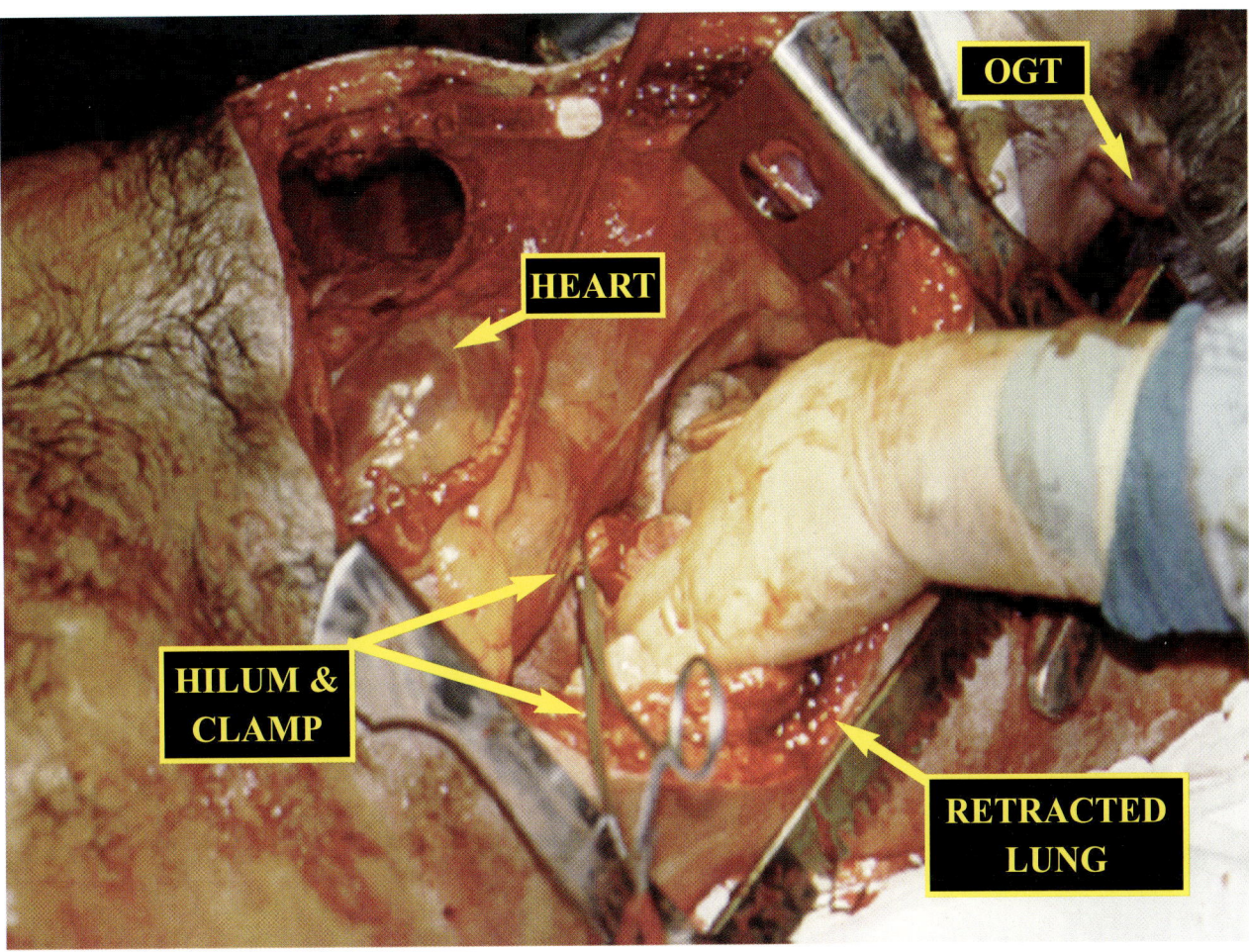

Postoperative Complications

Additional complications that may develop after cardiac injuries have been repaired include arrhythmias from myocardial ischemia or disruption of the conducting system. There may be injuries to the valves, the chordae tendineae, or the papillae. These injuries can lead to valvular incompetence.

A transesophageal echocardiogram may be indicated in order to assess for intracardiac injuries if the patient is hemodynamically unstable in the operating room. If the patient is stable, additional echocardiography, including a transthoracic echocardiogram and transesophageal echocardiogram, may be indicated once the patient arrives in the intensive care unit.

CARDIAC INJURIES

- Complications
  - conducting system injury
  - coronary vessel injury
  - valve injury

- Follow up echo
  - transthoracic echocardiogram

  - transesophageal echocardiogram

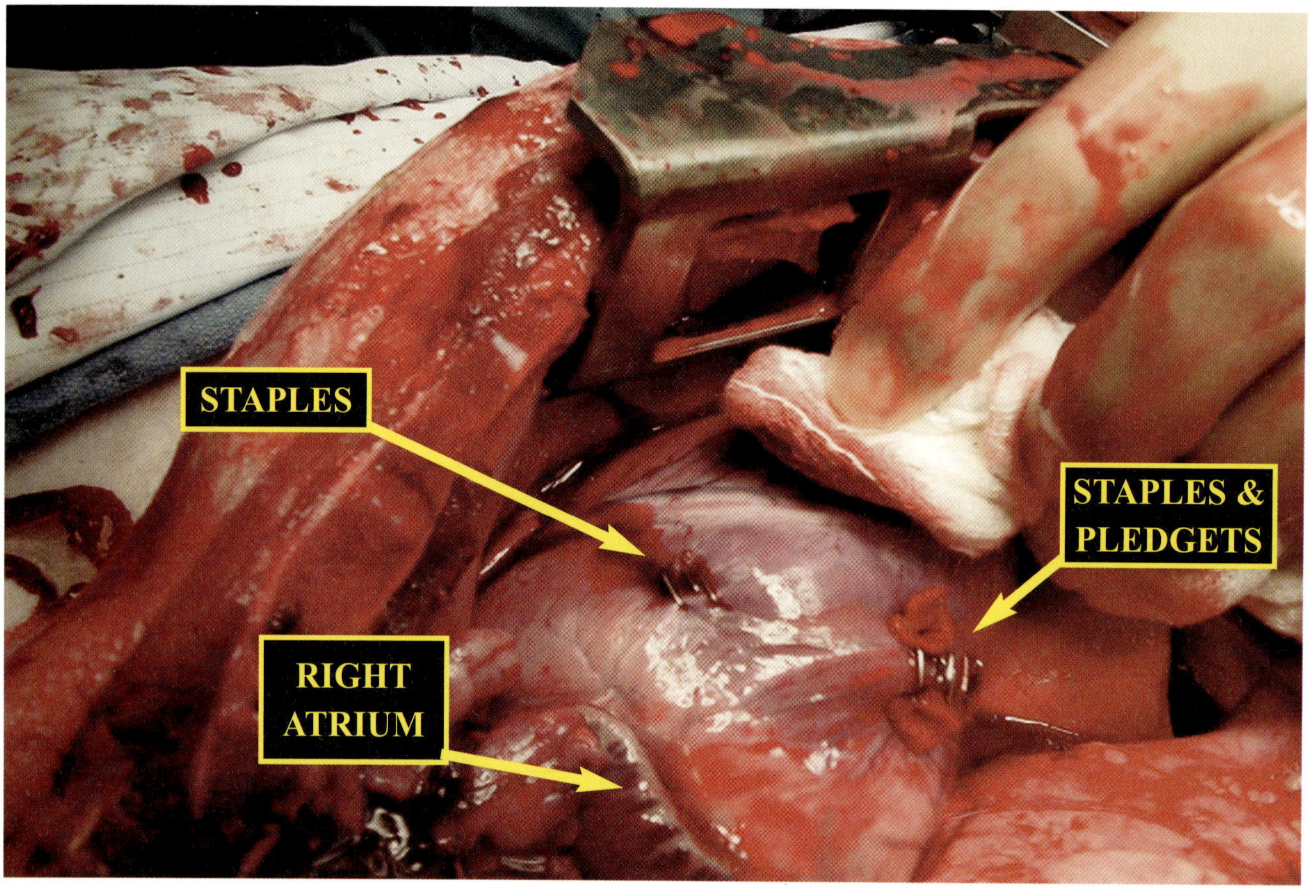

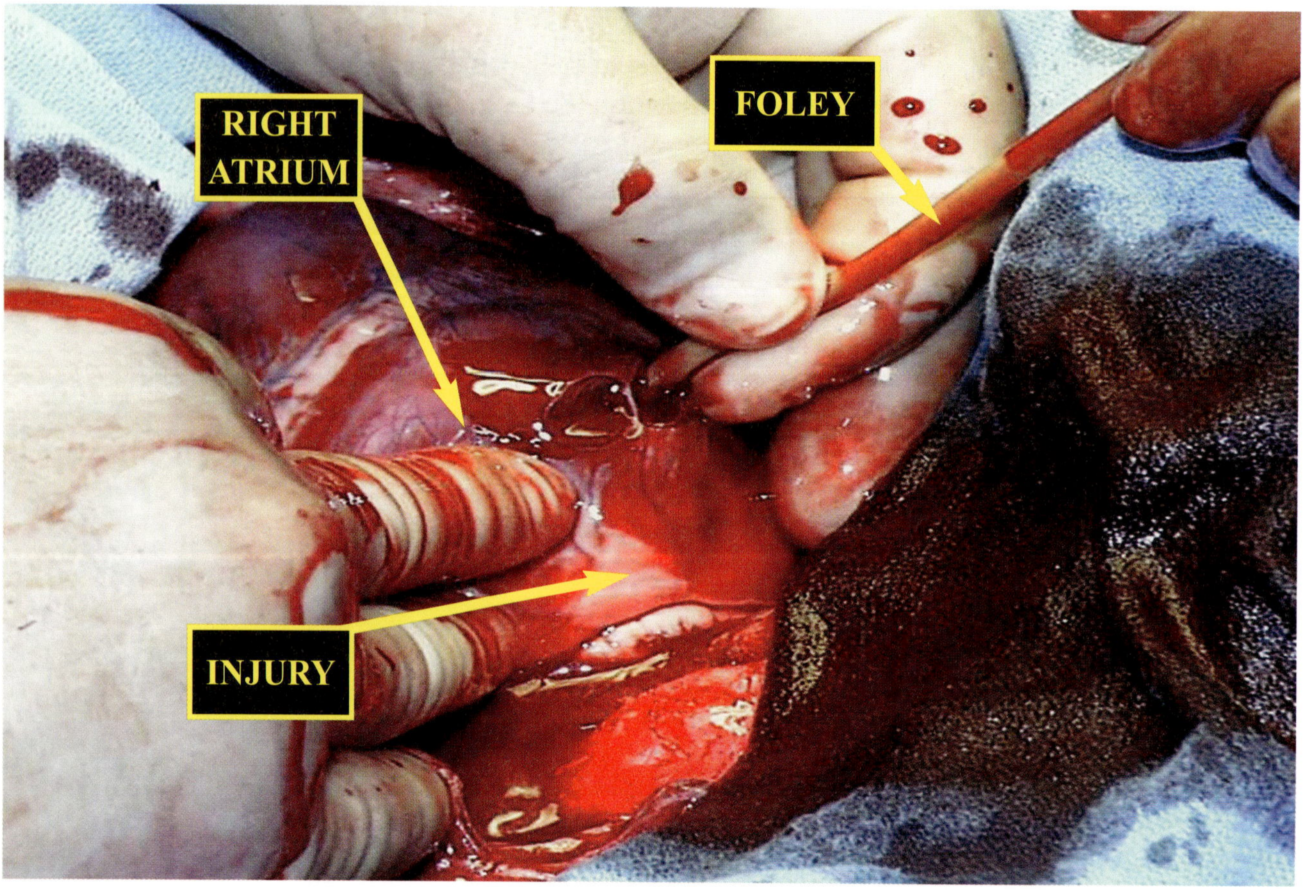

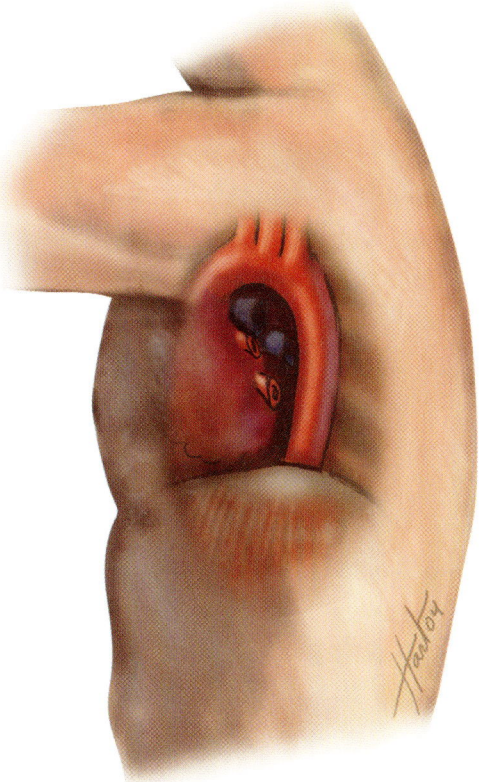

Injuries to the aorta commonly occur within the superior and posterior mediastinum.

Aortic Injuries

Mechanisms of Blunt Aortic Injury

A blunt aortic injury caused by a deceleration mechanism is usually located distal to the ligamentum arteriosum and the takeoff of the left subclavian artery. Disruption of the ascending aorta may be caused by the water hammer stress effect, which forces blood against a closed aortic valve. Compression, torsion, and shearing of the ascending aorta as the sternum is compressed against the center of the vertebral column may cause transection.

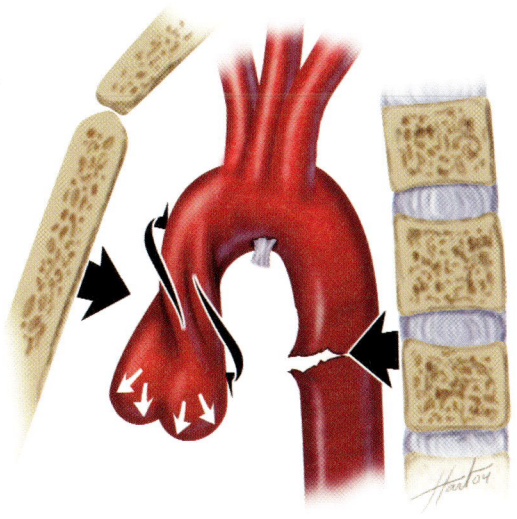

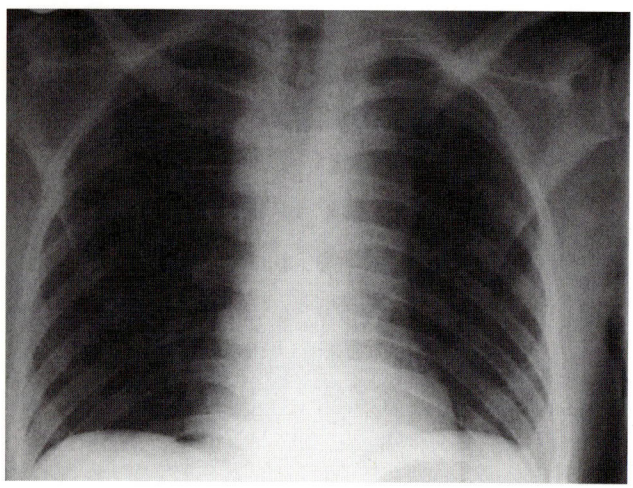

Diagnosis

The diagnosis of a transected aorta can be facilitated by a number of signs seen on chest x-ray, including a widened mediastinum. Other signs include, but are not limited to, an orogastric tube or nasogastric tube shifted to the right, an apical cap, and the absence of rib fractures with a left hemothorax.

Surgical Repair

It is important to gain proximal and distal control before entering the hematoma surrounding the injured vessel. This holds true for any vascular injury and aortic injuries.

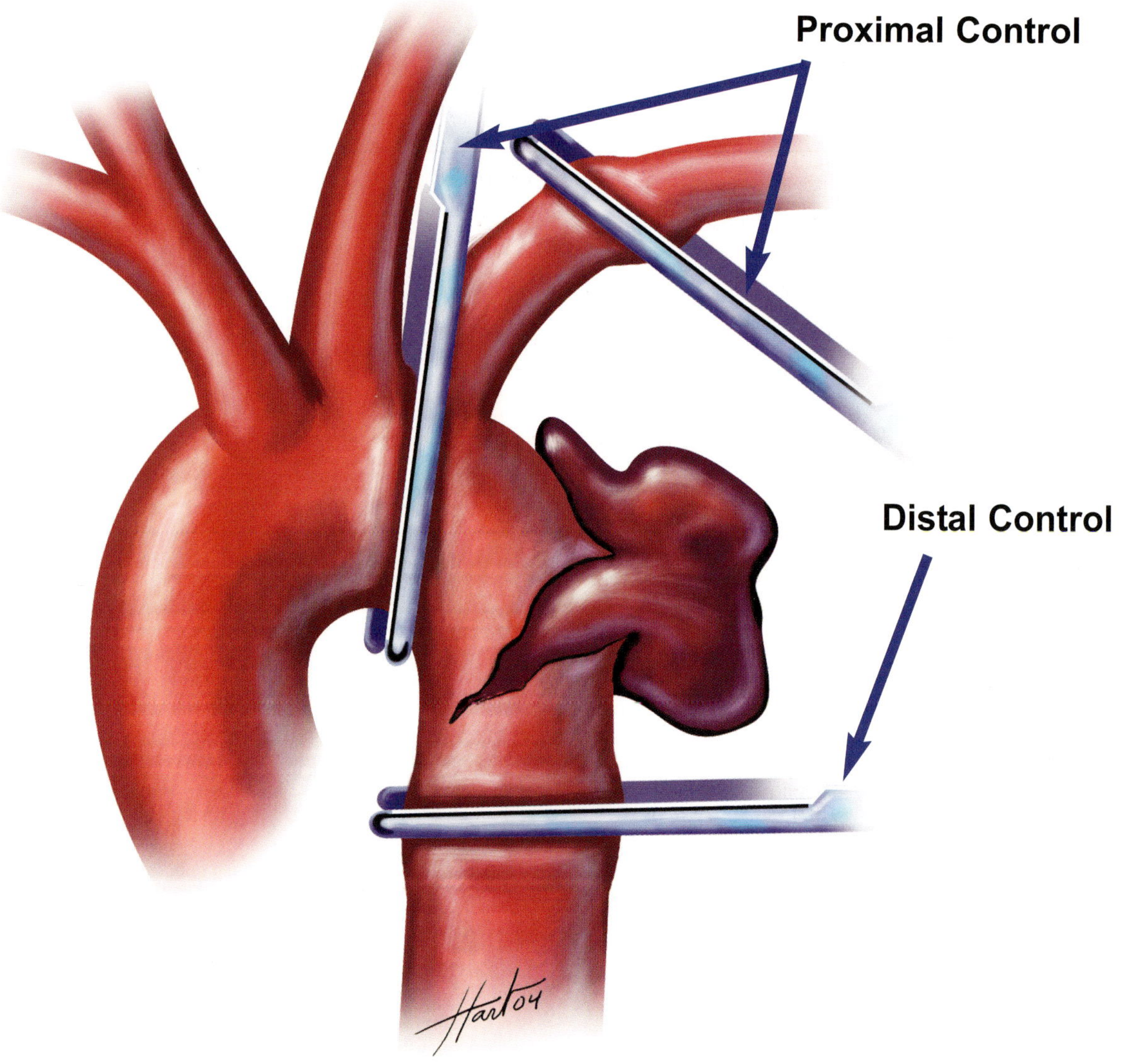

Proximal Control

Distal Control

Clamp, Bypass or Shunt

The incidence of paraplegia may be as high as 30% if the cross clamp time is greater than thirty minutes in patients undergoing repair of blunt aortic injuries. This is secondary to spinal cord ischemia.

Profusion of the artery of Adamkiewicz, which supplies blood to the spinal cord, may be enhanced with a roller pump. The use of passive shunts such as Gott shunts, which bypass the injured segment of the aorta, has also been successful.

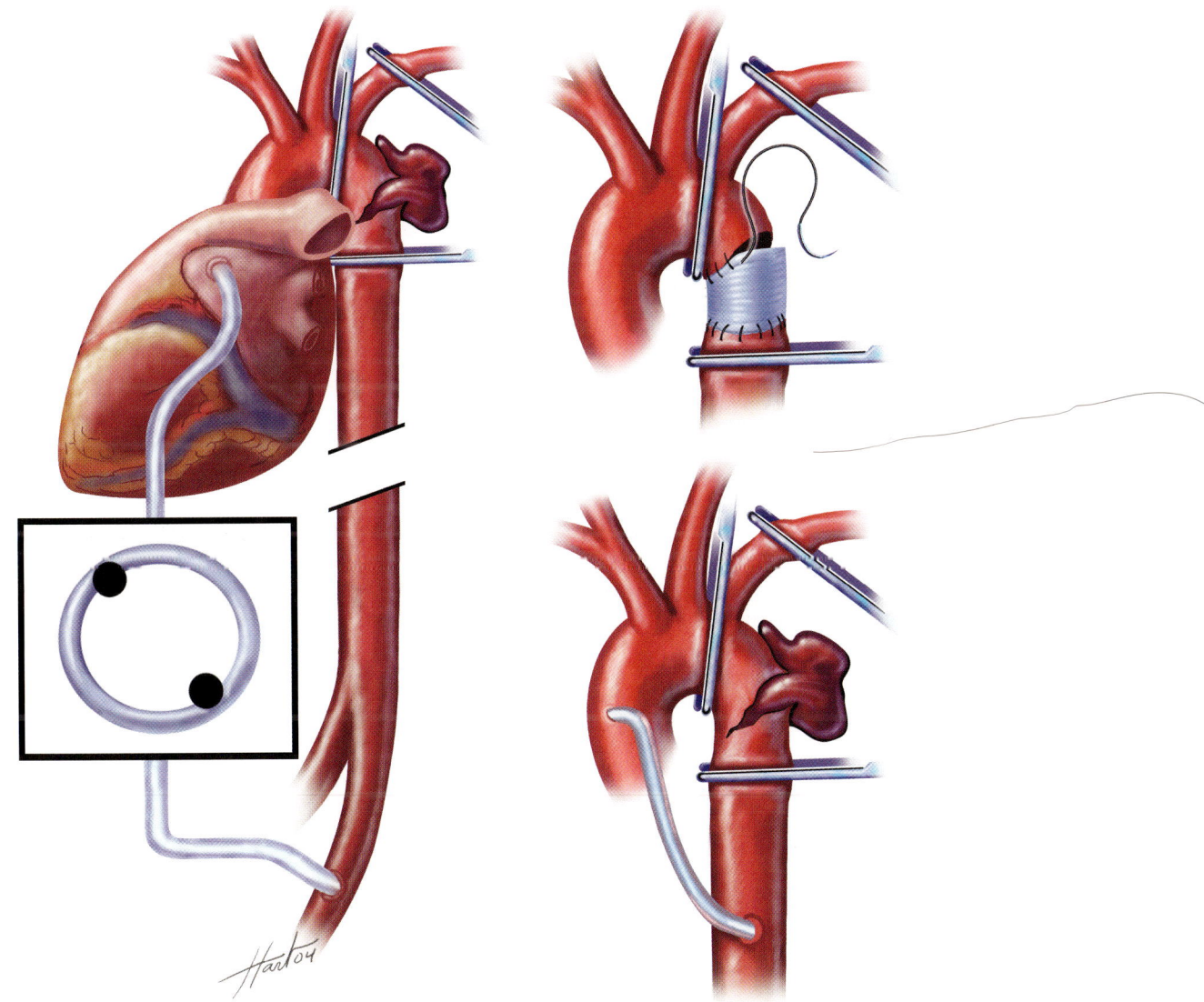

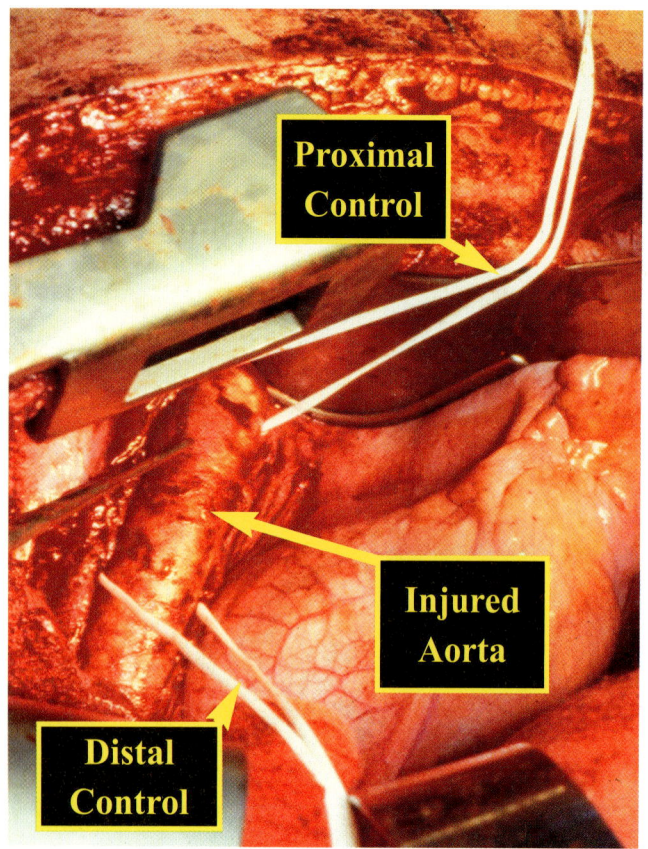 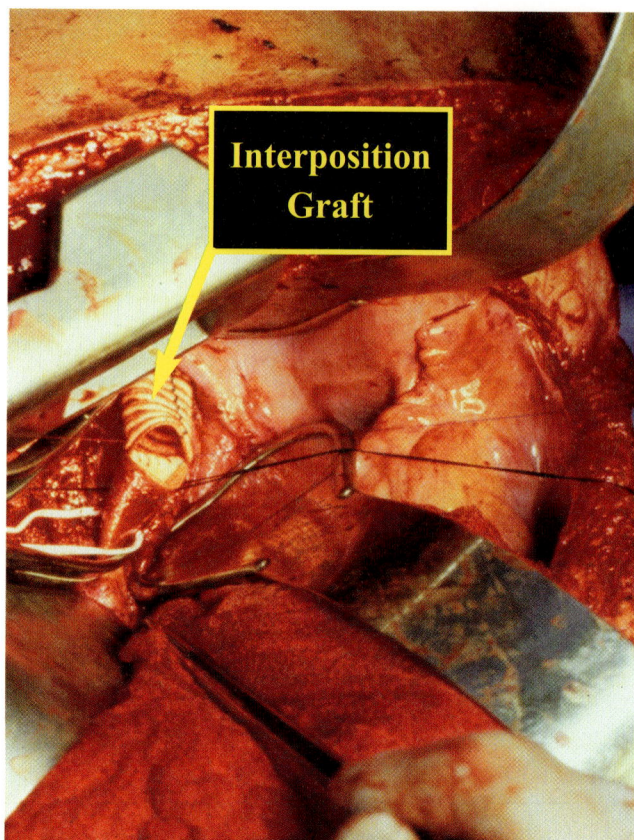

Aortic Injury
The damaged vessel is resected and the interposition graft sutured in place after achieving proximal and distal control of the injured area of the aorta.

Completed Aortic Repair
The aortic repair is completed when the damaged vessel has been resected and the interposition graft is in place.

COMPLETE TRANSECTION

- Injured vessel resected
- Dacron interposition graft

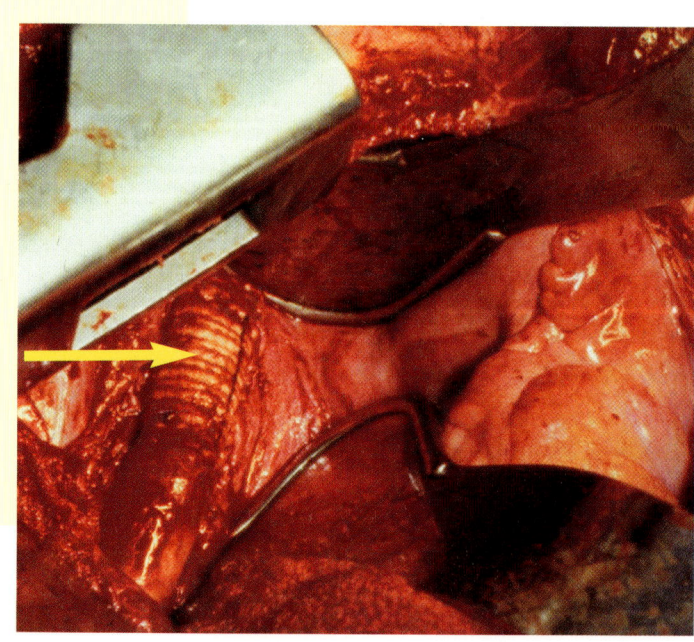

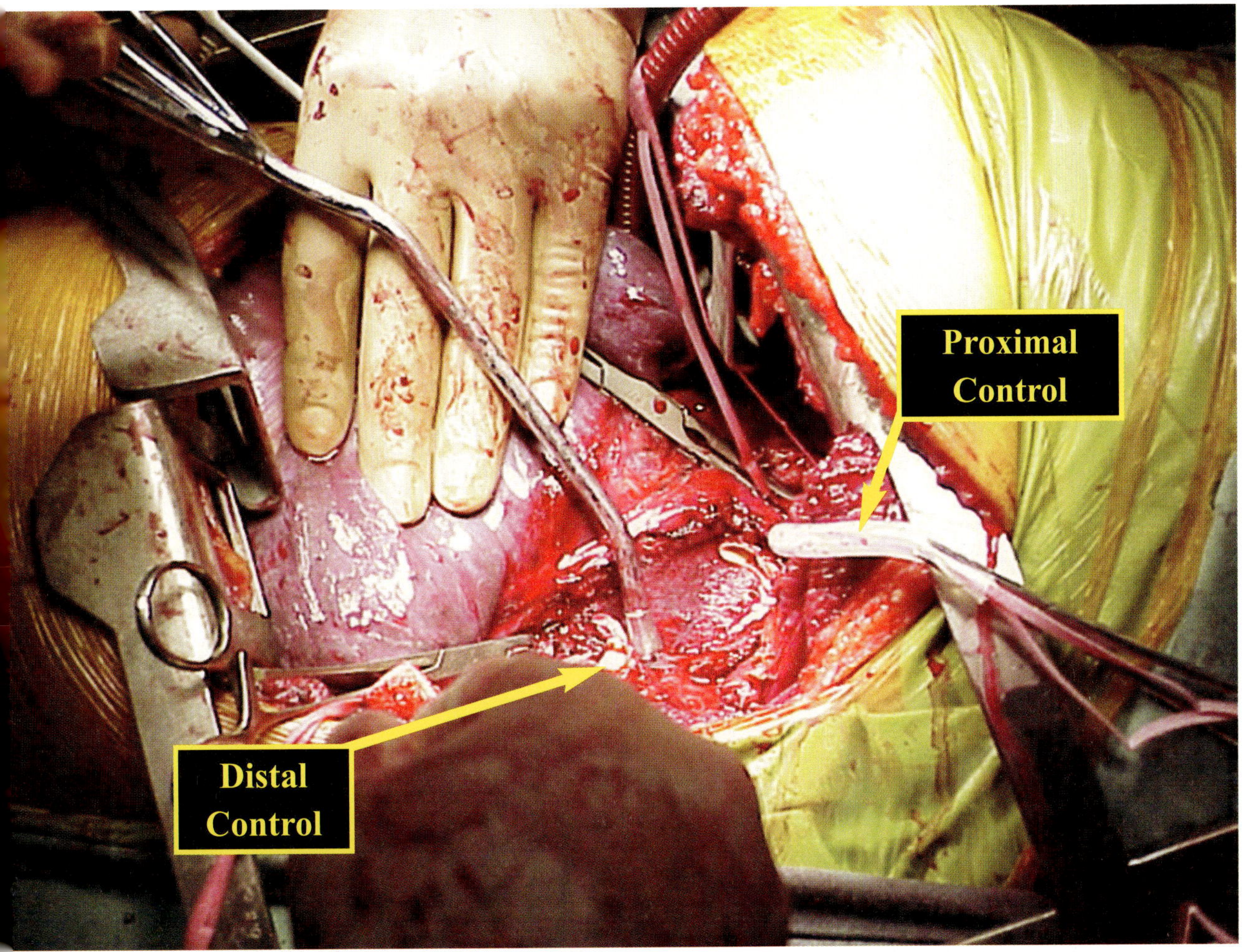

Proximal and distal control of the resected injured aorta can be seen in an open chest.

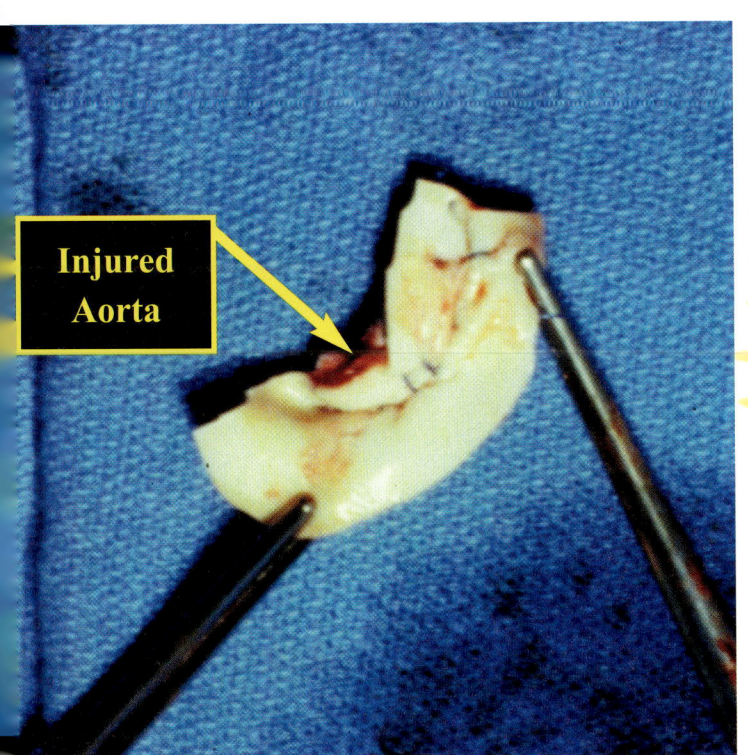

Attempted Primary Repair

This picture shows the inside surface of an injured vessel with externally applied Prolene sutures that were unable to control the hemorrhage. This vessel was subsequently resected, and an interposition graft was put in place.

Complications

The mortality rate may be as high as 50% for patients with a transected aorta. This high rate is most common among patients with multisystem organ failure.

Paraplegia, caused by alteration of blood flow through the artery of Adamkiewicz to the spinal cord, is another complication. It occurs in up to 30% of patients who are cross clamped for more than thirty minutes. Infection, fistulas, and occlusion may also occur.

COMPLICATIONS

- Operative mortality: 0 to 54%
- Paraplegia: 8 to 30% if cross clamping >30 minutes
- Infection
- Aortic venous fistulae
- Aortic enteric fistulae
- Thrombosis and occlusion

RETROPERITONEAL HEMATOMAS

- Zone I: Centromedial
   - duodenum
   - pancreas
   - major abdominal vasculature

- Explore in both penetrating and blunt injury

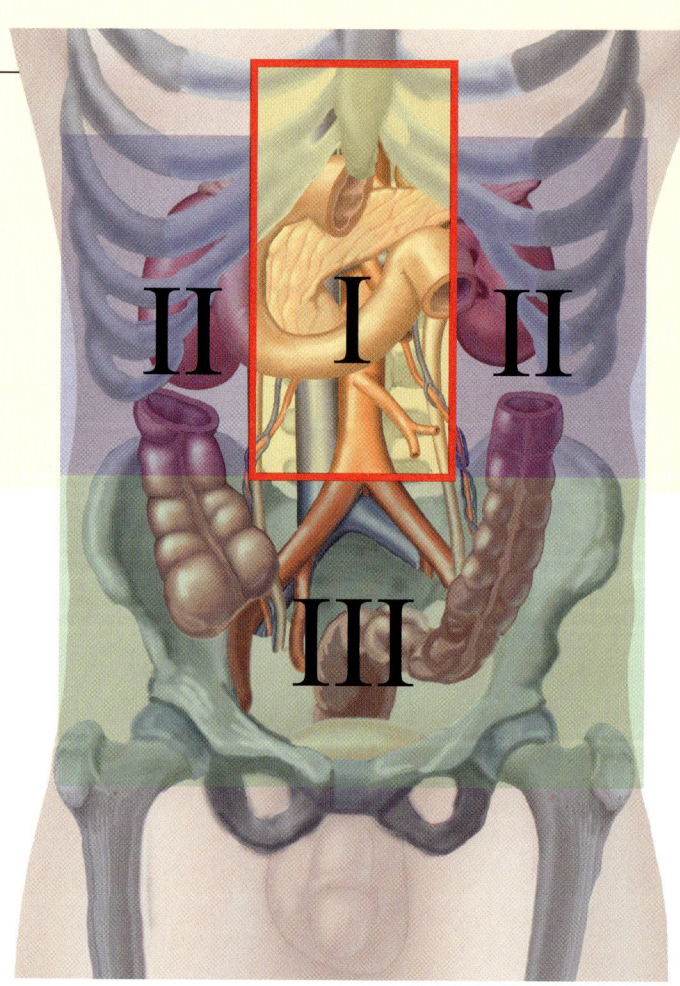

Chapter Six - The Cardiac & Vascular System

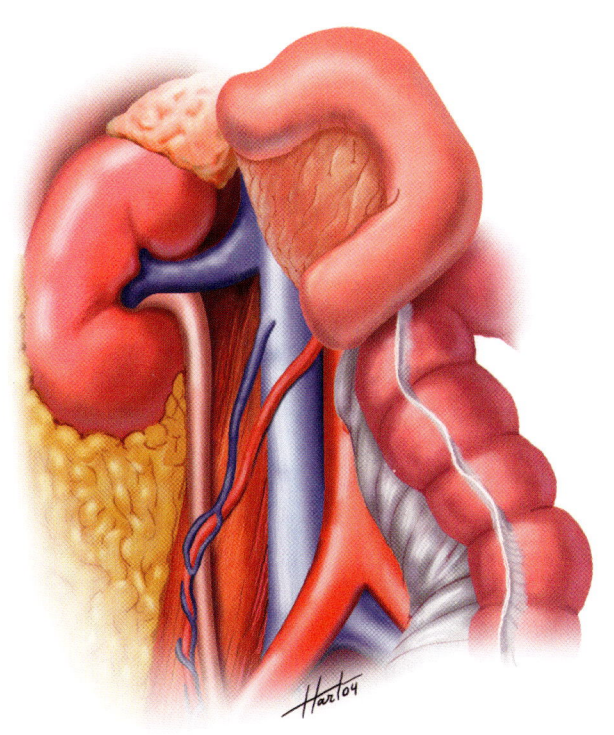

Infrahepatic Inferior Vena Cava (IVC) Injuries

Retroperitoneal Hematomas

Injuries resulting in a hematoma in Zone I of the retroperitoneum may involve major abdominal vasculature and the duodenum and pancreas. Exploration of hematomas in Zone I of the retroperitoneum is mandatory in both blunt and penetrating injuries.

IVC Exposure

Mobilization of the hepatic flexure and an extended Cattel Braasch maneuver optimize exposure of the infrarenal IVC. Once medial visceral rotation of the right and proximal transverse colon has been accomplished, the Kocher maneuver, which dissects the duodenum from its retroperitoneal attachments, and medial rotation of the duodenum and head of the pancreas allow outstanding visualization of the infrarenal IVC.

RETROPERITONEAL HEMATOMAS

- Cattel Braasch maneuver
    - right side medial visceral rotation
- Kocher maneuver

INFRAHEPATIC IVC INJURIES

- Hemorrhage control
    - direct pressure
    - proximal and distal control
    - balloon catheters

- Must know if the injury is:
    - suprarenal
    - infrarenal

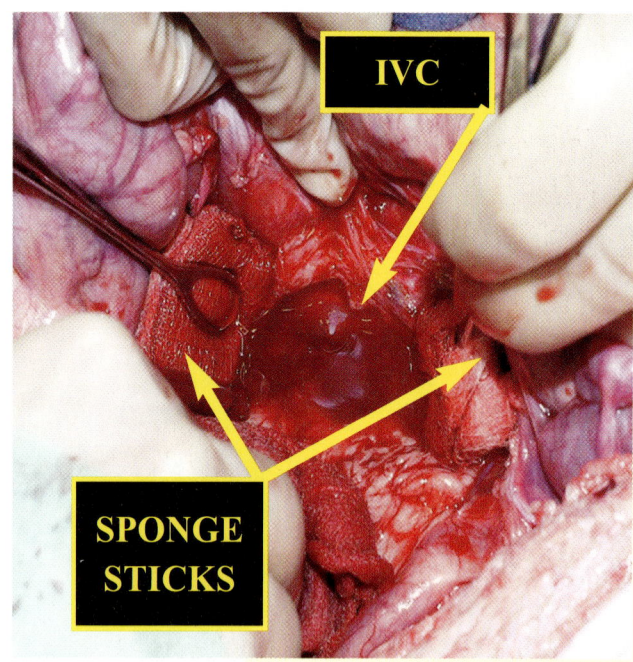

An IVC injury and hematoma, with sponge sticks in place.

CONTROL OF HEMORRHAGE

- Digital control
- Sponge sticks

Infrahepatic IVC Injuries

Initial control of infrahepatic IVC injuries can be achieved using direct digital pressure or sponge sticks to gain proximal and distal control of the injured segment. Severe hemorrhage can be controlled effectively using vascular clamps above and below the injured area, or a Satinsky clamp that includes the injured segment of the IVC. A balloon catheter can be introduced and inflated to tamponade bleeding and allow the surgeon to identify the extent of the injury.

CONTROL OF HEMORRHAGE

- Manual control
- Complete IVC dissection
- Vascular control with clamps

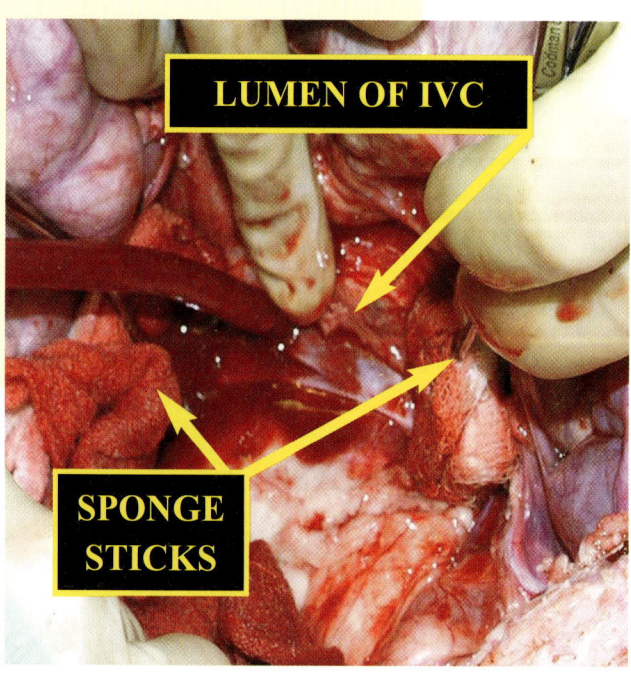

Manual control and exposure of the injury.

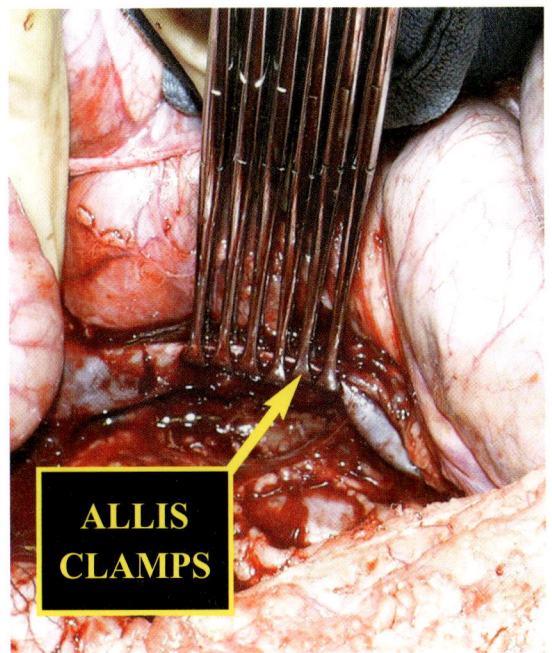 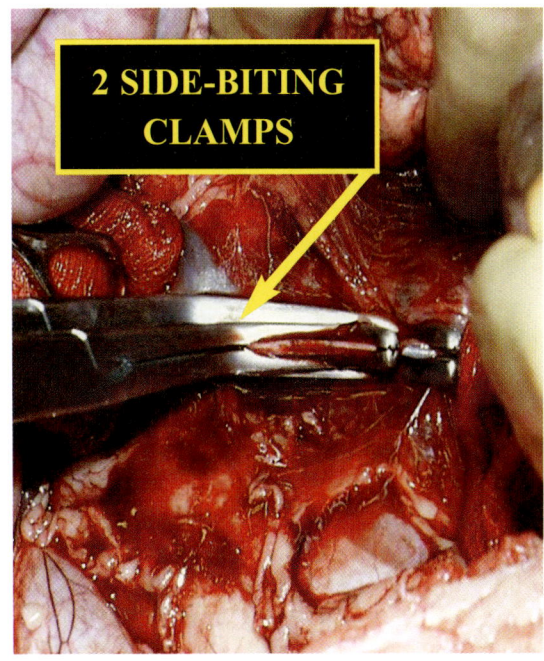

IVC Control and Exposure

As mentioned earlier, direct digital pressure can be used to achieve initial control of an infrahepatic IVC injury.

Allis clamps can be placed next to each other sequentially to control bleeding. Placement of two side-biting clamps can also be used to isolate the injury. Both methods allow venous return while isolating the injured area for repair.

Infrahepatic IVC Injuries

Injuries to the posterior wall of the IVC can be closed in a continuous running fashion through the injured anterior wall. The anterior wall can then be repaired using a continuous running 5-0 Prolene suture. If the repair results in significant narrowing of the IVC, the surgeon can perform a patch angioplasty with either autologous vein or synthetic material. Although these techniques preclude narrowing of the injured IVC, they are time consuming and technically challenging.

Ligation is an option if the injury is suprarenal and damage to the IVC is extensive enough to preclude repair.

IVC INJURIES

- Posterior wall closure
- Anterior wall closure
- Patch angioplasty
- Ligation of suprarenal IVC requires reconstruction

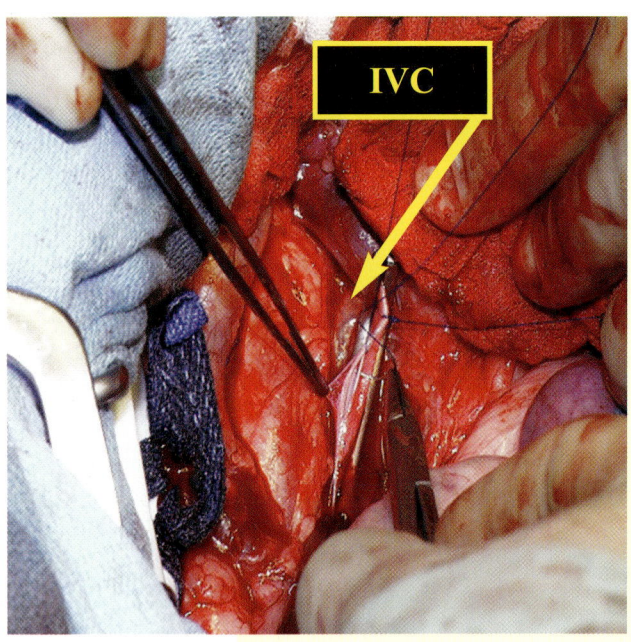

OPTIONS FOR REPAIR

- Primary closure with 5-0 Prolene

- Graft

- Transluminal repair for posterior injuries

- Infrarenal ligation

However, it requires immediate reconstruction of venous return. Collateral venous drainage through the retroperitoneum and the left gonadal vein will provide adequate venous return if the infrarenal IVC has been ligated.

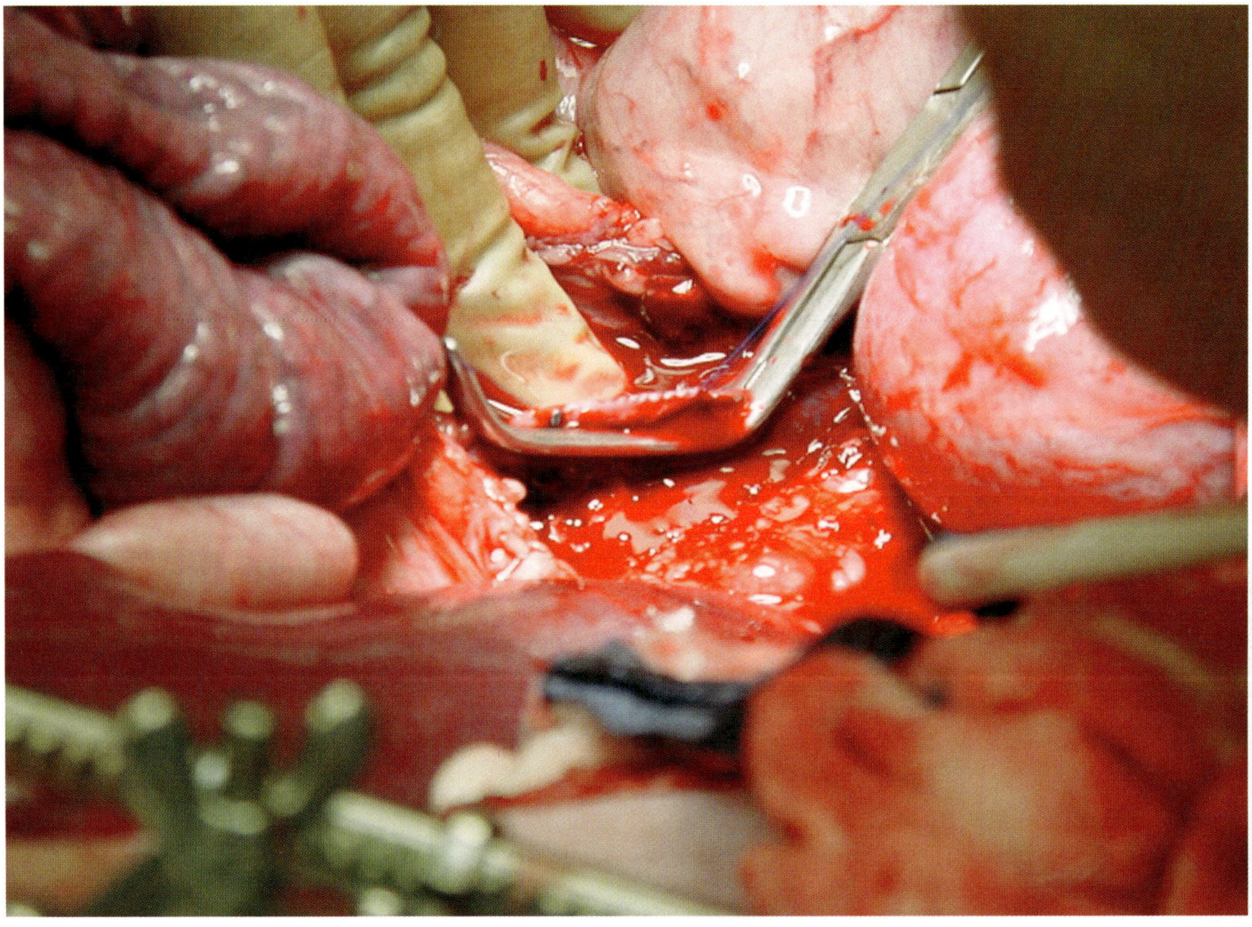

Side-biting clamp and a completed suture line.

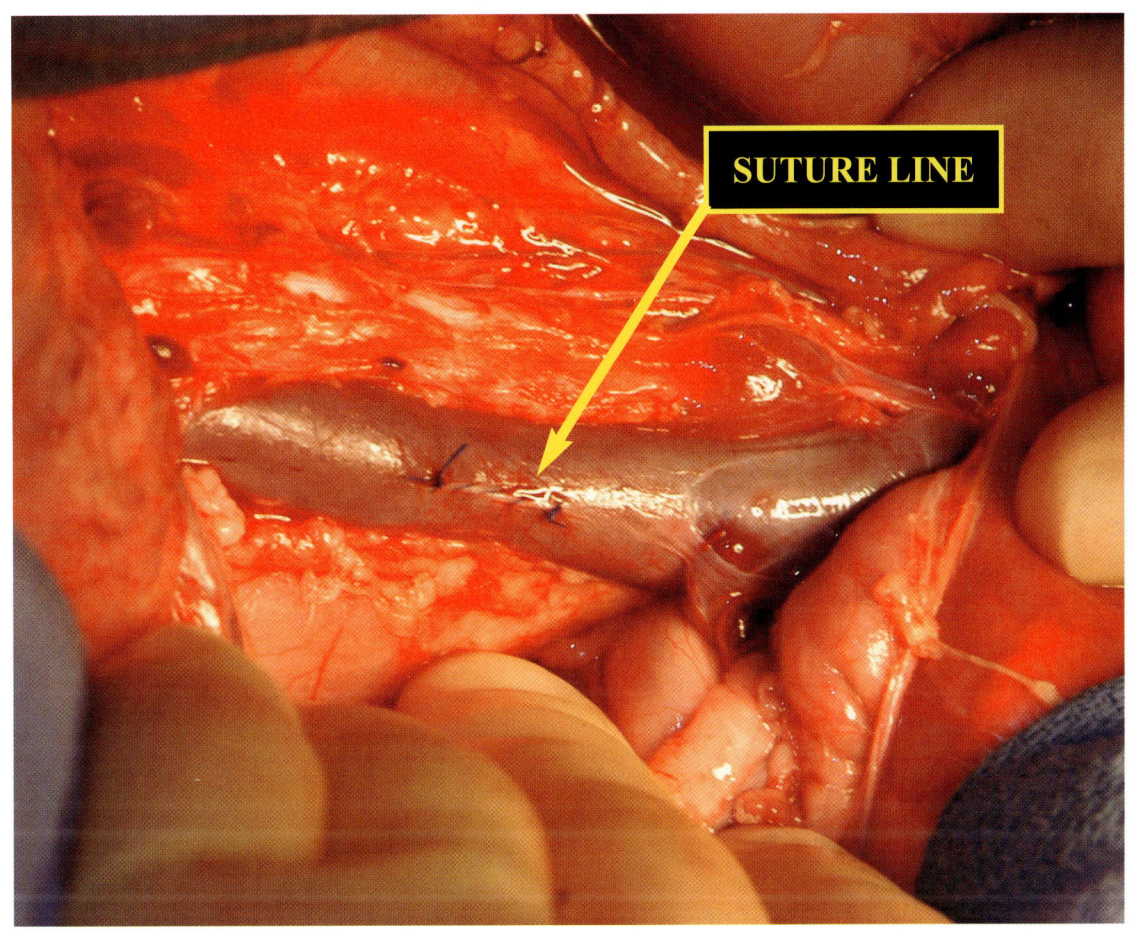

IVC Primary Repair

Optimal primary closure of the injured IVC can be achieved with a continuous 5-0 Prolene suture.

COMPLICATIONS OF IVC INJURIES

- Compartment syndrome
- Edema
- Emboli

As mentioned earlier, an injury to the infrarenal IVC anterior wall can be repaired with a continuous 5-0 Prolene suture. The lumen shown in this picture is slightly narrow secondary to venospasm and surgical repair. This degree of narrowing is acceptable.

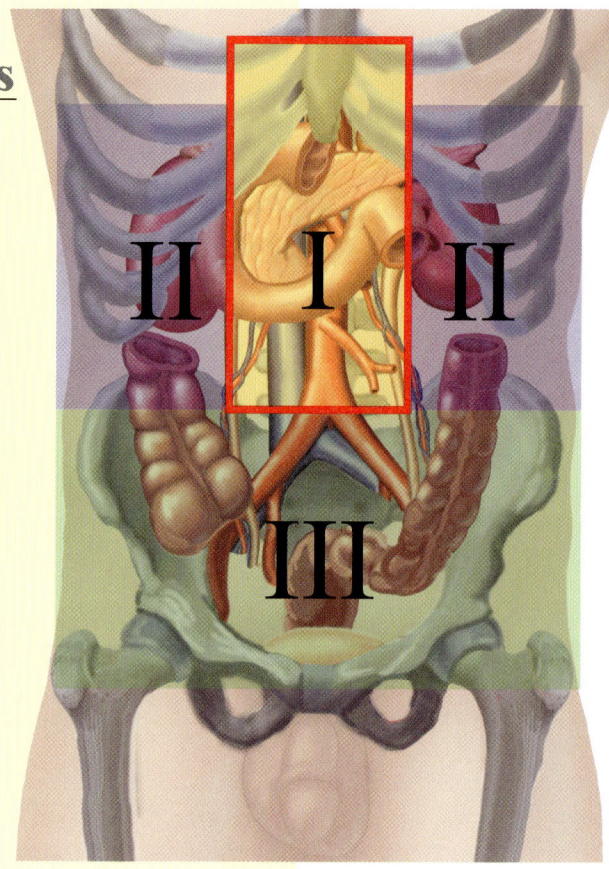

Retroperitoneal Hematomas

- Difficult to expose
- Transection of the right common iliac artery
- Exposure and repair of the vein injury
- Reconstruct right common iliac artery
- Also applies to the internal iliac artery

Infrahepatic IVC Injuries

Postoperative complications that can develop secondary to infrahepatic IVC injury repair include compartment syndrome of the legs, acute and chronic edema, and emboli.

Exposure of Common Iliac Vein Injuries

Surgical exposure of the right common iliac vein is difficult because of its location posterior to the common iliac artery, which limits exposure. This makes it difficult to repair injuries involving the common iliac vein on the right side.

Transection of the right common iliac artery may provide exposure to the injured common iliac vein. Once the vein has been repaired, reanastomosis of the transected common iliac artery is completed using a continuous or interrupted 5-0 Prolene suture. This technique can also be used to repair the left common iliac vein.

ADVANCED TRAUMA OPERATIVE MANAGEMENT

Selected Readings

Chapter 6 - The Cardiac & Vascular System

Mattox KL et al. Clamp/repair: a safe technique for treatment of blunt injury to the descending thoracic aorta. Ann Thor Surg. 1985;40:456-463.

Sweeney MS et al. Traumatic aortic transactions: eight year experience with the "clamp-sew" technique. Ann Thorac Surg. 1997;64:384-389.

Rozycki et al. The role of surgeon-performed ultrasound in patients with possible penetrating cardiac wounds: A prospective multicenter study.
J Trauma 1999;45:190.

Buckman RF et al. Juxtahepatic venous injuries: A critical review of reported management strategies. J Trauma 2000;48:978-984.

Mattox KL. Heart. In: Thal ER, Weigelt JA, Carrico CJ. Operative Trauma Management: An Atlas. 2nd Edition. McGraw-Hill. 2002:140-153.

Perry MO. Injuries to the Inferior Vena Cava. In: Thal ER, Weigelt JA, Carrico CJ. Operative Trauma Management: An Atlas. 2nd Edition. McGraw-Hill. 2002:316-321.

Mangram A et al. Blunt cardiac injury that requires operative intervention: An unsuspected injury. J. Trauma 2003;54:286-288.

Moldovan S et al. Bilateral temporary aortoiliac shunts for vascular damage control. J Trauma 2003;55:592.

Ivatury RR. The injured heart. In: Moore EE, Feliciano DV, Mattox KL, eds. Trauma. 5th ed. 2004 McGraw-Hill:555-569.

Tips From the Masters

There are a number of safe methods to manage blunt and penetrating trauma in the operating suite. The following technical surgical tips have been successfully used by the authors to deal with difficult or challenging operating situations.

Chapter 6: The Cardiac & Vascular System

TABLE OF CONTENTS

Exposure of the Aorta in the Abdomen 303
Kenneth Boffard, MD

The Mattox Maneuver 305
Kenneth L. Mattox, MD

Abdominal Vascular Injuries, Exposures, and Management 307
Juan A. Asensio, MD

Cricothyroidotomy: Precise Anatomic Aide to Dissection Technique 310
Paul R. G. Cunningham, MD

Flail Chest – Internal Fixation 311
Donald D. Trunkey, MD

Management of Trapped Lung Syndrome (Retained Hemothorax) 313
David L. Ciraulo, DO

Pulmonary Tractotomy 316
Edward E. Cornwell, MD

Exposure in Management of an Atrial Laceration 318
J. Wayne Meredith, MD

Repair of Laceration of the Right Ventricle 320
Lenworth M. Jacobs, MD

Repair of Stab Wound (1.5 cm) to Right Ventricle 323
Glen Tinkoff, MD

Stapled Repair of Cardiac Laceration 325
Robert Mackersie, MD

**Exposure Management of a 1.5 cm Stab Wound
to the Right Ventricle** 328
J. Wayne Meredith, MD

Control of the Aorta Through The Left Chest 330
Aurelio Rodriguez, MD

**Supraceliac Aortic Control and
Skin Only Closure After Damage Control** 332
Michael Rotondo, MD

Gunshot Wounds to the Abdominal Aorta 334
Demetrios Demetriades, MD

**Exposure and Management of a 2 cm Laceration
to the Infrarenal Abdominal Aorta** 335
David V. Feliciano, MD

Injury to a Major Vein 337
Donald D. Trunkey, MD

Repair of the Inferior Vena Cava 339
Lenworth M. Jacobs, MD

Stab Wound to the Inferior Vena Cava 342
Blaine L. Enderson, MD

Repair of the Inferior Vena Cava 344
Thomas M. Scalea, MD

Penetrating Injury to the Vena Cava 346
Susan Briggs, MD, FACS

**Exposure and Management of a 2 cm Laceration
of the Infrarenal Portion of the Inferior Vena Cava** 348
L.D. Britt, MD

**Laceration of Infrarenal Inferior Vena Cava
with Hypotension and Massive Hemorrhage** 350
Rao Ivatury, MD

Gunshot Wound to the Left Common Iliac Artery 352
Norman McSwain, MD

Celiac Trunk Injury 354
Eric R. Frykberg, MD

Laceration of the Vena Cava 2 Centimeters Distal to the Renal Vessels 356
Norman McSwain, MD

**Emergency Department Resuscitative Thoracotomy
and Management of Cardiopulmonary Injuries** 358
Juan A. Asensio, MD

**Exposure and Repair of the Celiac Trunk
and/or Superior Mesenteric Artery** 361
David V. Feliciano, MD

TECHNICAL OPERATIVE PROCEDURES:
HOW I DO IT

Exposure of the Aorta in the Abdomen

Kenneth D. Boffard, MB, BCh, FACS

Scenario

A 22-year-old man was stabbed in the epigastrium and had a rapidly distending tense hemoperitoneum. He was hypotensive and tachycardic. At exploration he had a large pulsating retroperitoneal hematoma in Zone II of the abdomen. There was an injury to the aorta.

Management

"The treatment of bleeding is to stop the bleeding!" The management of an aortic injury revolves around immediate access to and control of hemorrhage.

A single dose of pre-operative antibiotic with broad-spectrum aerobic and anaerobic coverage was given. The patient was prepared from sternal notch to the knees. In all vessel injury, proximal and distal control is essential, and may necessitate a left lateral thoracotomy to gain access to the thoracic aorta, and groin incisions to control the iliac vessels. Autotransfusion should be considered in all cases.

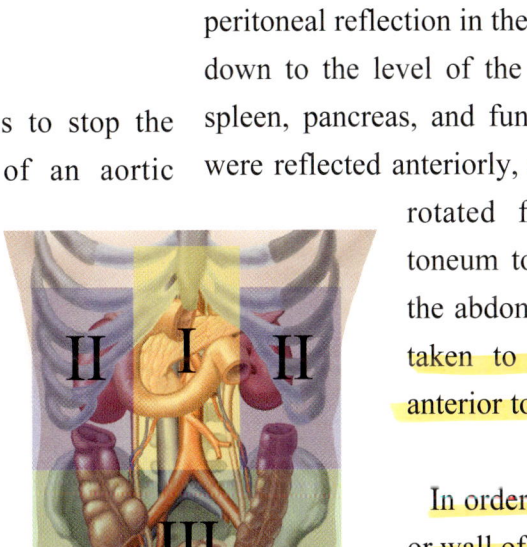

A long incision, the full vertical length of the abdomen was used. To expose the potential sites of arterial bleeding in the upper midline region of the retroperitoneum, medial visceral rotation was performed. This entailed mobilization of the splenorenal ligament, dividing of any ligaments or adhesions between the spleen and the diaphragm, and incision of the peritoneal reflection in the left paracolic gutter, down to the level of the sigmoid colon. The spleen, pancreas, and fundus of the stomach, were reflected anteriorly, and the organs were rotated from the retroperitoneum towards the center of the abdomen. Care should be taken to remain in a plane anterior to Gerota's fascia.

In order to reach the posterior wall of the aorta, the kidney can be mobilized as well, and rotated medially on its pedicle, taking great care not to cause ischemia or further injury.

Aorta

The entire abdominal aorta and the origins of its branches are exposed by this technique. This includes the celiac axis, the origin of the superior mesenteric artery, the splenic artery and vein, the left renal artery and vein, and the iliac vessels. The dense and fibrous superior mesenteric and celiac nerve plexuses, however, overlie the proximal aorta and need to be sharply dissected in order to identify the renal and superior mesenteric arteries.

Control of the aorta can be achieved at several different levels depending on the site of injury. The supraceliac aorta can be exposed by incising the gastrohepatic ligament, and retracting the left lobe of the liver superiorly and the stomach inferiorly. A window is then made in the lesser omentum and the peritoneum overlying the crura of the diaphragm is divided. The fibers of the crura are separated by blunt dissection. The esophagus is then mobilized to the left in order to reach the abdominal aorta at the diaphragmatic hiatus. The aorta can be clamped or compressed at this point. This is for control, as exposure for repair is not ideal with this approach, and better exposure can be obtained by performing a left medial visceral rotation procedure.

The distal aorta can be approached transperitoneally by retracting the small bowel to the right, the transverse colon superiorly, and the descending colon to the left. The aorta below the left renal vein now can be accessed by incising the peritoneum over it and mobilizing the third and fourth part of the duodenum superiorly. Both iliac vessels can be exposed by distal continuation of the dissection. The ureters should be identified and carefully preserved, especially in the region of the bifurcation of the iliac vessels

- The dense structures overlying the aorta need to be sharply dissected
- The fibers of the crura of the diaphragm are separated by blunt dissection
- Suture of the aorta should never be attempted while it is under pressure

Repair

The aorta is repaired using a continuous suture of 4-0 Prolene. Suturing should never be attempted while the aorta is under pressure, and it should first be controlled proximally and distally before suturing is attempted. If the defect is large, a graft, usually of Dacron is helpful. Drains are not normally used.

References

Luchette FA, Borzotta AP, Croce M, et al. Practice Management Guidelines for prophylactic antibiotic use in penetrating abdominal trauma.

EAST Practice Management Guidelines Work Group. 2001; Online. Available: http://www.east.org 2004.

Boffard KD Ed. Definitive Surgical Trauma Care (DSTCTM). DSTCTM Course of the International Association for the Surgery of Trauma and Surgical Intensive Care. Arnold. London. 2003.

TECHNICAL OPERATIVE PROCEDURES:

HOW I DO IT

The "MATTOX" Maneuver

Kenneth L. Mattox, MD, FACS

Medial rotation of the viscera is an extremely valuable maneuver to expose the retroperitoneum, especially in the left upper quadrant of the abdomen. Because such an extensive dissection has the potential for injury to the kidney, renal arteries, segmental arteries off the aorta, the adrenal gland, and other structures, one should not proceed with a Mattox maneuver unless there is clear suspicion that a major retroperitoneal vascular injury exists. The decision that a suprarenal aortic injury exists is made soon after one enters the abdomen, because of a large, usually reddish, upper abdominal midline hematoma.

The surgeon on the right hand side of the operating room table bluntly divides the lateral attachments of the descending colon in the left lower abdomen. This blunt dissection is then carried bluntly down to the psoas muscle and carried upward toward the spleen. As the dissection is carried medially and upward, care is taken to stay BEHIND the kidney fascial compartments, and behind the tail of the spleen. With this dissection, the spleen, stomach, tail of pancreas, and left kidney are swept toward the midline and onto the right side of the open midline incision. A large sterile towel is placed over these viscera. Attachments of the spleen, stomach, or colon to the left diaphragm are divided sharply. As this dissection proceeds, the surgeon encounters the retroperitoneal hematoma. At this point the surgeon should be as high in the abdomen, near the diaphragm, as possible. Should brisk bleeding be encountered, the surgeon controls the bleeding with his hand, as dissection continues to the aorta and esophageal hiatus. Should the bleeding be near the hiatus, a finger is inserted in the left lateral crus and it is sharply cut with heavy scissors, carrying the diaphragmatic incision out radially. Through this medial opening in the diaphragm, the descending thoracic aorta can be exposed as high as T6. A vascular clamp can be applied for proximal control.

With a vascular clamp applied for proximal control, and digital pressure over any active aortic bleeding, the surgeon, or first assistant continues the dissection immediately on the adventitia of the aorta along the posterolateral wall of the aorta. At the area of the celiac axis, the surgeon encounters dense fibrous nerve

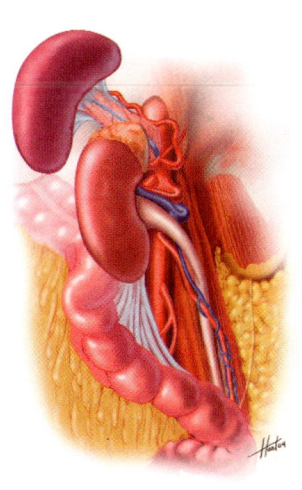

tissue and this should be initially swept anteriorly. Care must be taken not to injure the segmental arteries, which come off the aorta posterolaterally. Care must also be taken not to injure the left renal artery, which at this point is stretched out and attenuated, as well as being displaced anteriorly. A vascular clamp is placed distally on the infrarenal abdominal aorta. The bleeding is now reassessed and the clamps brought closer together close to the area of injury. The surgeon then determines the most appropriate method of reconstruction and/or damage control.

- Care must be taken not to injure the posterolateral sequential arteries which come off the aorta

- Care must be taken with the left renal artery as when mobilized it is stretched out and attenuated

Several rules of thumb exist:

The initial dissection for a Mattox maneuver is accomplished with the surgeon being on the right side of the operating room table.

- The dissection is most easily accomplished when a periaortic hematoma has already accomplished the dissection

- Care must be taken to stay in a dissection plane immediately anterior to the psoas muscle

- The safest site for arterial dissection is immediately on the adventitia

- The surgeon can perform reconstructive procedures better from the left side of the operating room table

- The aorta from T6 through the bifurcation and even the external iliac artery can be exposed via the Mattox maneuver

TECHNICAL OPERATIVE PROCEDURES:

HOW I DO IT

Abdominal Vascular Injuries, Exposures and Management

Juan A. Asensio, MD, FACS

Technique

In the operating room the patient's entire torso, from neck to midthigh, is prepared and draped. The area of the midthighs is quite important should the necessity arise to obtain an autogenous saphenous vein graft. There must be sufficient units of blood in the operating room for immediate transfusion via rapid infusion technology. Prevention of hypothermia can be accomplished by placement of a warming blanket in the operating room, covering the patient's lower extremities with a circulating warm air mattress, covering the head to prevent heat loss, increasing the ventilator cascade temperature to 42°C and an ample supply of microwave heated irrigation fluids. In addition, the availability of auto transfusion apparatus and cell saving technology is of great value.

A midline incision extending from xiphoid to pubis is performed. Immediate control of life threatening hemorrhage followed by immediate control of sources of gastrointestinal spillage is performed. The next step in the management of abdominal injuries consists of thorough exploration of the abdominal cavity. Since the abdominal vasculature resides in the retroperitoneum, a thorough exploration of these structures must be performed utilizing a systematic approach to the anatomic zones of the retroperitoneum.

The first and most important goal to achieve in the management of abdominal vascular injuries is hemorrhage control. As in all vascular injuries proximal and distal control of the hemorrhage is ideal. However, in exsanguinating abdominal vascular injuries, achieving this rapidly can be quite difficult.

Frequently these patients experience severe and profound hypotension, therefore cross clamping of the aorta is the first maneuver to stop life threatening hemorrhage. If the patient arrives profoundly hypotensive or experiences cardiopulmonary arrest in the operating room an immediate left anterolateral thoracotomy with aortic cross clamping is performed prior to proceeding with laparotomy.

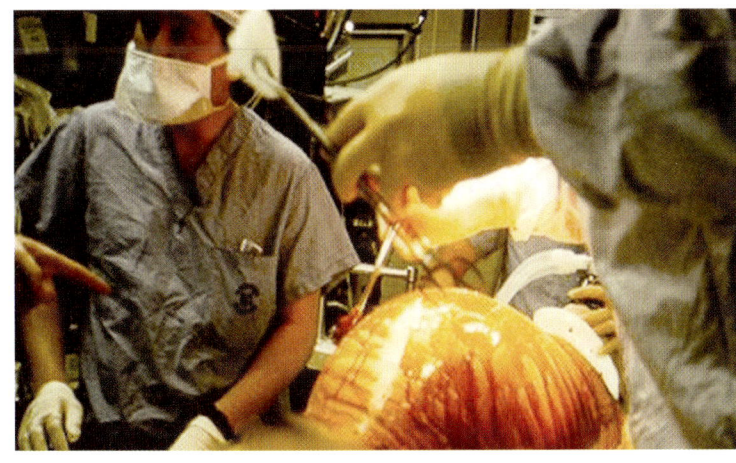

In the case in which the patient arrives with some degree of hemodynamic stability, but decompensates during laparotomy, the abdominal aorta can be controlled either digitally at the aortic hiatus, by the use of an abdominal aortic root compressor or by placement of a cross clamp. Placement of a cross clamp in this area can be difficult, as the abdominal aorta is surrounded by the crura of the diaphragm, which may require transection.

Procedure: *Right-sided visceral rotation*

An extended Kocher maneuver is performed to mobilize the duodenum and the head of the pancreas medially. The avascular line of Toldt of the right colon is dissected. This maneuver mobilizes the right colon, hepatic flexure, duodenum and head of the pancreas to the level of the superior mesenteric vessels. The loose retroperitoneal tissue to the left of the inferior vena cava is carefully dissected. This maneuver exposes the suprarenal abdominal aorta between the celiac axis and the superior mesenteric artery. A disadvantage is that the exposure obtained is below the level of any injury to the supraceliac aorta and the aorta at the hiatus.

Maneuvers used to expose inframesocolic injuries in Zone I include displacing the transverse colon and mesocolon cephalad, eviscerating the small bowel to the right, locating the ligament of Treitz, transecting it along with the loose retroperitoneal tissue alongside the left of the abdominal aorta until the left renal vein is located. This exposes the infrarenal aorta. To expose the infrarenal inferior vena cava the avascular line of Toldt of the right colon is transected along with a Kocher maneuver, sweeping the pancreas and duodenum to the left and incising the retroperitoneal tissues that cover the inferior vena cava.

Exposure to the right and left Zone II depends as to whether the perirenal hematoma or active bleeding is located laterally or medially. If active bleeding is found medially or if there is an expanding hematoma, vascular control of the vessels of the pedicle is preferable. Vessel loops should be used for control; alternatively a Henley clamp may also be used. On the right, this is achieved by mobilizing the right colon and hepatic flexure as well as performing a Kocher maneuver, exposing the inferior vena cava infrarenally and continuing the dissection cephalad by incising the tissues directly over the suprarenal infrahepatic inferior vena cava. This is continued until the right renal vein is encountered. Further dissection superiorly and posteriorly to the right renal vein will locate the right renal artery.

On the left side, the left colon and splenic

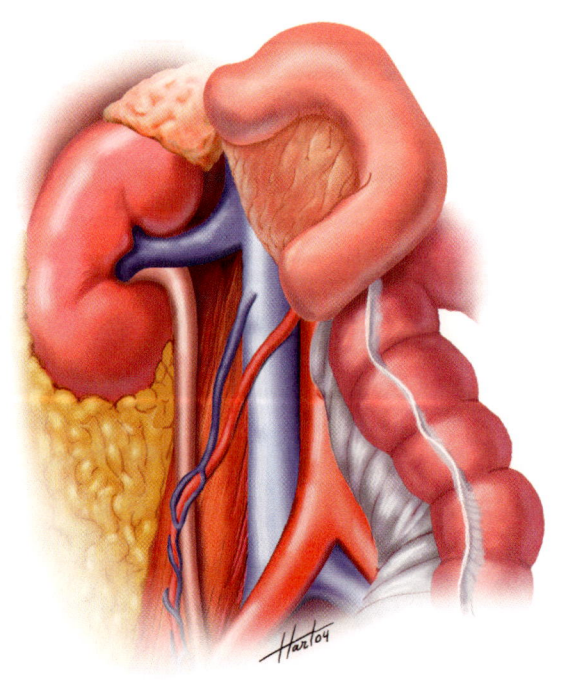

flexure are mobilized. The small bowel is then eviscerated to the right. The ligament of Treitz is located and the transverse colon and mesocolon are displaced cephalad. This should locate the infrarenal abdominal aorta. Cephalad dissection will locate the left renal vein as it crosses over the abdominal aorta. The left renal artery will also be found superiorly and posteriorly to the left renal vein. Alternatively, if a perirenal hematoma or bleeding is found laterally with no extension into the hilum of the kidney, the lateral aspects of Gerota's fascia can be incised and the kidney elevated and displaced medially to locate the hemorrhage.

Exposure to the vessels in Zone III can be achieved by taking down the avascular line of Toldt of both the right and left colons and displacing them medially. Utilizing a combination of blunt and sharp dissection, the common iliac vessels will be located. Meticulous attention must be paid to locating the ureter as it crosses the common iliac artery. Avoidance of devascularization of the urethra's blood supply is a must. A vessel loop should be passed around the ureter to retract it. Dissection is then extended in a caudad direction opening the retroperitoneum over the vessels.

The management of inferior mesenteric artery injuries is usually by ligation, as they rarely require reconstruction. The management of injuries to the infrahepatic suprarenal inferior vena cava, as well as the infrarenal inferior vena cava will consist of lateral venorrhaphy whenever feasible. If through-and-through injuries are found in these vessels, both anterior and posterior aspects of the vessel must be repaired. This can prove to be quite challenging.

Whenever I perform an abdominal vascular repair, serious consideration is given to second look operations to assess for bowel viability. This is of particular importance after repair of any of the portions of the superior mesenteric artery and can also be considered after repair or ligation of the portal vein or superior mesenteric vein. Whenever possible all grafts either autogenous or prosthetic should be reperitonealized. Similarly, for all vascular repairs adjacent to gastrointestinal suture lines an effort should be made to interpose viable tissue, generally omentum between the suture lines to prevent vascular-enteric fistulas or anastomotic dehiscence and blowouts.

> - Kocher maneuver exposes the duodenum and the head of the pancreas
>
> - Expose the suprarenal aorta between the celiac axis and the superior mesenteric artery
>
> - Exposure of vessels in Zone III is achieved by taking down the avascular line of Toldt of both the ascending and descending colon

TECHNICAL OPERATIVE PROCEDURES:

HOW I DO IT

Cricothyroidotomy: Precise Anatomic Aide to Dissection Technique.

Paul R. G. Cunningham, MD, FACS

Background

Cricothyroidotomy remains an accepted and useful technique in reliably accessing the airway in the critically injured patient. The success of this procedure is predicated on precise localization of the cricothyroid membrane and creation of an incision, based on this determination.

This surgery is typically completed under suboptimal conditions, including lighting and positioning of the patient. There is a need for alacrity, and even though this is a well-accepted procedure, for any one practitioner, the frequency of actually performing this maneuver for airway control is relatively low. This lack of familiarity may lead to an increased opportunity for loss of precision and confidence in execution.

Recommended Technique

1. Palpate the cricothyroid membrane in the neck, just inferior to lower border of thyroid cartilage.

2. Positively localize the position of this membrane, by percutaneously transfixing the structure in the midline with an 18 gauge hypodermic needle.

3. Maintain the needle in place with one hand and with the other hand, create a transverse incision immediately next to the metal shaft, first through the subcutaneous tissues, and then into the airway.

4. Remove the needle, and insert a gloved finger into the airway for dilation. Further dilate with forceps if necessary.

5. Immediately replace the gloved finger for an appropriate sized #6 or #7 cuffed endotracheal tube. (Note: No retractor or other implements are required to complete this technique successfully.)

Rationale

By transfixing the cricothyroid membrane with a large bore needle, the likelihood of creating an aberrant incision is minimized. This maneuver will allow efficient, safe, and reliable access to the cricothyroid membrane and airway, even under the most challenging emergency circumstances.

- The cricothyroid membrane is transfixed with an 18 gauge needle

- This maneuver provides safe and reliable access to the airway

TECHNICAL OPERATIVE PROCEDURES:

HOW I DO IT

Flail Chest – Internal Fixation

Donald D. Trunkey, MD, FACS

Scenario

A 24-year-old logger is loading his truck when the chain breaks, and the log rolls onto his chest. He has severe right-sided chest pain and physical examination shows decreased breath sounds and obvious paradoxical motion of the right lateral chest.

Management

Almost three-fourths of rib fractures associated with flail chest can be managed with appropriate analgesia. My preference is for epidural analgesia in those patients who have multiple fractures. Twenty to twenty-five percent of patients with flail chest will benefit from operative fixation of their rib fractures. Reconstructed views of the CT of the chest will show the surgeon the degree of flail, the degree of comminution and serves as a road map for operative fixation.

In addition to rib fractures, I also prefer to fix all sternal fractures that are associated with severe pain, including those with a stepoff or subluxation of one fragment onto the other. The principles of operative management of rib fractures and sternal fractures are no different than internal fixation of extremity and pelvic fractures, which will also reduce pain.

Many patients with flail chest will have associated injuries such as closed head injury that may require ventilatory management. If the patient will be on the ventilator for protracted periods (>18 days), operative management of the flail chest is usually not indicated.

- Wait 24 to 48 hours postinjury for fixation

- Then entire flail segment has to be bridged with the plate

- Ventilator management can be discontinued 24 to 48 hours after internal fixation

- It is not necessary to remove the wires or plates

Procedure

For patients with flail chest, I generally wait 24 to 48 hours postinjury until the patient has been resuscitated, life-threatening injuries cared for, and a complete secondary examination has been carried out. If the patient's primary reason for being on the ventilator is management of the flail chest and pain, or in patients with severe pain without ventilator management, I prefer internal fixation of the rib fractures. My personal choice is to use the Arbeitgemeinschaft Osteosynthesefragen reduction plate (AO Plate). The 3.5 mm reduction plate comes in many lengths. It can be curved to conform to the circumferential curve of the chest and the curve upwards of the ribs as they go from anterior to posterior. The entire segmental fracture has to be bridged with the plate. My personal choice is to use wire sutures to stabilize both ends of the plate to the rib. I usually center the incision in the chest wall over the middle of the flail, and in some instances, it may require two incisions if the flail extends over six to eight ribs. If the ribs are very comminuted, I would plate each rib, but if they are simple segmental fractures, it may be necessary only to plate every other rib. Most patients will require temporary pleural drainage; and since a foreign body is implanted, I usually give a preoperative antibiotic, such as a first generation cephalosporin. In my experience, ventilator management can usually be discontinued 24 to 48 hours after operative internal fixation.

Fixation of sternal fractures is done through a median incision, carrying the incision down to the fracture site in the sternum and exposing the sternum two inches above and two inches below the fracture. Using a bone hook or towel clip, the fracture is reduced, and then using an AO reduction plate, this is placed vertically over the fracture site and wired to the sternum on both sides of the fracture. A preoperative dose of cephalosporin is given.

In my experience, it has not been necessary to remove the wire or plates. These are well tolerated.

TECHNICAL OPERATIVE PROCEDURES:

HOW I DO IT

Thorascopic Management of Trapped Lung Syndrome (Retained Hemothorax)

David L. Ciraulo, DO, FACS

Scenario

A patient presenting with a traumatic hemopneumothorax is at risk for incomplete drainage of that thoracic cavity resulting in a retained hemothorax.

Management

Complete drainage of the hemothorax should be obtained. In the event that chest radiographs continue to demonstrate a retained effusion, a CT scan of the chest is ordered. A CT scan of the chest determines the location of the trapped hemothorax, the size of the loculated fluid, and the potential for complicated loculations demonstrating air fluid levels which could be indicative of an empyema. Once the determination for surgery is made, consent should be obtained for diagnostic and therapeutic thoracoscopy, as well as the potential for an open thoracotomy. The patient should be counseled regarding potential complications to include hemorrhage, air leak, injury to major vascular structures, and the potential need for lung resection.

Procedure: *Thorascopic removal of a retained hemothorax*

Adequate IV access must be obtained. A minimum of two 16 gauge peripheral lines are initiated. It is helpful to have an arterial line placed prior to the positioning of the patient to allow for accurate continuous measurements of arterial pressure. The patient's airway should be managed by a double lumen endotracheal tube, allowing for single lung ventilation and continuous or intermittent collapsing of the affected side. Confirmation of endotracheal tube placement should be completed by anesthesia with fiberoptic brochoscopy. Assessment of occlusion of the bronchial lumen allows for confirmation of collapse of the lung in the thoracic cavity.

The patient is placed in the lateral position for a standard thoracotomy. A 'bean bag' device is utilized to provide adequate support of the patient on the operative table. A Mayo stand is placed at the level of the patient's head to allow the arm on the operative side to be placed superiorly and forward of the operative thoracic site. The use of pillows to support the arm on the Mayo stand as well as the use of tape to secure the arm in this position is recommended. A roll is placed under the axilla of the dependent side of the patient's thorax. The patient's legs should be padded and flexed at the knee with a pillow being placed between the knees to protect them. The chest is prepared for thoracoscopic exploration.

The first trocar should be placed in the position that would allow for the safest access of the thoracic cavity, based upon an assessment of the CT scan. A mid-axillary placement of the first trocar at the fourth to fifth interspace is usually the most efficacious, allowing one to visualize and inspect the thoracic cavity. This location is equidistant from the apex and the base of the cavity. Trocar placement is accomplished with an open technique and bluntly dissecting and entering the chest with the use of a hemostat. Once the thoracic cavity is entered, a finger should be placed into the portal and swept in a 360° fashion to assure that there are no parenchymal adhesions. Following this, a camera should be placed into the thoracic cavity for determination of subsequent trocar placements. Depending upon the extent of the pathology, a three-trocar approach, utilizing two dissectors/graspers/irrigators is preferred, with a single portal being utilized for the video camera. All trocar portals should be of the same size, appropriate for the introduction of the camera into all portal sites. Both 5 mm and 10 mm cameras have been found to be useful in this procedure. The lung is collapsed on the operative side. It is appropriate to assess the need for possible insufflation with CO_2 to facilitate more effective compression of the lung parenchyma which will allow better visualization and inspection of the thoracic cavity. Care must be taken to assure that cardiopulmonary compromise is not created by the insufflation of CO_2. Pressures of 10 to 14 mmHg have been found to be appropriate, resulting in no cardiopulmonary instability. The surgical procedure should first address the issues of visualization with attention being given to lysis of adhesions and removal of large fibrinous clotted material. Secondly, diagnostic considerations to the need for partial or complete decortication must be addressed. The lung can then be ventilated to visualize for unrestricted expansion of the lung. If the lung expands completely, decortication may not be necessary. If decortication is necessary, meticulous dissection and mobilization of the scar tissue must be performed to avoid a pulmonary injury and an air leak. Instruments found to be helpful include; thoracoscopy lung clamps, Maryland dissectors, and expandable fan retractors.

Following the evacuation of the thoracic cavity it should be copiously irrigated with saline. With the lung completely collapsed, the placement of the chest tubes should be performed under direct visualization. It may be possible to use one or both of the trocar sites for the chest tube portals, decreasing

- Double lumen endotracheal intubation allows for single lung ventilation

- Bronchial intubation should be confirmed with bronchoscopy

- Make sure there are no pleuropulmonary adhesions

- Meticulous dissection of scar tissue avoids pulmonary injury the surgical morbidity and the number of sites requiring closure. A two chest tube evacuation is performed utilizing a straight 40 Fr. chest tube placed posteriorly and superiorly to the apex and a 36 Fr. right angle chest tube placed in the costophrenic angle. The reexpansion of the lung should be observed with the scope.

With the portals closed and the chest tube secured with #2 silk, the patient is allowed to return to a supine position on the operating table. With the patient in this position a therapeutic bronchoscopy is performed to remove any secretions that may have developed in the collapsed lung, as well as the dependent lung. If the patient presented to the operative arena intubated, the double lumen endotracheal tube should be replaced with a single lumen endotracheal tube prior to returning to the intensive care unit. If the patient presented to the operative arena without intubation, there is no reason why they should not be able to be adequately extubated postoperatively.

Postoperative Care

Postoperative care includes initially monitoring the patient's O_2 saturation, an assessment of the chest x-ray to assure adequate expansion of the lung parenchyma on both sides, and to confirm good placement of the chest tubes. Twenty-four hours of negative suction on the chest tube drainage devices, monitoring for air leaks, as well as adequate drainage of the thoracic cavity is indicated. The chest tube should be removed when drainage is less than 100 cc per 24-hour period. A followup chest x-ray should be taken after the chest tube is removed.

TECHNICAL OPERATIVE PROCEDURES:
HOW I DO IT

Pulmonary Tractotomy

Edward E. Cornwell, III, MD, FACS

Scenario

A 20-year-old man has been stabbed with a large knife in the mid-axillary line in the third interspace of the left chest. The injury is confined to the mid-zone of the lung with profuse exsanguinating hemorrhage. The patient is hypotensive despite aggressive resuscitation.

Management

Injury to the lung and hilar vessels are a common cause of traumatic hemothorax requiring life-saving thoracotomy. Systemic air embolism is an under appreciated and potentially devastating sequela to patients undergoing thoracotomy for penetrating injuries to the lung. The recipe for this disaster is afforded by: 1) the ongoing hemorrhage that leads to depressed intravascular volumes and pressure; 2) a bullet or knife tract that has disrupted the pulmonary parenchymal architecture, and; 3) endotracheal intubation that completes the resulting scenario of high positive airway pressure combined with low intravascular pulmonary pressures in the face of abnormal communications between these components of the pulmonary anatomy created by the knife or the bullet. Care should be taken to minimize the length of time that these conditions exist by rapid transport to the operating room. If possible this should occur before intubation.

On arrival to the operating room, the patient should be positioned, rapidly prepared and draped. He should then be intubated close to the point of the actual incision. In injuries to the left chest advancing the endotracheal tube into the right mainstem bronchus and keeping the left lung collapsed may be of benefit if the patient can tolerate it. Once the left hemithorax is entered, occluding the pulmonary hilum with a vascular clamp or the surgeon's fingers can impede the passage of air into the pulmonary veins, the left atrium and ultimately cerebral and other systemic circulations.

- One arm of the stapler is placed through the entrance and exit wounds
- When the stapler is fired, the track is exposed
- Direct control of vessels and bronchi

Procedure: *Pulmonary tractotomy*

Pulmonary tractotomy for hemorrhage control has become one of the major advances in thoracic trauma surgery. With the lung clamp placed on either side of the tract created by the knife or bullet, the gastrointestinal anastomosis (GIA) stapling device is positioned so that one arm is placed through the entrance and exit wound of the lung, the other arm is placed over top of the lung parenchyma. When the stapler is fired, the bullet or knife tract is fully exposed, allowing the surgeon to suture directly bleeding vessels and transected bronchi. Figure-of-eight sutures with 3-0 Dexon or Vicryl facilitates direct hemorrhage control. The use of stapled pulmonary tractotomy has dramatically reduced the necessity for segmental resection or a pneumonectomy in the management of penetrating lung injuries.

TECHNICAL OPERATIVE PROCEDURES:

HOW I DO IT

Exposure in Management of an Atrial Laceration

J. Wayne Meredith, MD, FACS

Atrial lacerations can be vexing to repair. In general, right atrial lacerations can often be approached and repaired through a median sternotomy incision whereas a left atrial laceration due to its posterior location, invariably requires a left thoracotomy for repair. Right atrial lacerations often occur in isolation whereas left atrial lacerations generally are associated with other major injuries either to the lung, pulmonary veins, or heart, once again due to its secluded nature posteriorly in the mediastinum. For heart lacerations a double lumen endotracheal tube is not a necessity. A bronchial blocker tube can be of use but it is quite acceptable to repair the laceration to the heart through a thoracotomy with ventilation being provided through a single lumen normal endotracheal tube. Upon completion of the lateral or posterior lateral thoracotomy the pericardium is opened parallel and anterior to the phrenic nerve taking care to avoid injury to this important structure.

- Right atrial lacerations – median sternotomy
- Left atrial lacerations – left thoracotomy
- Grasp edges with an Allis clamp
- Apply a curved Satinsky
- Avoid the right coronary artery
- Repair with running horizontal mattress suture
- Oversew with simple sutures

Procedure: *Repair of atrial lacerations*

An atrial appendage injury is easily repaired by ligating the base of the atrial appendage. This is particularly easy on the left where the appendage often has a very narrow base. Alternatively, a vascular staple can be applied across the base of the atrial appendage to control bleeding lacerations of the atrial appendage. More commonly the laceration is to the body of the atrium. I prefer to control this bleeding initially by placing a finger over the laceration. I then grasp the edges of the laceration with Allis clamps and hold the two clamps together to approximate the edges and control the bleeding. A curved Satinsky clamp is then applied to the atrium incorporating the entire laceration with enough cuff to provide good exposure for closing the laceration. At this stage it's also important to avoid incorporating the right coronary artery in the clamp and compromising blood supply to the ventricle. I prefer to repair atrial lacerations without pledgetted suture, though that is a perfectly acceptable technique and is commonly utilized.

My preferred technique is to repair the laceration with a running horizontal mattress suture then an oversewing simple suture just superficial to the running horizontal mattress. The horizontal mattress suture provides strength through a broad base of contact with the atrium that will not pull through, as a simple suture will. The simple suture line provides hemostasis. It is important to avoid allowing air to enter particularly the left atrium as it is likely that it will subsequently become embolized and cause organ ischemia. The pericardium is generally closed over an angled chest tube and the thoracotomy is closed in layers with one or two pleural chest tubes.

TECHNICAL OPERATIVE PROCEDURES:

HOW I DO IT

Repair of Laceration of the Right Ventricle Foley/Staple/Pledget Technique

Lenworth M. Jacobs, MD, MPH, FACS

Scenario

A 40-year-old man is stabbed in the epigastrium. He presents to the emergency department with distended neck veins, a blood pressure of 90/60 and says he thinks he is going to die.

Management

The patient is intubated and has a 14 gauge intravenous line started in each antecubital fossa. Crystalloid is rapidly infused to increase preload. An ultrasound confirms pericardial tamponade. The patient is transported to the operating room

Procedure: *Foley/staple/pledget cardiac repair*

He is widely prepared and draped from the neck to the groin and bilaterally to the posterior axillary line. An incision is made from the xiphoid for three inches inferiorly. The fascia is opened but the peritoneum is left intact. The dissection is carried cephalad to expose the pericardium. Two thin Deaver retractors are placed and the base of the heart is exposed. A bulging pericardium is observed. I gently palpate the pericardium and discern a boggy hematoma and an ill-defined cardiac impulse. This confirms the diagnosis of pericardial tamponade. No attempt is made to open the pericardium since this will produce significant hemorrhage. It is very difficult to visualize and deal with the laceration in the myocardium if hemorrhage is coming from the base of the wound.

The sternum is then opened in the midline with a sternal saw or a Lebsche knife. A Finochietto retractor is introduced and the sternum is spread open. The pericardium is seen to be bulging.

A 14 Fr. Foley catheter with a 10 mL balloon is obtained and the balloon tested for competence. A skin stapler is procured and 3-0 Prolene with a large curved needle (MH) and Teflon pledgets are placed on a surgical towel. The handle of the retractor and the entire field is draped with surgical towels.

The pericardium is opened vertically taking care to avoid the phrenic nerve. The 1 cm laceration in the right ventricle medial to the left anterior descending coronary artery is identified. A pulsatile stream of blood is observed. The length of the column of blood confirms that there is an injury to the relatively low pressure right ventricle and not the high pressure left ventricle.

I place the index finger of my left hand over the laceration in the right ventricle and then quickly introduce the tip of the Foley catheter into the right ventricle. The catheter is then advanced for a distance of 3 cm, and the balloon is inflated with saline not air. A Kelly clamp is placed on the end of the Foley catheter after blood starts to come from the open end. It is important to vent all the air from the Foley catheter before clamping it to prevent an air embolism.

If the blood pressure falls to zero or if an arrhythmia immediately occurs, it is because the balloon of the catheter is located in the pulmonary valve or in the main pulmonary artery. This phenomenon creates a NO cardiac output situation. The balloon should be deflated and the catheter withdrawn 1 cm and then the balloon should be reinflated. It is important not to remove the catheter from the heart. The catheter and the balloon are then gently retracted against the myocardium.

I like to keep just enough tension to only have a minimal amount of hemorrhage occur with each systolic beat. There is no need for complete hemostasis. In fact, it is not indicated since this means that the balloon is being forcefully pulled against the myocardium. If there is an extra systole, there is a likelihood that the balloon will pull out of the myocardial wound and increase the size of the laceration. The results can be catastrophic.

Once reasonable hemostasis is ensured, the catheter is pulled to one side of the laceration and a staple is placed to partially close the laceration. A second or third staple is then

- The sternum is opened in the midline

- The pericardium is opened vertically to avoid the phrenic nerve

- Primary digital control of the myocardial laceration

- Foley catheter occlusion of the laceration

- Staples around the catheter

- Pledgeted buttressing of the stapled repair

placed very close to the first. The catheter is then pulled in the opposite direction toward the staples. A staple is then placed on the other end of the laceration. The staples will have made the walls of the myocardium fit snugly to the Foley catheter. The catheter is then removed. There should be no bleeding or only minimal ooze from the area from which the Foley catheter was removed. A last staple is placed to bring the edges of the laceration together.

A Teflon pledget is then used to buttress the staple line. I use 3-0 Prolene sutures on a large curved needle and place a horizontal mattress suture. It usually requires two or possibly three Teflon pledgets to completely buttress the laceration. The staples are left in situ permanently.

Care must be taken to avoid stapling the Foley catheter into the myocardium. The Foley catheter balloon must be avoided when suturing the pledget.

At the end of the repair the right ventricle is inspected for normal myocardial contractions. A finger is placed on the heart at the pulmonary outflow tract to palpate for a thrill. This would indicate pulmonary valvular incompetence. The cause of this may be due to picking up the chordae tendinea or the valve itself with the suture. If this is the case, it is wise to seek cardiac surgical assistance. If the patient is hemodynamically stable, it is preferable to formally evaluate valvular function by echocardiogram or with contrast imaging prior to contemplating any formal intervention.

The pericardium is then loosely closed and the sternum closed with wires. The skin is then closed.

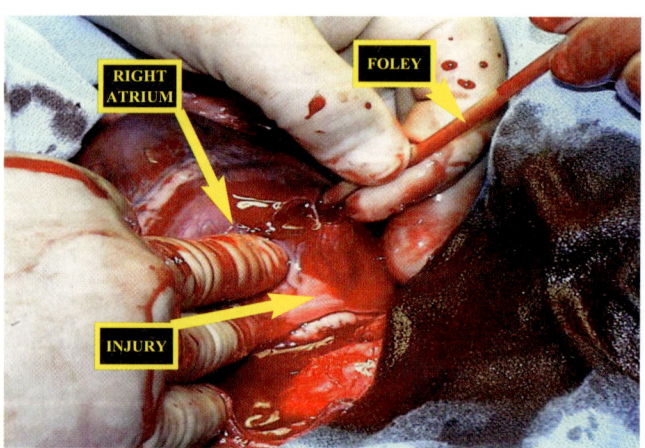
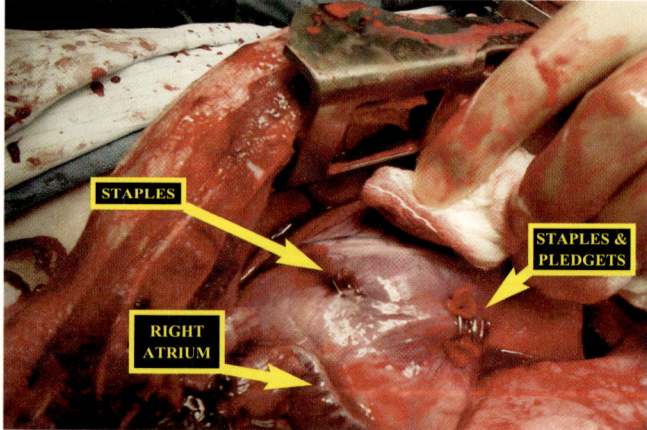

TECHNICAL OPERATIVE PROCEDURES:

HOW I DO IT

Repair of Stab Wound (1.5 cm) to Right Ventricle

Glen Tinkoff, MD, FACS

Scenario

A 25-year-old male presents with a stab wound to the precordium. He has a systolic blood pressure of 90 and distended neck veins.

Initial Management

Management of patients with the possibility of a penetrating cardiac wound must begin with rapid initial assessment based on ATLS principles. A primary survey should proceed rapidly with simultaneous resuscitation. The airway must be maintained, ventilation assured, and venous access for volume resuscitation obtained.

Although present in this scenario, the clinical signs of Beck's triad, jugular venous distension, muffled heart sounds and hypotension, are infrequently encountered in acute trauma. A patient presenting with a wound in the precordium must be approached with a high index of suspicion for a cardiac injury. Diagnostic assessment should include a FAST exam utilizing subxiphoid and/or parasternal windows for the assessment of pericardial effusion. This finding appears as an anechoic area separating the ventricular myocardium from the pericardium.

If ultrasound is unavailable or equivocal, pericardiocentesis can be performed utilizing a 16 gauge Angiocath (preferred) or an 18 gauge spinal needle. The needle with syringe is inserted below the xiphoid process at a 30° angle to the skin and directed toward the left shoulder. As the needle is advanced, the syringe is aspirated continuously until blood is aspirated. Hemodynamic improvement usually is immediate. The patient should be monitored for abrupt changes in rhythm or ST or T wave changes indicating injury to the myocardium.

- Once open, the pericardial space is evacuated of blood and clots

- Direct digital control of the laceration

- Suture with 3-0 polypropylene placed beneath the occluding finger in a figure-of-eight fashion

Given this patient's presenting symptoms, further diagnostic studies such as subxiphoid pericardial window are unwarranted. Even in the face of equivocal ultrasound or pericardiocentesis findings, this patient should be taken to the operating room for further diagnostic and therapeutic intervention.

Operative Technique

After induction of general anesthesia, the patient is prepped from shoulders to anterior thighs. A left anterior thoracotomy should be performed. A median sternotomy is also an option. The incision is carried through the fifth intercostal space and the left chest is entered. A rib spreader is then inserted and opened exposing the pericardial sac. If additional exposure is necessary the sternum can be incised transversely using a Lebsche knife. The left lung is then retracted cephalad with a hand or broad retractor.

The pericardial sac is secured with either forceps or a clamp and incised longitudinally anterior and parallel to the phrenic nerve. Once open, the pericardial space is evacuated of blood and thrombus. The wound to the right ventricle is identified and controlled digitally. Once hemorrhage is controlled, the patient should be transfused with crystalloid to restore normotension before suture repair.

Most cardiac injuries of this size (1.5 cm) can be managed by direct suturing using 3-0 polypropylene placed beneath the occluding finger in figure-of-eight fashion. An alternative technique would be a running repair with a knot tied at either end or a double row by running down and back with the knot at a single end. In situations where the myocardium is friable, Teflon pledgets should be utilized with horizontal mattress technique. In injuries near the coronary artery, care should be taken to avoid iatrogenic occlusion by passing the suture beneath the coronary artery and around the injury in pledgeted horizontal mattress fashion.

After completion of the repair, time should be given to further resuscitate the patient and correct acidosis, hypothermia and coagulopathy prior to closure. Chest tubes should be inserted through separate stab wounds and positioned anterior and posterior in the left thorax. The thoracotomy incision can be closed using several #1 PDS sutures to encircle the ribs. The overlying muscle fascia should be closed with a running 3-0 absorbable suture. Skin can be reapproximated with staples.

TECHNICAL OPERATIVE PROCEDURES:

HOW I DO IT

Stapled Repair of a Cardiac Laceration

Robert C. Mackersie, MD, FACS

Scenario 1: *Mild/moderate impairment of cardiac function*

A 28-year-old male is involved in an altercation during which he sustains a stab wound to the anterior chest. He arrives in the emergency department approximately 20 minutes after the reported event and a short ambulance transport with two intravenous lines in place. He is breathing spontaneously with a field blood pressure reported at 100 systolic and a heart rate of 110 per minute.

Management

On arrival in the emergency department, he is awake and alert with a Glasgow Coma Score of 15, a blood pressure of 94/60, a heart rate of 120, and a respiratory rate of 24. A quick evaluation shows an isolated 3 cm stab wound just to the left of the sternum and at approximately the level of the nipples without active bleeding. Breath sounds are clear and neck veins are distended. A chest x-ray shows no mediastinal hematoma, a normal cardiac silhouette and clear lung fields without hemothorax and pneumothorax. A FAST exam shows a large pericardial effusion, but a negative abdominal evaluation. The patient receives an immediate 2 liters of crystalloid solution. His blood pressure increases to 106/82 with no change in his heart rate. He is

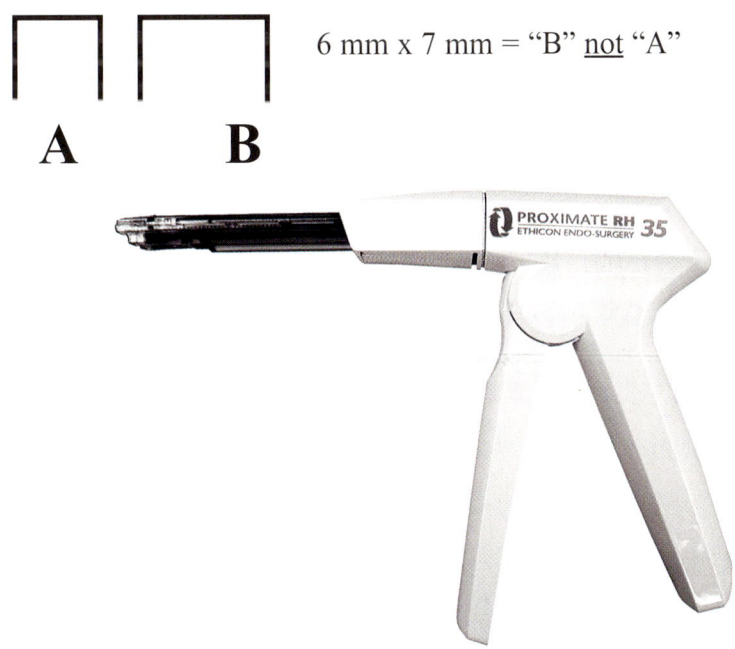

Figure 1: Long-neck skin stapler with ~6mm staples.

taken immediately to the operating room with a presumed diagnosis of pericardial tamponade and a cardiac laceration.

Procedure: *Repair of cardiac injury*

The patient remains hemodynamically unchanged through the very short transport to the operating room. He is placed in the supine position, widely prepped and draped for a median sternotomy prior to the beginning of induction of general anesthesia. Large bore resuscitation lines had been established and blood was available. The surgical team is scrubbed, gowned, and ready to perform either a median sternotomy, an emergency decompressive subxiphoid pericardial window, or an anterolateral emergency resuscitative left thoracotomy in the event the patient deteriorates during induction.

During the rapid sequence induction, the patient's blood pressure dips into the 80's and returns to the low 90's. Heart rate remains elevated at 120 to 130. A median sternotomy incision is made and an oscillating saw used to divide the sternum. The pericardium is tensely distended and during sternal retraction, the patient's systolic pressure drops into the high 60's. The pericardium is quickly opened in its anterior portion and the pericardial tamponade is relieved with approximately 300 cc of blood and clot removed. There is a large amount of active bleeding from a full thickness right ventricular laceration approximately 2 cm in length.

- The cardiac wound is initially digitally controlled

- Staples are placed 5 mm apart

- Pledgeted horizontal mattress sutures buttress the repair

- The pericardium is loosely closed

The cardiac bleeding is initially controlled with digital pressure only. The myocardium is irritable with multiple premature ventricular contractions, and myocardial contractility is thought to be possibly impaired. The heart is moderately full and all fluids are cut back to minimal. With evidence of myocardial ischemia and good control of bleeding digital pressure is carefully maintained for several minutes during which the PVC's resolved.

Using continued gentle digital compression, the cardiac wound is then repaired first using a skin stapler (extended head, pistol grip with 6 mm wide staples, Figure 1) placed 5 mm apart. This effects complete control of bleeding from the right ventricular laceration.

The heart is then allowed to further recover over the next 15 to 20 minutes with resolving acidemia and improvement of ventricular contractility. Double armed, double loaded Teflon pledgeted horizontal mattress sutures of 3-0 Prolene are then placed at the border of the staple line and tied carefully into position. The staples are then removed using a conventional staple remover.

The pericardium is irrigated gently and the remaining clot and blood removed. The heart is carefully inspected for additional wounds. Transesophageal echo may be used intraoperatively to evaluate cardiac function and any potential valvular injury or irregularities. The pericardium is loosely closed. A 36 Fr. straight chest tube is placed for drainage underneath the sternum and the sternum closed in the conventional manner.

Scenario 2: *Severe impairment of cardiac function - near cardiac arrest*

A 32-year-old man is delivered to the emergency department entrance by private vehicle. The patient is unconscious. He is placed on a gurney and found to have no palpable pulse and a weak, ventilatory activity. He arrives in the trauma room with CPR in progress. His isolated injury appears to be a stab wound to the left anterior chest just above the left nipple. Intravenous access is established concurrently with endotracheal intubation and an immediate left thoracotomy. There is an anterior non-bleeding lung laceration and an obvious anterolateral pericardial wound with tense pericardial tamponade. The pericardium is opened longitudinally but anteriorly to the phrenic nerve. Organized cardiac activity is present and a heart rate of about 100. There is a very large amount of active bleeding from a 2+ cm right ventricular stab wound. Bleeding is inadequately controlled with digital pressure alone. A large skin stapler (Figure 1) is used to control the bleeding in conjunction with digital control maintained during stapling. The bleeding is completely controlled with the stapler, and the blood pressure is now 88/60. The wound is covered and resuscitation continued in the operating room.

Comment

Cardiac stapling is technically simple, safe, very rapid, and quite effective for most cardiac injuries. Staples can be used to effect immediate control of cardiac hemorrhage and for more difficult posterior cardiac wounds where elevation of the heart is poorly tolerated. Staples help reduce the manipulation of an ischemic, irritable myocardium, and reduce the incidence of needlestick injuries when suturing cardiac lacerations under digital control. Since the pistol-grip stapler can be placed snugly against the heart and allowed to move along with the beating myocardium, ensuring accurate staple placement is often less difficult than suturing.

Although staples have been used as a definitive means for cardiac wound closure, placement of pledgeted sutures in the operating room, after complete resuscitation of the ischemic heart, is recommended. The staples may be left in place, if desired, after suture placement. Stapling should be used very carefully in cases where cardiac wounds are in close proximity to coronary vessels in order to avoid difficult-to-repair staple injuries to these delicate vessels or staple occlusion and myocardial ischemia.

Reference

Macho JR, Markison RE, Schecter WP: Cardiac stapling in the management of penetrating injuries of the heart: rapid control of hemorrhage and decreased risk of personal contamination. J Trauma. 1993 May;34(5):711-5.

TECHNICAL OPERATIVE PROCEDURES:

HOW I DO IT

Exposure Management of a 1.5 cm Stab Wound to the Right Ventricle

J. Wayne Meredith, MD, FACS

Scenario

A 20-year-old man is involved in an altercation and sustains a stab wound just to the right of the sternum, presenting with hypotension and distended neck veins.

Management

The diagnosis of a patient such as this can generally be made on clinical findings. The patients usually will present with evidence of cardiac tamponade. If the rent in the pericardium is sufficiently large to allow easy egress of blood to the pleural space, the patient may present in hemorrhagic shock. If imaging is needed to confirm the diagnosis, it is best performed with a FAST exam. If the FAST is equivocal or unavailable, it is acceptable to confirm the diagnosis with a pericardial window. It is not necessary or appropriate to delay treatment in patients in whom the diagnosis can be made by physical examination and who are in shock.

Most anterior "mantel" stab wounds can be best approached and repaired via a median sternotomy incision. The rare exceptions for these stab wounds are for a very lateral stab wound on the left. Gunshot wounds typically require thoracotomy. Prophylactic antibiotics are usually administered prior to making the incision. It is valuable to listen to the precordium for abnormal heart sounds indicative of a ventricular septal defect (VSD) or valvular insufficiency as a consequence of the laceration prior to operation. The operation to release tamponade and control the laceration should not be delayed due to these findings. It is also valuable to prep the patient prior to induction since many patients experience cardiovascular collapse with induction of anesthesia.

Procedure: *Exposure management of a 1.5 cm stab wound to the right ventricle*

Most cardiac surgeons today prefer to divide the sternum from superior to inferior. This technique allows a smaller incision to be used and provides a better cosmetic result. For

- Control the laceration with gentle digital pressure

- Repair with felt pledgeted monofilament sutures

- Use horizontal mattress sutures

- Place sutures 1 cm apart and 0.5 cm from the edge of the laceration trauma or for less experienced surgeons, I recommend a longer incision that extends slightly above the sternal notch and 3cm to 5 cm below the xiphoid process dividing the linea Alba but not entering the peritoneum. I believe it is safer, although it requires a larger incision, to then perform the sternotomy from inferiorly to superiorly. This is accomplished by first mobilizing the xiphoid as one would for a subxiphoid pericardial window. The xiphoid itself is split with scissors and the pericardium is mobilized from the posterior surface of the sternum. The dense ligaments between the insertions of the sternocleidomastoid along the very top of the sternal notch are divided and the substernal plane is established bluntly superiorly and then the sternum is divided with a saw.

The thymus is mobilized from the superior pericardium taking care to avoid the innominate vein which lies at its base. The pericardium is opened vertically in the midline and may be 'T'd' at its base. In most cases it is useful to suspend the edges of the pericardium with sutures. Time does not usually allow this maneuver in a trauma situation. I prefer to control the laceration with gentle, digital pressure. Many authors describe placing a Foley catheter into the laceration, inflating the balloon and placing gentle outward traction to control the bleeding. This is a perfectly acceptable technique, but I personally prefer the control that the finger provides. This approach also lessens the likelihood of the assistant pulling the balloon through the laceration and extending the laceration. It also lessens the chance of unintentionally bursting the balloon or capturing the catheter itself with a suture.

The laceration is repaired with felt pledgeted 2-0 monofilament sutures. I prefer an MH needle. The suture is applied in a horizontal mattress fashion. It is best to plan where the sutures will enter the epicardium and position the suture on the pledget exactly that distance apart as well. Placing the sutures more narrowly on the pledget than in the pericardium causes a tendency to have tearing of the epicardium. Placing the suture too widely on the pledget tends to buckle the pledget, making it more difficult to get a secure application to the epicardium. Usually these sutures are placed about a centimeter apart and a half a centimeter back from the edge and are full thickness through all layers of the ventricle. If the laceration is near the left anterior descending coronary artery or other major coronary artery the suture should be placed deep to the vessel so as not to encircle it with a suture causing ischemia distally. It is valuable to feel the ventricle, atrium, and pulmonary artery for thrills upon completion of the repair to get some notion as to the presence of a VSD or valvular insufficiency. These are not generally repaired initially at the time of emergency operation unless the patient has florid heart failure. It may be valuable to check oxygen saturations on blood drawn from the atrium and ventricle simultaneously to look for a step up if a VSD is expected. Generally one chest tube is first placed in the pericardium at the base, generally an angled chest tube and a substernal chest tube is placed prior to closure of the sternum. The sternum is closed with sternal wires. A secure sternal closure is extremely important to prevent subsequent sternal wound difficulties.

TECHNICAL OPERATIVE PROCEDURES:
HOW I DO IT

Control of the Aorta Through The Left Chest

Aurelio Rodriguez, MD, FACS

Scenario
A 25-year-old man was involved in a motor vehicle crash. The vital signs in the field were a blood pressure of 80 systolic and a pulse of 140. On arrival to the trauma center, the pulse and blood pressure were absent.

Management
After the establishment of an endotracheal tube, simultaneous infusion of two liters of crystalloid through two large intravenous lines and closed cardiopulmonary resuscitation was initiated. It is decided to perform an emergency resuscitative thoracotomy.

Procedure: *Control of the aorta through the left chest*
Povidone (Betadine) solution is generously poured over the anterior left and right chest. A right chest tube thoracostomy and a FAST examination are performed concomitantly to the opening of the left chest. The incision is performed below the nipple, approximately at the level of the fourth intercostal space from the midsternal line to the posterior axillary line. The incision is deepened to the subcutaneous tissue and anterior chest wall muscles. The intercostal space is pierced with the scalpel and totally opened in the landmarks previously established with the help of a curved Mayo scissors.

A Finochietto chest retractor is placed and opened with the transverse bar toward the sternal area. The following maneuvers should be followed.

The inflation of the left lung is inspected to assure that the endotracheal tube is in the correct position. The anesthesiologist is notified if the lung is not moving with respiratory ventilation.

Closed heart massage with the pericardium intact is performed for a few seconds. The pericardium is opened to the phrenic nerve with a Metzenbaum scissors. A generous incision is used to allow for adequate visualization of the myocardium.

Bimanual cardiac massage is initiated after inspection of the heart and exclusion of a cardiac injury that needs to be surgically addressed. The assistant retracts the left lung with his/her hands gently towards the right side of the patient. The descending aorta is palpated with the left hand thumb in its location at the left paraspinal area.

The aorta is expeditiously bluntly dissected from the parietal pleura. A Satinsky vascular clamp is used to occlude the aorta. The aorta is directly visualized to confirm that the clamp is correctly placed. The esophagus is identified to confirm that the structure in the clamp is indeed the aorta. The left lung is returned to its normal position.

Cardiac massage is continued during the clamping procedure. The assistant can help perform compression of the heart against the sternum.

- Incision at the fourth intercostal space from the midsternal line to the posterior axillary line

- The left lung is retracted towards the right side

- The aorta is directly visualized

- The esophagus is visualized

- A Satinsky clamp occludes the aorta

TECHNICAL OPERATIVE PROCEDURES:

HOW I DO IT

Supraceliac Aortic Control and Skin Only Closure After Damage Control

Michael F. Rotondo, MD, FACS

Scenario

The patient is a 40-year-old male who presents with a stab wound to the midepigastric region. The wound is located 6 cm above the umbilicus in the midline. Patient was transported having been found after an unknown period of time with a temperature of 34°C and a blood pressure of 80 systolic.

Management: *Initial resuscitation and damage control laparotomy*

The need for operation is immediately recognized upon discovery of the midline penetration in the presence of hypotension. After obtaining large bore peripheral intravenous access, blood is obtained for type and crossmatch. After an abbreviated neurologic examination, the patient undergoes rapid sequence induction and intubation for immediate airway control. Resuscitation is initiated with warm crystalloid solution and universal type O blood. The patient is fully exposed and examined for additional penetrations and no other injuries are identified. A rectal examination is completed, which reveals gross blood. A Foley catheter is placed and a nasogastric tube is placed, both of which reveal no gross blood. The initial temperature is 34°C. The total resuscitation time is 12 minutes. He is taken to the operating room for exploratory laparotomy. It is clear from the information available that the patient has a torso injury confined to the abdomen and likely to involve large intestine and a major vascular structure. Due to the wounding mechanism and the abnormal physiology on presentation, the patient should immediately be identified as a candidate for damage control.

Procedure: *Supraceliac aortic control*

The patient is persistently hypotensive and a supraceliac aortic clamp is placed. The surgeon on the right side of the table performs this by first retracting the stomach inferiorly and to the patient's left, identifying and bluntly incising the hepatogastric omentum. The supraceliac aorta is palpated with the left hand through the right crus. With the aortic pulsation stabilized between the thumb and first finger of the operating surgeon's left hand, the fibers of the right crus of the diaphragm are incised using a very long Metzenbaum scissors to admit the index finger of the surgeon's left hand to the aorta and digital dissection using the thumb and first finger is performed to isolate the aorta in the supraceliac position. A long Satinsky clamp is then placed on the aorta at this level utilizing digital guidance. It is important that this clamp is placed securely and the time of the clamp application should be noted. This procedure should take no longer than two to four minutes. Four quadrant and central retroperitoneal packing then ensues. The Bookwalter retractor is set up for general exposure. As the blood pressure is normalized, the supraceliac aortic clamp may be removed one click at a time as tolerated.

Only moderate bleeding is noted with the aortic cross clamp in place. The aortic cross clamp is slowly removed. Bleeding is identified at the base of the hematoma at the origin of the middle celiac artery, which is controlled using a 0-silk free tie after a right angle clamp has been applied. A series of venous and small arterial bleeders are similarly controlled. The aortic cross clamp is then successfully removed from both a hemodynamic and hemorrhage control standpoint.

- Control the aorta with the thumb and first finger of the left hand

- Incise the crus of the diaphragm

- Use digital dissection to isolate the aorta

- Place a Satinsky clamp using digital guidance

- Remove clamp one click at a time

TECHNICAL OPERATIVE PROCEDURES:

HOW I DO IT

Gunshot Wounds to the Abdominal Aorta

Demetrios Demetriades, MD, FACS

Scenario

A 30-year-old man sustains a .32 caliber gunshot wound to the left upper quadrant. The abdomen is distended and tense. The patient is hypotensive. Following resuscitation he is brought to the operating room. There is an injury to the aorta immediately distal to the superior mesenteric artery. There is a large pulsating retroperitoneal hematoma in the superior abdomen.

Management

The abdomen is entered through a long midline laparotomy incision. Once the large Zone I retroperitoneal hematoma is identified, a vascular injury should be suspected and proximal and distal control should be obtained. Generally, proximal control can be obtained by dissecting the aorta just below the diaphragm. This maneuver can be facilitated by dividing the left crus of the diaphragm at two o'clock. However, in large supramesocolic hematomas infradiaphragmatic control of the aorta might not be possible. In these cases a left thoracotomy and supradiaphragmatic aortic cross clamping may be necessary. The distal aorta is exposed by medial rotation of the left colon and a vessel loop is placed around the aorta. Only after proximal and distal control should the hematoma be explored. A combination of direct dissection of the hematoma and medial rotation of the left colon, the tail of the pancreas and the spleen, should provide good exposure of the aortic injury. Depending on the site of aortic injury the left kidney may be rotated medially or left undisturbed.

The aortic injury may be repaired with continuous vascular sutures, although in most cases with gunshot wounds a prosthetic patch or even a graft may be necessary.

- Proximal control can be obtained by dissecting the aorta just below the diaphragm

- Divide the left crus of the diaphragm at 2 o'clock

- Obtain proximal and distal control

TECHNICAL OPERATIVE PROCEDURES:
HOW I DO IT

Exposure and Management of a 2 cm Laceration to the Infrarenal Abdominal Aorta

David V. Feliciano, MD, FACS

Overview

As in patients with injuries to the suprarenal abdominal aorta or its branches, almost all patients with injuries to the infrarenal abdominal aorta have associated injuries to the duodenum, small bowel, or colon. Of interest, this does not affect the choice of repair in most centers.

In contrast to injuries to the suprarenal abdominal aorta, the technique for exposure of an infrarenal aortic injury is the same whether a contained inframesocolic hematoma or hemorrhage is present.

Procedure: *Exposure of the infrarenal abdominal aorta*

After manual and suction evacuation of blood and gastrointestinal contents, the surgeon may once again complete rapid closures of large gastrointestinal perforations using a stapling device or one-layer closure with polypropylene suture when a midline retroperitoneal hematoma is present. The abdomen is then rapidly irrigated with a saline solution containing antibiotics. The transverse colon is retracted superiorly, and the small bowel is eviscerated to the surgeon's side of the operating table and covered with a moist towel. There are two types of inframesocolic hematomas surrounding an injury in the infrarenal abdominal aorta. Most commonly, there is a large midline hematoma appearing almost like a mountain in the retroperitoneum. A few patients with lateral perforations may have more of a diffuse hematoma approaching the left colon or encompassing the inferior vena cava on the right.

In patients with a mountain present, the anterior perforation in the infrarenal abdominal aorta is immediately under the apex of the mountain. When a more diffuse hematoma is present, the exact location of the perforation is unclear.

Should the apex of the mountain or the area of hemorrhage be adjacent to the transverse mesocolon? The inexperienced trauma surgeon may find it safest to rapidly cross clamp the suprarenal abdominal aorta through the lesser sac approach previously described for injuries to the suprarenal abdominal aorta. A more experienced trauma surgeon may simply divide the midline hematoma under the apex of the mountain and obtain manual control of the infrarenal abdominal aorta at the perforation. Further rapid dissection in the midline retroperitoneum will allow for application of DeBakey aortic clamps just below the left renal vein and distally beyond the injury. Should the surgeon misjudge the location of the aortic perforation and find that it is juxtarenal, division of the left renal vein and its lumbar branch will allow for proximal cross clamping of the juxtarenal or suprarenal abdominal aorta.

Procedure: *Vascular repair of the aorta*

A small aortic perforation is closed with a continuous 3-0 or 4-0 polypropylene suture, while two perforations are connected and a transverse closure performed. An extensive loss of tissue on one wall is closed with a tailored PTFE patch. Destruction of a segment of the infrarenal abdominal aorta is generally treated with débridement of both ends and insertion of a 12 mm, 14 mm, or 16 mm woven Dacron graft, albumin-coated Dacron graft or a PTFE graft - none of which require preclotting. Proximal and distal flushing prior to completion of the distal suture line is performed, and the proximal cross clamp is reapplied. As air is flushed out of the aorta by back bleeding from the distal end, the final suture is tied on the distal anastomosis. The proximal aortic cross clamp is then gradually removed by the surgeon as the anesthesiology team infuses blood or crystalloids and sodium bicarbonate to counteract hypotension and washout acidosis.

All repairs of the infrarenal abdominal aorta are completely covered with a viable pedicle of left-sided omentum to prevent a postoperative aorto-duodenal fistula. In patients undergoing a damage control procedure, the omental pedicle can be mobilized and placed at the first reoperation. Intravenous antibiotics, third generation cephalosporin, are continued for three postoperative days, though the data is unclear on whether this is better than one postoperative day.

- Aortic injury will be found directly below the peak of a well-contained mountain hematoma

- Best approach to aortic control in a patient with a well-defined retroperitoneal mountain hematoma is directly onto aorta through the hematoma

- Aortic control of a more diffuse retroperitoneal hematoma is best obtained proximal to the hematoma

- Division of left renal vein and its lumbar branch enables placement of a juxtarenal or suprarenal aortic cross clamp

- All repairs are covered with viable left-sided omental pedicle

TECHNICAL OPERATIVE PROCEDURES:

HOW I DO IT

Injury to a Major Vein

Donald D. Trunkey, MD, FACS

Scenario

A 24-year-old male has been stabbed with a bayonet in the right upper quadrant. The patient is hypotensive, is taken immediately to the operating room where a midline incision is performed. Three liters of blood are found in the abdomen.

Management

Preoperative antibiotics are given presumptively for a possible associated hollow viscous injury. After the packs are removed from the abdomen and exposure is obtained, there appears to be large retroperitoneal hematoma with a laceration at the root of the mesentery just below the third portion of the duodenum. The small bowel is transected in one area and nearly transected in another. These are closed with a staple gun. Blood coming from the rent in the retroperitoneum is dark, is partially controlled with two large sponge sticks, placed proximal and distal to the laceration in the peritoneum.

A presumptive diagnosis of injury to a major vein is assumed and a medial visceral rotation from the right side is carried out. This includes mobilizing the cecum, ascending colon, hepatic flexure and duodenum towards the midline. As this is done, the temporary tamponade with sponge sticks is released, and the entire mesentery is bluntly and sharply dissected off from the inferior vena cava. The sponge sticks are immediately reapplied after the visceral rotation

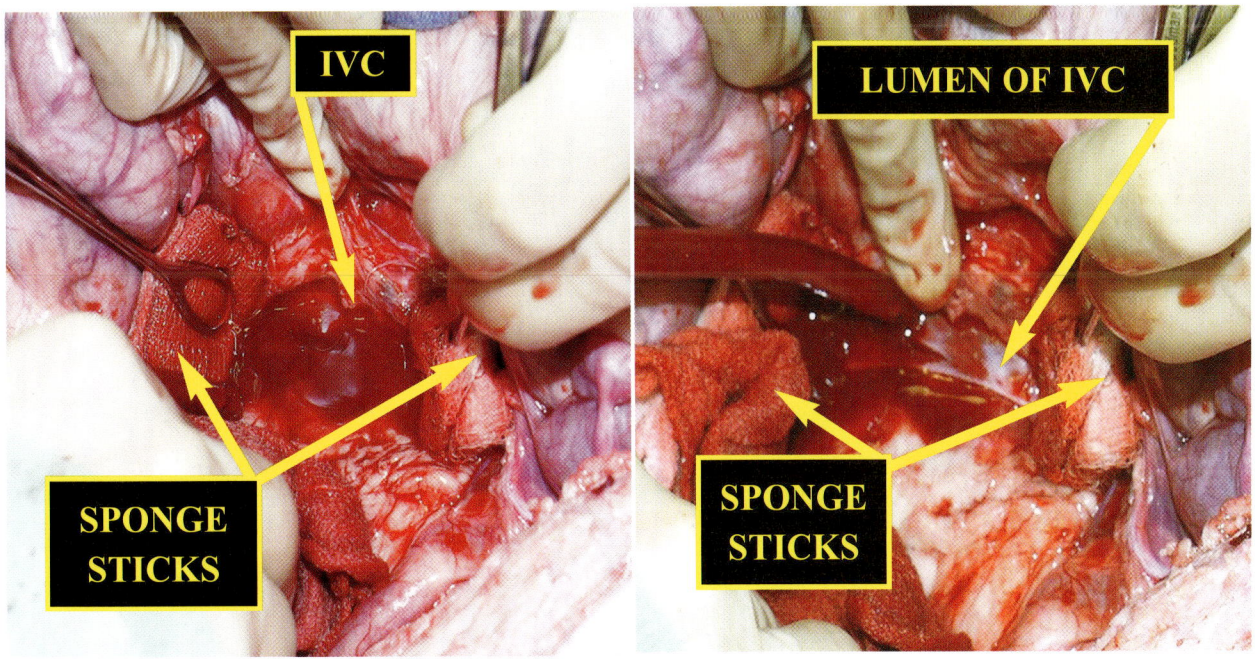

and this shows a 3 cm laceration of the anterior lateral surface of the inferior vena cava midway between the right renal vein on the right and the right iliac vein. With direct compression of the sponge sticks proximal and distal, the bleeding can be controlled. The laceration is repaired with 5-0 Prolene or silk in a running fashion. There is some oozing from behind the cava, which requires isolation of two separate pairs of lumbar veins, which are doubly ligated, and the inferior vena cava is retracted medially using sponge sticks by rolling the cava towards the left side of the patient. A 1 cm laceration is identified, which is repaired with 5-0 Prolene.

Both injuries to the small bowel are repaired with a two-layer anastomosis of 3-0 Vicryl and 3-0 silk inverting Lembert stitches.

A right medial visceral rotation will allow the surgeon to repair most injuries to the inferior vena cava from the iliacs to and including the right and left renal veins. If an error has been made and the infrarenal aorta is injured, this can be repaired through the same retroperitoneal approach. A left medial visceral rotation is indicated primarily for injuries to the suprarenal aorta. Injuries to the retrohepatic cava or the inferior vena cava above the renal veins will require complete mobilization of the right lobe of the liver and most often vascular isolation of the liver in order to achieve repair of the inferior vena cava and ligation of segment I branches, which are often avulsed.

- Temporary tamponade with sponge sticks is effective

- The laceration is repaired with a continuous 5-0 Prolene suture

TECHNICAL OPERATIVE PROCEDURES:

HOW I DO IT

Repair of The Inferior Vena Cava Double Satinsky Clamp Technique

Lenworth M. Jacobs, MD, MPH, FACS

Scenario

A 21-year-old man was stabbed with a 10 inch kitchen knife in the right periumbilical area. He was severely hypotensive and he had a tense hemoperitoneum.

Management

The patient was intubated and 14 gauge intravenous lines were placed in the right and the left antecubital fossa. A chest x-ray showed no hemopneumothorax and a FAST exam of the heart and abdomen were performed. The heart was normal with no evidence of a hemopericardium. There was a large amount of free blood in the abdomen. The temperature in the operating room was increased to 80°F. The blood bank was alerted and told to type and cross match ten units of blood and to be prepared to always have ten units of blood available for this patient. The autotransfusion device was available and anesthesia was alerted that this is a major trauma case. Broad spectrum antibiotics were given to cover gram negative and anaerobic organisms.

The abdomen was rapidly prepped from the neck to the midthigh and a large midline incision from the xiphoid to the pubis was performed. Blood was collected with the autotranfusion suction device and clots scooped out with the surgeon's hand into a large bowl. The small bowel was eviscerated and dark blood was seen to be rising from a rent in the retroperitoneum at the level of the fourth lumbar vertebra. The hemorrhage was audible.

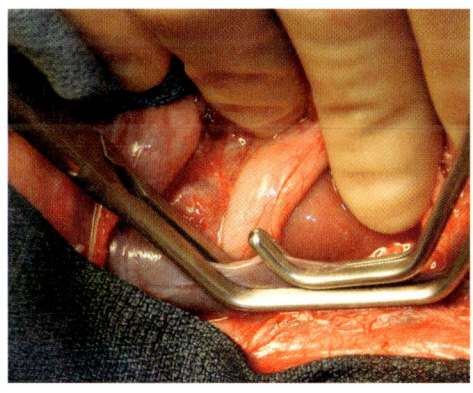
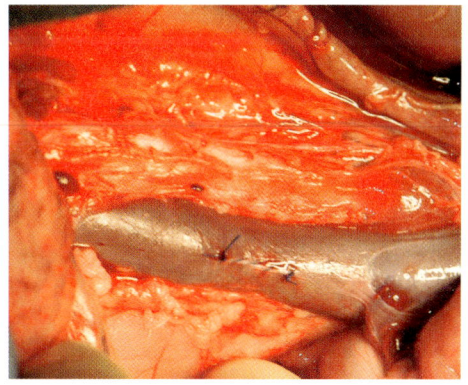

The suspicion was that this was a vena caval injury since the hemorrhage was profuse, nonpulsatile, and dark. I immediately palpated the bifurcation of the aorta and moved my hand laterally to compress the distal inferior vena cava. My other hand compressed the inferior vena cava at the level of the duodenum. These maneuvers slowed the hemorrhage. The entire small bowel with the mesentery was then swept to the left upper quadrant. This maneuver will usually expose the rent in the mesentery which leads to the laceration in the inferior vena cava. The mesentery and the peritoneum over the cava were carefully dissected taking care not to tear and enlarge the laceration in the vena cava. Iatrogenic injuries to the cava by rough manipulation can convert a salvageable injury into a fatal non-repairable laceration.

Two sponge sticks were then used to obtain proximal and distal control of the cava. The suction device was then used to visualize the extent of the laceration. If the retroperitoneal hematoma is extensive and it is difficult to visualize the laceration, the cecum and the ascending colon are mobilized by sharply dissecting the lateral attachments at the white line of Toldt. The entire ascending colon and the small bowel were then mobilized, swept medially and placed in the left upper quadrant. I find that the hematoma has usually created a plane and this entire dissection can be quickly and easily performed by blunt dissection with one's fingers (Cattel Braasch maneuver).

The bifurcation of the aorta, the vena cava, and the gonadal vessels were exposed. If the laceration extends up toward the renal vessels, the duodenum and the head of the pancreas are bluntly dissected and rotated medially (extended Kocher maneuver). The vena cava and the injury were visualized.

Procedure: *Double side biting Satinsky clamp inferior vena cava control*

I now take an angled Satinsky clamp and grasp the portion of the inferior vena cava that contains the laceration. The handles of the clamp were placed at the inferior portion of the abdomen. A second larger Satinsky clamp was opened and placed under the first clamp so that the entire laceration was contained within the basket of the Satinsky clamp. The handles of this clamp were placed at the superior porton of the abdomen. The handles rest on the viscera and the clamp is now balanced in the abdomen and should require minimal manipulation to maintain an optimal position to repair the laceration.

- Two sponge sticks are used to gain proximal and distal control of the inferior vena cava

- A second larger Satinsky basket clamp is placed under the first

- The laceration is then visualized and closed with a continuous 5-0 Prolene suture

- Vigorous transfusion through the superior vena cava will correct hypotension

A suction catheter was used to prepare the operative field and to identify if there was a posterior laceration or if a lumbar vein had been lacerated. The laceration was then closed with a 5-0 Prolene continuous suture. One millimeter bites should be taken on each side of the laceration of the vena cava to avoid narrowing the lumen.

One drawback of this method is that the second Satinsky clamp can capture enough of the vena cava that the flow through the inferior vena cava is significantly attenuated. This is not usually a major problem since there is adequate collateral circulation to bypass the inferior vena cava occlusion. In any event, the anesthesiologist should be alerted that the inferior vena cava is obstructed and this could be a cause of hypotension. Vigorous transfusion through the superior intravenous lines will correct hypotension.

If there is a posterior wall laceration, I dissect out, ligate and transect one or two lumbar veins and then roll the cava laterally to identify the posterior laceration. This is usually smaller than the anterior laceration. It is then closed with a running 5-0 Prolene suture.

I like to drape the handles of the Satinsky clamp and the bowel out of the field so that only the basket of the Satinsky clamp and the injury are exposed. This minimizes the chances that the suture will be caught in the handles of the clamp. Exclusion draping is very important since the procedure is being performed deep in the bottom of the operating field. It is essential to minimize any chance of technical misadventures.

The repair in the inferior vena cava was inspected and palpated for hemorrhage, narrowing or a venous thrill. A small degree of narrowing can be tolerated. If the narrowing is significant, a venous patch can be fashioned and sutured in place to increase the size of the lumen. I have not found this to be necessary. The bowel is then returned to its original position. A full exploratory laparotomy is then performed to look for other injuries. At the end of that procedure the inferior vena cava repair is then re-inspected and the abdomen closed.

TECHNICAL OPERATIVE PROCEDURES:

HOW I DO IT

Stab Wound to Inferior Vena Cava

Blaine L. Enderson, MD, MBA, FACS, FCCM

Scenario

A 36-year-old man is stabbed in the abdomen with an isolated through-and-through wound to the infrarenal inferior vena cava.

Management

Hemodynamically unstable patients with stab wounds to the abdomen should be taken directly to the operating room. Broad spectrum antibiotics should be given on the way to the operating room. High flow resuscitation lines should be placed above the level of the diaphragm and warmed fluids and emergency released blood available via rapid infusers to resuscitate the patient as the injury is controlled in the operating room. Use of a cell saver to reinfuse shed blood should be considered, but should not delay operative intervention or resuscitation.

The abdomen is rapidly entered through a generous midline incision. One member of the team can obtain control of inflow to the abdomen by manually compressing the aorta against the spine at the level of the diaphragm, while other team members rapidly pack the abdomen to control and identify the source of blood loss. Once the midline hematoma is identified, this can be controlled with direct pressure with lap pads to allow resuscitative efforts to catch up and to allow time to expose the injury.

Exposure of the inferior vena cava is best accomplished by medially rotating the right-sided abdominal viscera. The lateral attachments of the colon are taken down rapidly with cautery and the right colon and duodenum are mobilized medially, exposing the inferior vena cava. Direct pressure with sponge sticks can then be applied to the wound in the inferior vena cava, allowing control of bleeding, while proximal and distal control are obtained.

The inferior vena cava is carefully dissected circumferentially proximally and distally to the injury and a vessel loop is passed around the IVC to assist with control. Often there will be continued bleeding from lumbar veins. These can be carefully dissected and controlled with vessel loops as well, to allow evaluation of the injury to the IVC. Once a through and through

- Vessel loops are passed around the IVC to gain proximal and distal control

- Lumbar veins are also controlled

- IVC wounds are repaired transversely if possible

- With massive destruction of the IVC, ligation is an option injury is identified, these lumbar vessels can be divided to allow mobilization and rotation of this segment of the inferior vena cava to assist in the repair of the posterior injury.

The wounds in the IVC are repaired transversely, if possible, with a running 5-0 polypropylene suture. If it is too large to repair transversely, it can be closed longitudinally, understanding that there may be some narrowing and a risk of thrombosis. In general, stab wounds can be closed primarily. In some cases, with massive destruction of the IVC and severe instability of the patient, the IVC can be ligated.

TECHNICAL OPERATIVE PROCEDURES:

HOW I DO IT

Repair of The Inferior Vena Cava

Thomas M. Scalea, M.D., FACS, FCCM

Scenario

A 26-year-old male presents hypotensive with a gunshot wound to the right lower quadrant and a 2 cm laceration of the inferior vena cava.

Management

Identification of injuries to the IVC is a high priority, as these can be lethal. Particularly in a patient in shock, prompt management is necessary to maximize the chances of survival.

As with any patient who is hypotensive after injury, a midline incision should be made from the xiphoid to the pubis. The abdomen is quickly explored and ideally blood is aspirated into a cell saver system. The abdomen is then packed and then a rapid search is made for the source of hypotension.

Patients with injuries to the vena cava almost always have evidence of right-sided retroperitoneal hematoma. Often these injuries bleed massively into the abdomen, but the volume of bleeding slows when the patient develops hypotension. The sophisticated clinician should not be lulled into a false sense of security by the lack of active bleeding at the time of laparotomy.

If I suspect a caval injury, I do a complete medial visceral rotation of the right colon. I completely mobilize the right colon by incising the white line of Toldt. In order to get the best exposure, I mobilize the colon all the way around the hepatic flexure into the mid-transverse colon. In addition, I completely mobilize the cecum, appendix and terminal ileum. If the area in question is located more cephalad around the renal vein, I also perform a complete Kocher maneuver. I mobilize the duodenum in the head of the pancreas all the way over across the cava giving full exposure of the entirety of the infrahepatic vena cava.

Obtaining proximal and distal vascular control is ideal, but often impossible in patients particularly if they have sustained hypotension. After mobilization of the right colon and duodenum, it is relatively easy to identify the anterior wall of the vena cava. It is important to completely skeletonize the cava in order to identify the areas of injury. A number of techniques exist to control the caval injury temporarily including finger control, use of a vascular clamp or sponge sticks. I find all of these cumbersome and unfortunately, by the time the surgeon has enough control with clamps or sponge sticks, it is impossible to see anything else.

Even if one is able to obtain proximal and distal vascular control before unroofing the injury, it is difficult to obtain complete hemostasis. The large posterior placed lumbar vein is often a source of significant bleeding. This can prove to be quite frustrating when the surgeon has a clamp on the cava proximally and distally, but still sees large volume blood loss. Completely occluding the inferior vena cava is sometimes followed by a cardiac arrest, particularly in patients who are hypotensive. The IVC supplies approximately two-thirds of the venous return. In a patient who is in shock, abrupt loss of cardiac filling may result in cardiovascular collapse.

Procedure: *Repair of the vena cava*

I generally prefer to attack injuries to the vena cava directly. I often begin in the upper abdomen, identifying the cava at the level just distal to the renal veins and work my way down towards the iliac vein. I do not generally loop the cava, but instead quickly divide the retroperitoneal tissue overlying the cava. When I reach the area of injury, often there is usually significant bleeding for a short time. This is almost always controlled with digital pressure. I then dissect the cava.

I then begin to slowly pull my finger back until I can visualize the edge of the injured cava. I place an intestinal Allis clamp at this juncture and then continue slowly to retract my finger, stacking the clamps as I go. It is important to get both ends of the lacerated cava into the jaws of the Allis clamp. A 2 cm defect can generally be controlled with two or three Allis clamps.

When the defect is completely controlled, I lift the clamps up. This allows for preservation of venous return while completely controlling the injuries. This technique is useful anywhere in the cava, but I find it particularly useful on caval injuries adjacent to the renal vein or near the caval bifurcation. Controlling the renal vessels as well as the cava in order to control vascular inflow is technically challenging. The same is true in the pelvis. This technique obviates the need for any of these.

- Skeletonize the inferior vena cava to identify the injury

- Control bleeding initially with digital pressure

- Slowly pull the finger back to visualize the edge of the injury

- Place Allis clamps as the laceration is exposed

- Repair with 4-0 Prolene sutures

I generally repair the cava with 3-0 or 4-0 Prolene sutures. I place the suture at the apex of the wound adjacent to the first clamp and tie it down. The suture can be passed back and forth under the clamps, taking small bites just underneath the clamps. As the defect is repaired, the clamps can be removed sequentially. I then run the suture back and tie it to itself. Any small residual bleeding can be repaired with another interrupted suture or generally controlled with topical hemostatic agents.

TECHNICAL OPERATIVE PROCEDURES:

HOW I DO IT

Penetrating Injury to the Vena Cava

Susan M. Briggs, MD, MPH, FACS

Scenario

The patient is a young male with a stab wound to the right lower quadrant of the abdomen. Initial blood pressure prior to resuscitation with crystalloid is 60/40 with a pulse rate of 140 and a respiratory rate of 32. The patient is awake but intoxicated and unable to follow commands. Large bore intravenous lines are placed and blood sent for type and cross match.

No preoperative imaging is performed. The patient is taken urgently to the operating room for exploration. His blood pressure following two liters of crystalloid resuscitation is 80/40.

Management

The patient is intubated and the abdomen and chest are prepped and draped in the usual sterile manner. Because of the potential for major abdominal venous injury, lower extremity intravenous lines are avoided. The right lower extremity is included in the prep in the event harvesting of the saphenous vein is necessary. As the patient is hypotensive, 0+ uncrossed matched blood is sent to the operating room until type-specific blood can be obtained. Preoperative antibiotics are given to the patient. A nasogastric tube and Foley catheter are inserted. A cell saver is on standby in the event of an isolated vascular injury without associated peritoneal contamination from a hollow viscous injury.

Procedure

A midline incision extending from the xiphoid to below the umbilicus is performed. On entering the abdomen, a large Zone I inframesocolic hematoma to the right of the midline is identified. Minimal intraperitoneal blood is present. The abdomen is packed in four quadrants and no other significant bleeding or contamination is identified.

The aorta is identified and appears intact. The location of the hematoma is suspicious for injury to the vena cava. The vena cava is visualized by mobilizing the right half of the colon and C-loop of the duodenum, leaving the right kidney in situ by performing a Cattel Braasch maneuver or medial mobilization of right-sided intraabdominal viscera. This allows visualization of the entire vena cava from the confluence of the iliac veins to the suprarenal vena cava below the liver. Dissection distally to proximally along the anterior surface of the vena cava is performed until a 2 cm longitudinal laceration of the infrarenal vena cava is identified. Proximal and distal control is initially obtained with gauze sponges in straight sponge sticks.

Examination of the vena cava must include the possibility of anterior and posterior lacerations of the vena cava. The lumen was opened and an intact posterior wall was visualized. It is often necessary to extend the anterior laceration slightly if adequate visualization of the posterior wall cannot be obtained. It is often, but not always, possible to repair the posterior laceration from inside the vena cava. Collateral circulation and lumbar veins often make it difficult to rotate the vena cava to visualize the posterior wall, depending on how close the vena caval laceration is to the confluence of the common iliac veins or the caval junction with the renal veins. Atraumatic Allis clamps are applied to the walls of the vena cava laceration to allow placement of a Satinsky vascular clamp. The vascular repair is performed with continuous 5-0 Prolene suture. Hemostasis was satisfactory and the lumen appeared adequate.

In this patient, satisfactory proximal and distal control was easily achieved. In more difficult locations of injury to the vena cava, direct compression or the use of balloon occlusion catheters may be necessary. Complex injuries to the infrarenal vena cava may require ligation or the use of autogenous saphenous vein patch or synthetic patches.

Postoperative anticoagulation is not utilized. Postoperative venous imaging studies are not helpful in identifying and preventing long-term complications of vena cava stenosis or occlusion.

- Dissection distally to proximally on the anterior surface exposes the IVC laceration

- Proximal and distal control with sponge sticks

- Repair with continuous 5-0 Prolene

TECHNICAL OPERATIVE PROCEDURES:

HOW I DO IT

Exposure and Management of a 2 cm Laceration of the Infrarenal Portion of the IVC, Allis Clamp Control of Laceration of the Vena Cava

L.D. Britt, MD, MPH, FACS

Scenario

During a domestic altercation, a 22-year-old man sustains a stab wound to the anterior abdomen to the right of the umbilicus. He presents to the trauma bay alert and hemodynamically stable. However, physical examination demonstrates evisceration of the omentum.

Management

Crystalloid resuscitation is initiated with two 14 gauge intravenous lines. The remaining physical examination is unremarkable. The patient is taken to the operative theater for abdominal exploration.

With adequate exposure being the sine qua non of all surgery, a long midline vertical incision from the xiphoid process to the symphysis pubis is still the mainstay incision of choice in the emergency trauma setting. However, care must be taken not to inappropriately enter the bladder or inadvertently decompress an expanding pelvic hematoma. The general steps in abdominal exploration in this hemodynamically stable trauma patient include the following: evisceration of the small intestine; removal of gross blood and clots; temporary control of active bleeding/packing of the four quadrants; temporary control of intestinal spillage careful removal of packs one-by-one, from the least suspicious quadrant to the most suspicious one and identify all retroperitoneal, mesenteric and organ hematomas; examination of the diaphragm for perforations; and prevention of cross-cavity contamination.

The timing of the definitive closure of the diaphragmatic rent depends on the hemodynamic status of the patient and the higher priority management of an actively bleeding vascular injury; establishment of definitive control of bleeding, and definitive control of bleeding takes precedence over definitive management of gastrointestinal injuries.

- Allis clamps are used to close the laceration

- Continuous 5-0 polypropylene sutures close the laceration transversely to avoid narrowing

Procedure: *Allis clamp control of laceration of the vena cava*

With respect to specific exposure and management of a 2 cm laceration of the infrarenal inferior vena cava, optimum exposure is obtained by incising the lateral peritoneal reflection of the right colon, with subsequent mobilization to the left of the colon, mesentery, and C-loop of the duodenum (i.e. right to left medial visceral rotation). The loose retroperitoneal tissue is removed from the vena cava by sharp dissection in order to localize the actual laceration. An anterior laceration of the infrarenal cava is found. Allis clamps are applied to close the perforation site to get control of the bleeding prior to definitive repair. For a more extensive injury, such as a through-and-through perforation, proximal and distal control can be achieved by applying gauze sponge sticks above and below the level of the laceration. The definitive venorrhaphy is done using a continuous 4-0 or 5-0 polypropylene suture in a transverse manner to avoid unnecessary narrowing of the vein. The abdominal cavity is carefully re-inspected for any active bleeding and occult injuries. The abdomen is subsequently closed.

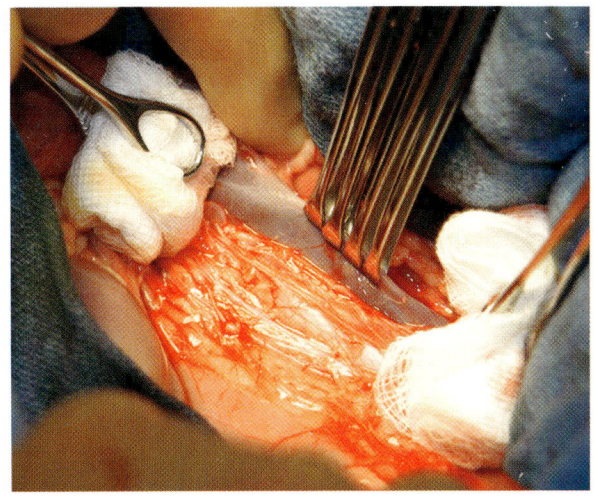

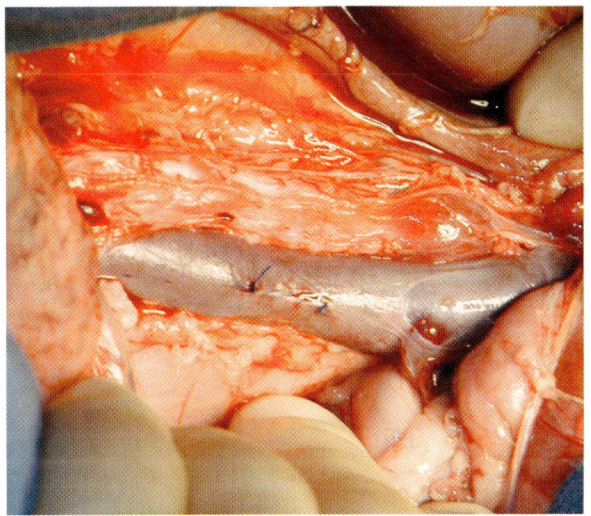

TECHNICAL OPERATIVE PROCEDURES:

HOW I DO IT

Laceration of Infrarenal Inferior Vena Cava With Hypotension and Massive Hemorrhage

Rao Ivatury, MD, FACS

Scenario

A 30-year-old man is stabbed in the periumbilical area with a kitchen knife. He presents with hypotension and a rapidly distending abdomen.

Management

I make a long midline incision from the xiphoid to the pubis. I suspect a major venous injury by identifying intraperitoneal hemorrhage and a large hematoma lifting up the duodenum and right colon.

Before trying to expose the injury, I consider the following:
- Abdominal aortic occlusion just under the diaphragm by an assistant
- Prepare for massive transfusion
- Prepare the anesthesia team for massive blood loss

I rapidly mobilize the right colon by incising the white line of Toldt on the right side. I then use finger dissection which is usually very easy because the blood has already dissected out the planes. I then reflect the entire colon and the duodenum utilizing the Kocher maneuver to the midline.

At this point, I am greeted with torrential blood loss, which can be controlled by tamponade with my fist or lap pads. I now suspect that there is an IVC injury by the site, amount, and color of the bleeding. If temporary compression can accomplish reduction in bleeding, I give the anesthesiology team a chance to replace blood. Once relative stability is achieved, I try to narrow down my compression to the point of hemorrhage by removing the packs quickly and tamponade the point of hemorrhage with finger compression. This will

- Primary hemorrhage control with finger compression

- Vascular loops and upward traction reduced hemorrhage enough to precisely identify the extent of the injury

- If the laceration is close to the renal veins, they also have to be controlled with vascular tapes

- Laceration closed with a running suture

allow me to mobilize the vena cava below and above the injury.

I get around the IVC with vascular tapes and by applying traction upwards on the tapes, the hemorrhage may be reduced enough to identify the laceration. If the laceration is close to the renal veins, I may have to isolate them in tapes as well.

I am very careful in doing these maneuvers, that I do not lacerate the lumbar veins that can increase the blood loss. If this proves difficult, one other option is to apply pressure on the IVC with sponge-sticks above and below the laceration.

Now I have several options to control the laceration: 1) I can apply a Satinsky clamp across the anterior wall of the cava; 2) I can rapidly occlude the laceration by applying Allis clamps serially to the edges of the lacerations.

Now I have controlled the hemorrhage. Once again, I will take a few moments to allow for resuscitation. The laceration can then be sutured rapidly with a running 5-0 Prolene suture.

I always make sure there is no posterior laceration. If present, the easiest way to repair this is through the anterior perforation. At times, the adjacent lumbar veins may be clipped and divided, the IVC rotated and the posterior laceration repaired.

The IVC may appear to be significantly narrowed after repair. This usually causes no post-operative sequelae. Once the hemorrhage is reasonably under control, I consider resuscitation and damage control celiotomy. If the IVC has a complex, ragged laceration, I consider ligation as a life saving measure.

TECHNICAL OPERATIVE PROCEDURES:
HOW I DO IT

Gunshot Wound to the Left Common Iliac Artery

Norman McSwain, MD, FACS

Scenario
A 27-year-old male with a gunshot wound to the left common iliac artery and vein with significant hemorrhage and hypotension.

Management
As in any hypotensive patient, resuscitation is initiated in the resuscitation bay and continued in the operating room. The cell saver should be ready before the abdomen is opened

Proximal and distal control of the vessel is obtained prior to the opening of any contained hematoma. If the hematoma is already open and bleeding freely into the abdomen, direct pressure is placed on the area with the hand of the assistant directly into the lumen of the vessels or with a small but tightly applied compression dressing over the injury while proximal and distal control is obtained. Proximal and distal control is obtained using pseudo Rommel tourniquets placed directly around the aorta and vena cava above and the iliac vessels below. The entire area is then opened.

If the hematoma is not open and freely bleeding, one should not enter a retroperitoneal hematoma until one is sure all of the intra-abdominal components of the hemorrhage are under control. Once this has been obtained, attention can be turned to the retroperitoneal hematoma.

Procedure: *Repair of the left common iliac artery*
The aorta and vena cava are identified above the hematoma by mobilizing the right or left colon across the midline, depending on which iliac vessel in injured.

The white line of Toldt is cut sharply using the Metzenbaum scissors from the cecum, or the sigmoid flexure to several centimeters above the hematoma. Once the colon is freed the upper portion is mobilized medially above the hematoma to visualize the vena cava and aorta. Once one has pseudo Rommel tourniquets placed proximal and distal on the aorta and vena cava, one may address the iliac hematoma.

The lower ends of the iliac vessels are then exposed below the hematoma below the inguinal ligament if necessary and a pseudo Rommel tourniquet is placed on the iliac artery and vein. Then dissection is carried into the hematoma, opened, and the extent of the injury is identified.

Repair
Bulldog clamps are placed proximal and distal to the injured segment. The injured vessel is mobilized for at least 6 cm proximal and distal to the injury. Most injuries to the

vessels can be repaired primarily if less than 1 cm in length. If longer then interposition grafting is necessary. My preference is to use a synthetic graft on the artery and a vein on the vein. The vein should be repaired primarily in the iliac region if possible. Edema of the leg is much more common with iliac vein injuries than with injuries to the vena cava. A running suture of 4-0 or 5-0 Prolene is used on the vessel with or without a graft.

- Proximal and distal control is obtained prior to opening the hematoma

- Pseudo Rommel tourniquets are used for control

- Direct pressure applied to the laceration

- Bulldog clamps isolate the injured segment

- Repair the laceration with running 5-0 Prolene

TECHNICAL OPERATIVE PROCEDURES:
HOW I DO IT

Celiac Trunk Injury

Eric R. Frykberg, MD. FACS

Scenario

A young male suffered a small caliber gunshot wound to the epigastric region of the abdomen. On laparotomy for hemodynamic instability, a large pulsatile hematoma was found in the lesser sac, pushing up the stomach and transverse colon. It appears to be tense and red. The patient had a blood pressure of 70 systolic.

Management

The patient is prepped and draped with an operative field extending from the chin to the mid thigh. Preoperative antibiotics are infused to cover enteric flora. A urethral bladder catheter is inserted. Attention should be focused on avoiding hypothermia by warming the operating room and all administered fluids as well as covering the patient's head and unprepped portions of the extremities. During the case, warm fluid should be infused through nasogastric tube and any other body cavity tubes present. Antibiotics should be redosed at a frequency consistent with the severity of hemorrhage to maintain therapeutic serum levels. The surgeon should confirm that an autotransfusion apparatus is available if possible and that thoracotomy tray, vascular clamps and aortic compressor are available.

A generous midline laparotomy incision is made from over the lower portion of the sternum to the pubis. Occasionally it may have been necessary to do an emergency room thoracotomy to cross clamp the aorta for patients who have arrested from abdominal hemorrhage prior to arriving in the operating room. This maneuver should not be performed electively prior to laparotomy if the patient is able to be brought to the operating room without losing his vital signs. After entering the abdomen, all blood should be evacuated as quickly as possible, and any obviously bleeding organs should be packed off with sterile sponges. All perforations of bowel should be clamped with Babcocks and packed off. In the presence of a pulsatile, red and expanding supramesocolic hematoma, immediate proximal control of the aorta should be obtained above the hematoma right at the aortic hiatus by digitally dissecting through the gastrohepatic omentum, retracting the esophagus to the left, and compressing the aorta manually. An aortic compressor should then be applied to this area for initial proximal control of any ongoing hemorrhage. The hematoma should not be entered until all necessary instruments are ready, the autotransfuser has been prepared, blood is available, and volume has been infused as much as possible to stabilize the patient.

It is best not to directly enter a supramesocolic hematoma anteriorly, as the possible major vascular injuries to the supra-renal aorta, celiac trunk and superior mesenteric artery are best exposed from a lateral direction. This should be done by performing a left-sided medial mobilization maneuver. This is performed by incising the left lateral peritoneal reflection, white line of Toldt, down into the pelvis and up to any splenic attachments to the diaphragm and retroperitoneum. This will allow manual mobilization of all bowel, the spleen and the distal pancreas medially. The left kidney is best left in place with the mobilization sweeping above it. The left aortic hiatus crus should then be incised sharply for about 2 cm to allow full visualization and formal vascular clamp control of the aorta at this level. Active bleeding should be controlled with digital compression until a distal clamp can be applied on the aorta or branch vessel to fully

- An aortic compressor is useful for initial proximal control

- Perform a left medial rotation maneuver

- Primary repair should be avoided

- Definitive repair after resuscitation and metabolic normalizationsss

control the point of bleeding. Vessel loops may be used to control backbleeding from branch vessels.

A perforation at the level of the celiac trunk or any of its branches is best managed by ligation. The collaterals supplying the spleen, stomach and liver will generally allow these to be perfused without problem, as long as the ligation is very proximal. Any perforation of the aorta should then be primarily sutured using 3-0 Prolene.

In this scenario the patient is virtually always in a state of profound hemorrhagic shock, coagulopathy, hypothermia and acidosis. Therefore, attempts at primary repair of injuries in this area should be avoided, and damage control principles should be instituted. Any concomitant bowel injuries should quickly be stapled off with no attempts at definitive repair or anastamosis. Once this is done and active bleeding has been controlled, packing should be performed for temporary abdominal closure and the patient sent to the intensive care unit as soon as possible to allow resuscitation from all metabolic derangements. The patient could then be brought back in 24 to 48 hours to investigate any mesenteric ischemia that may have resulted from the ligation of the celiac trunk and to perform definitive repairs of any bowel injuries. Any injuries to the pancreas could also be addressed at this time, generally by distal pancreatectomy. Although gastric, hepatic and splenic ischemia is very unusual with ligation of the celiac trunk, any necrosis of these organs can be addressed either by resection or a formal bypass between the aorta and celiac trunk at a second procedure. Again, this should be carried out only in the setting of a fully stabilized patient at a second look operation.

The method of abdominal closure after the second look procedure depends on the severity of bowel edema. Definitive fascial closure should be carried out if allowed without undue tension, otherwise one of the many forms of temporary closure should be considered. In this case, suturing of an absorbable mesh to the fascial edges would be the best option if primary closure cannot be performed, and the resulting ventral hernia then electively repaired at a later date.

TECHNICAL OPERATIVE PROCEDURES:
HOW I DO IT

Laceration of the Vena Cava Two Centimeters Distal to the Renal Vessels

Norman McSwain, MD, FACS

Scenario

A 27-year-old man presents with a gunshot would to the mid abdomen, just above the umbilicus. On opening the abdomen, a retroperitoneal hematoma is noted along the bullet pathway. The blood is dark rather than bright red.

Management

As in any hypotensive patient, resuscitation is initiated in the resuscitation bay and continued in the operating room.

Generally, retroperitoneal hemorrhage is self-contained and therefore one should address intraabdominal hemorrhage before addressing retroperitoneal hemorrhage. One should not enter a retroperitoneal hematoma until one is sure all of the intraabdominal components of the hemorrhage are under control. Once this has been obtained then attention can be turned to the retroperitoneal hematoma. Proximal and distal control should be obtained before the hematoma is opened as usual with any vascular injury.

Procedure: *Repair of the inferior vena cava*

The abdomen is opened rapidly from xiphoid process to symphysis pubis. As the linea Alba is opened and the peritoneum is visualized, one gets the initial impression as to whether there is a large amount of blood in the abdominal cavity or not. The peritoneum is then opened using blunt dissection with the fingers or sharply using the Metzenbaum scissors.

On opening the peritoneal cavity the trajectory of the bullet is followed. Laparotomy packs are NOT put in all four quadrants of the abdomen. This takes up space in the abdomen and makes it more difficult to define the bleeding point. Packs and cell saver suction can be used to remove excessive hemorrhage, but not left in the abdomen.

- Proximal and distal control by pseudo Rommel tourniquet

- Visualize both the anterior and posterior injury

- After the repair, Surgicel soaked in thrombin is wrapped around the laceration for complete hemostasis

As in any vascular hemorrhage, the hematoma itself, which is containing the blood loss should not be entered until proximal and distal control have been obtained. In a lesion that is 2 cm below the renal vessels, proximal and distal control is obtained by clamping or placing a pseudo Rommel tourniquet around the vessels to prepare for later occlusion.

My preference is to use a pseudo Rommel tourniquet rather than vessel loops doubled around the vessel since a pseudo Rommel tourniquet can be immediately pushed down on the vessel without having to stretch the vessel loops and clamp it to an unstable platform such as the drapes. My preference is to use a straight hemostat on the arteries and a curved hemostat on the veins. This will allow one at a glance to identify which tourniquet to tighten.

The aorta and vena cava is identified above the hematoma by mobilizing the right or left colon across the midline. It is my preference to use the ascending left colon, mobilize it across the midline, simply because it is easier.

The white line of Toldt is cut sharply using the Metzenbaum scissors from the cecum to the hepatic flexure. Once the colon is freed the upper portion is mobilized medially above the hematoma to visualize the vena cava and aorta.

Once one has pseudo Rommel tourniquets placed proximal and distal on the aorta, vena cava, iliac artery and vein, then dissection is carried into the hematoma. Open it, and determine the extent of the injury. In a vena cava injury such as described above, I perform a vascular repair using a running suture.

The vena cava is mobilized sharply for at least 4 cm cephalad and caudad. The vessel is cleaned to ensure a tight closure. In most gunshot wounds of the IVC, there is both an anterior and posterior injury. Therefore the mobilization must visualize both. Smaller vessels that branch from the vena cava must be ligated.

The edges of the vessel are approximated with Allis clamps. A running suture of 4-0 Prolene is placed starting either proximally or distally and run along the edges. As the repair advances to the Allis clamps each it removed in turn.

There will be some constriction of this vessel and it will have somewhat of an hourglass shape when both the entrance and exit wounds in the vena cava have been closed.

An alternative which is particularly attractive when there are multiple other injuries that have produced a lot of hemorrhage is simply to ligate the vena cava on either side of the injury. There is some morbidity associated with this.

After completion of the repair, Surgicel soaked in thrombin is wrapped around the vessel to control the minor bleeding from the suture holes.

TECHNICAL OPERATIVE PROCEDURES:
HOW I DO IT

Emergency Department Resuscitative Thoracotomy and Management of Cardiopulmonary Injuries

Juan A. Asensio, MD, FACS

Technique

Emergency department thoracotomy should be performed simultaneously with the initial assessment, evaluation and resuscitation. Immediate endotracheal intubation coupled with immediate venous access and the simultaneous use of pressure driven fluids via rapid infusion complements the resuscitative process.

The left anterolateral thoracotomy remains the incision of choice for the management of patients that arrive in extremis. This incision is most often used in the emergency department for resuscitative purposes. It is also the incision of choice in patients undergoing celiotomy that deteriorate secondary to unsuspected cardiac injuries. The left anterolateral thoracotomy can be extended across the sternum as bilateral anterolateral thoracotomies if the patient's injuries extend into the right hemithoracic cavity. This is the incision of choice in a patient who is hemodynamically unstable or for injuries that have traversed the mediastinum. It allows full exposure of the anterior mediastinum and both hemithoracic cavities. It is important to note that upon transection of the sternum, both internal mammary arteries are sacrificed and must be ligated at the completion of the procedure.

Patients are transferred to the emergency department gurney upon arrival. The left arm is elevated and the entire thorax is prepped rapidly with an antiseptic solution. A left anterolateral thoracotomy commencing at the lateral border of the left sternocostal junction and inferior to the nipple is carried out and extended laterally to the latissimus dorsi. In females, the breast is retracted cephalad. This incision is rapidly carried through skin and subcutaneous tissue and the serratus anterior

- Left anterolateral thoracotomy is the incision of choice

- Vertical incision in the pericardium

- Avoid the phrenic nerve

- Immediate digital control of a myocardial laceration

- Monofilament mattress sutures for repair

- Teflon pledgets buttress sutures

- Definitive inspection and closure of the chest in the operating room muscles until the intercostal muscles have been reached. Muscles are sharply transected with Metzenbaum scissors. The pleura is then opened. Occasionally, the left, fifth or fourth costochondral cartilages are transected to provide greater exposure. A Finochietto retractor is then placed to separate the ribs. At this time, the extent of hemorrhage present within the left hemithoracic cavity is evaluated.

The left lung is then elevated medially and the descending thoracic aorta is located immediately as it enters the abdomen via the aortic hiatus. The aorta should be palpated. It can be temporarily occluded digitally against the bodies of the thoracic vertebrae until it can be cross clamped.

Prior to cross clamping the descending thoracic aorta, a combination of sharp and blunt dissection commencing at both the superior and inferior borders of the aorta is performed, so that the aorta may be encircled between the thumb and index fingers, in order for the aortic cross clamp be safely placed. A previously placed nasogastric tube can serve as a useful guide in differentiating the esophagus from an empty thoracic aorta.

Often the pericardium is inspected. If it is tense and bluish, a cardiac injury is present. A vertical incision on the pericardium is then made superior to the phrenic nerve and extended longitudinally. The phrenic nerve must be preserved. Injudicious opening of the pericardium with a knife may iatrogenically lacerate the underlying epicardium. The pericardium is grasped with two Allis clamps to stabilize it prior to making a 1 cm to 2 cm incision with a knife. The pericardium is opened longitudinally with Metzenbaum scissors.

After opening the pericardium, clotted blood is evacuated. The type of underlying cardiac rhythm, as well as the location of the penetrating injury or injuries is observed. Immediate digital control is imperative. An attempt must be made to trace the trajectory of the wounding agent, as missiles often enter one area and migrate to adjacent areas, such as the contralateral hemithoracic cavity. The blood volume remaining within the cardiac chambers is estimated. Reliable predictors of poor outcome are empty coronary arteries and the presence of air in the coronary veins signifying air emboli.

Digital control of penetrating ventricular injuries prevents further hemorrhage. I use monofilament sutures such as 2-0 Prolene and employ mattress sutures to repair these injuries. Lacerations of the atria can be controlled with a Satinsky partial occlusion vascular clamp prior to definitive cardiorrhaphy. If the injury or injuries are quite large, balloon tamponade utilizing a Foley catheter can temporarily arrest the hemorrhage.

Teflon pledgets may need to be used to buttress sutures when myocardial tissues are unable to hold sutures. I do not recommend the use of skin staplers to temporarily occlude lacerations of the cardiac muscle in anticipation of definitive cardiorrhaphy. In my experience, staples do not effectively control hemorrhage, tend to enlarge the original cardiac injury, and prove rather difficult to remove.

In patients surviving these injuries, the pericardium may not be able to be closed due to distension of the heart. If this is the case, it should be left open.

If associated pathology is encountered in the contralateral hemithoracic cavity, the sternum is transected sharply and the left anterolateral thoracotomy is then converted to a bilateral anterolateral thoracotomy. If the patient is successfully resuscitated, immediate transportation to the operating room is mandated for definitive inspection and closure of the chest.

TECHNICAL OPERATIVE PROCEDURES:

HOW I DO IT

Exposure and Repair of the Celiac Trunk and/or Superior Mesenteric Artery

David Feliciano, MD, FACS

Overview

The majority of patients with injuries to the arteries in the upper midline retroperitoneum are victims of gunshot wounds, and almost all will have associated injuries to the liver, stomach, transverse colon and pancreas. The technique of exposure for the vascular injury will depend on whether a contained retroperitoneal supramesocolic hematoma or active hemorrhage is present.

- Medial visceral rotation only appropriate as initial maneuver for supra mesocolic hematoma, NOT active hemorrhage

- Medial visceral rotation done with surgeon exerting traction from the right on organs while assistant performs sharp dissection from the left

- Divide aortic hiatus at the two o'clock position if necessary to gain control

- Second-look operation is 8 to 12 hours for persistent acidosis in patients where aorto-superior mesenteric artery graft was necessary

All patients undergoing an emergency laparotomy for abdominal trauma have their arms placed at their sides to allow for attachment of large self retaining retractors, particularly for upper abdominal exposures, and for easy access to all thoracic incisions.

Procedure: *Exposure if supramesocolic hematoma present*

After the long midline incision has been completed, free blood and gastrointestinal contents are removed using laparotomy pads, warm saline irrigation and a suction device. In the absence of overt bleeding from the midline supramesocolic hematoma, any perforations in the overlying stomach or transverse colon are closed with a stapling device or one-layer full thickness closure using 3-0 or 4-0 polypropylene sutures. Active hemorrhage from the liver or pancreas is controlled with selective vascular ligation.

All left-sided intraabdominal viscera are then mobilized to the midline. This starts with the sigmoid colon and continues with the descending colon, splenic flexure, left kidney, spleen, tail of pancreas, and fundus of the stomach. This maneuver is most easily performed if the surgeon on the patient's right uses manual traction over laparotomy pads on the organs to be mobilized as the assistant on the patient's left performs the sharp dissection with scissors. This maneuver takes four to five minutes and is completed by mobilizing the celiac ganglia and lymphatics of the supraceliac abdominal aorta from left to right in or just below the aortic hiatus of the diaphragm. If the hiatus is particularly long and obscures the area of injury or the area where proximal control is to be obtained, the hiatus is divided with the electrocautery at the two o'clock position. Proximal control of the supraceliac aorta with a DeBakey aortic clamp is obtained in the hiatus or above in the descending thoracic aorta.

Procedure: *Exposure if hemorrhage present*

Injuries to the gastrointestinal tract may have to be temporarily controlled with Glassman, Babcock or Allis clamps. The esophagus and lesser curve of the stomach are retracted to the left, the lesser omentum is manually opened outside the nerves of Latarjet, and the surgeon attempts to put his or her left second and third fingers inside the muscle fibers of the aortic hiatus to reach the spine posteriorly. Failure to complete this maneuver may mandate division of the muscle fibers of the hiatus at the two o'clock position with the electrocautery.

Procedure: *Vascular ligation or repair*

With proximal control of the supraceliac aorta in place, dissection on the upper edge of the aorta proceeding inferiorly should expose the nearly V shaped origin of the celiac and superior mesenteric arteries. Transection of the celiac axis is treated with ligation of both ends in the unstable patient. On occasion, the hepatic artery can be salvaged with a lateral repair or interposition graft. A major injury to the superior mesenteric artery at its origin or beneath the pancreas is best treated with proximal ligation and insertion of a saphenous vein or PTFE bypass graft. This graft goes from the infrarenal abdominal aorta, end-to-side, to the distal uninjured superior mesenteric artery, end-to-end or end-to-side, through the mesentery of the small bowel. A viable omental pedicle is used to cover the origin of the graft off the infrarenal abdominal aorta, and mesenteric tissue is closed around the suture line on the superior mesenteric artery. A second-look operation is appropriate in eight to twelve hours to assess viability of the midgut if the patient's metabolic acidosis does not resolve in the postoperative period.

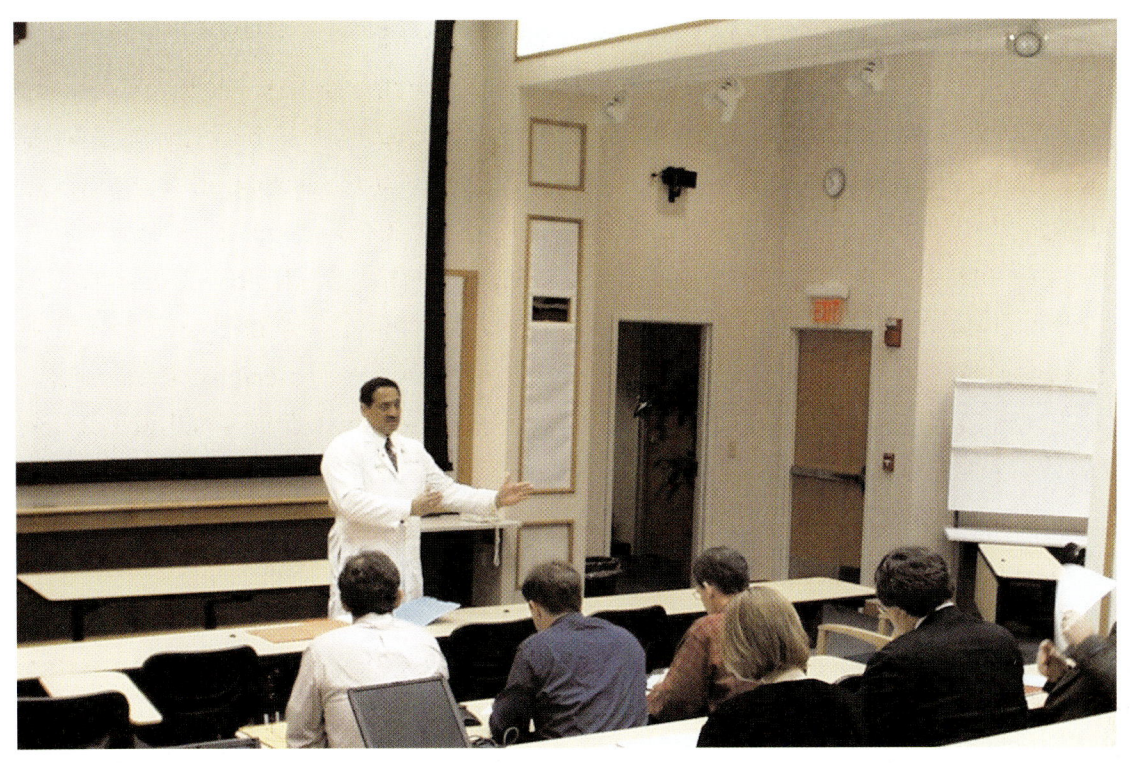

ATOM Evaluation: Participant & Course Evaluation

7

Theoretical Framework

Social Cognitive Theory guides the educational activities of the ATOM course, as well as the evaluation methods of the course.[1] A central construct of Social Cognitive Theory is self-efficacy. Self-efficacy is concerned with "people's judgments of their capabilities to organize and execute courses of action required to attain designated types of performances."[1] (p.391) The ATOM course is grounded in self-efficacy because it affords the "most comprehensive understanding of the interplay of cognition, affect, and behavior."[2] (p.5) All three of these domains must be considered in order to best achieve learning.

Self-efficacy judgments are best made for clearly defined tasks.[1] High levels of perceived self-efficacy for a particular task are related to successful and enduring performance. Conversely, low levels of perceived self-efficacy are related to avoidance of the task or, if attempted, a poor performance.[1] Affective attributes such as self-efficacy can be measured in a consistent manner by instruments designed to quantify latent constructs.[2]

Educational Activities

Educational activities should be directed at increasing self-efficacy for the desired behaviors. Self-efficacy can be strengthened by four methods.[1] The most powerful way to increase self-efficacy is by having students actually perform the desired tasks and achieve success. This is known as performance accomplishment. Another way is by vicarious experience or witnessing someone else being effective. A third way is by getting verbal encouragement from others. A fourth route to increased self-efficacy is through interpretation of physiologic cues. Physiologic cues can hinder the ability to execute appropriate actions such as when one becomes so nervous that performance is fumbled. Conversely, the physiology can remain in a relaxed state and contribute to optimal performance.

In order to increase students' self-efficacy, teaching activities should: 1) have the students perform the desired tasks and successfully accomplish them; 2) offer opportunities for observational learning by having students witness others performing tasks correctly; 3) provide verbal encouragement regarding the expectation for success; and 4) eliminate disabling physiologic stress.

ATOM provides all four sources of efficacy information. The laboratory experience gives students an opportunity to practice skills and successfully accomplish tasks. In addition to the CD-ROM, the laboratory experience offers observational learning by having students witness the repair of injuries on the CD-ROM and also see faculty in the laboratory demonstrate techniques. ATOM instructors act as advocates of the students' successes by offering assurance that mastery of the tasks is achievable. Finally, ATOM instructors act to redirect physiologic cues that may hinder the students' performances. This may be accomplished through stress management techniques, verbal encouragement, and breaking tasks down into smaller more manageable steps to permit success. Table 1 summarizes these important teaching behaviors.

ATOM as a Simulation

As ATOM is a simulation education experience, the course is structured to adhere to the principles that guide this type of learning experience.[3] First, the learning objectives of the course must be clear and the critical behaviors that must be successfully performed by the students identified. The laboratory experience in the ATOM course delineates precisely what must be done to identify each injury, develop a treatment plan, and competently repair the injury. Second, students need to be prepared for the simulation. ATOM does this by having the students view the CD-ROM before they come to the course. Next, the simulation must represent true life as much as possible. In the porcine laboratory, ATOM uses true-to-life clinical scenarios of penetrating injury. The laboratory completely replicates the human operating room environment and mimics the human environment with visual and auditory cues of real-life experiences. Additionally, ATOM identifies student and teacher roles so that everyone has clear expectations of what is to happen in the course and the behaviors that are appropriate. Finally, ATOM offers debriefing and feedback sessions for each student during which time the experience is assessed and strengths and weaknesses are identified. Debriefing is necessary to help students reflect upon their performance so that they may integrate the experience and identify areas for future learning.[3]

Evaluation of ATOM Participants

Evaluation of ATOM participants includes assessments of learning in the affective, cognitive, and psychomotor domains.[4] For the affective domain, a 25-item self-efficacy instrument was developed. It asks participants to rate their level of confidence for performing the surgical procedures taught in ATOM on a 5-point Likert scale. A response of 1 on the self-efficacy instrument indicates very little confidence, and a response of 5 indicates quite a lot of confidence (see Table 2).

The self-efficacy instrument was validated by a technique commonly referred to as "known groups." With this technique, the instrument is administered to groups of individuals known to have high or low amounts of the attribute of interest. Scores are examined to determine if the groups scored as predicted. The ATOM self-efficacy instrument was administered to anesthesiologists, emergency department physicians, junior surgical residents, senior surgical residents, trauma fellows, surgical attendings, and expert traumatologists. It was hypothesized that the anesthesiologists and emergency physicians would score the lowest and the surgical practitioners would score according to their level of training or practice. Results confirmed these hypotheses and lend support for the validity of the ATOM self-efficacy instrument.[4]

For the cognitive domain, a 25-item multiple-choice test assesses knowledge of the content areas taught in the course. Each content area is equally represented. The questions consist of a stem and five options. Only one option is correct. The answers to the questions were validated by a national panel of expert traumatologists and are supported with annotated references from the literature.[4]

ATOM participants complete the knowledge test and the self-efficacy instrument online before taking, and immediately after completing, the ATOM course. Data from the first 50 participants have shown substantial gains in both knowledge and self-efficacy after taking the ATOM course.[4]

Psychomotor skill in the laboratory is evaluated on a 3-point scale that reflects the degree of assistance needed by the student to complete each task (see Table 3 and Table 4). For each injury, students must: 1) identify the injury; 2) develop a treatment plan, and; 3) repair the injury (see Table 4). Critical behaviors to accomplish these essential skills for each injury are posted in the laboratory for easy reference. The content of the operative performance evaluation was evaluated by the national panel of expert traumatologists. A score of 1 point indicates that the student could not complete the required task, 2 points indicates that the student needed help, and 3 points indicates that the student performed independently. After completion of the laboratory session, the students are given feedback from the instructor as to the strengths and weaknesses of their performance. This is done in a collegial manner to promote a positive experience and stimulate future learning by the student.

After completing ATOM, results of the pre- and post-course tests are available on the ATOM Web site. Students can access the site and see their standing relative to those of other students who have taken the ATOM course. While personal grades are available to each individual, other students' results are listed anonymously. Standing can be compared based upon the level of training.

Evaluation of ATOM by Participants

Immediately upon completion of the ATOM course, students are asked to complete a course evaluation and an instructor evaluation. The course evaluation asks students to rate their level of agreement to eight items on a 5-point Likert scale. A response of 1 indicates strong disagreement, and a response of 5 indicates strong agreement. The items reflect the objectives of the course to improve knowledge, confidence, and psychomotor skill for identifying injuries, and to develop treatment plans and repair injuries. Three items ask for written comments to address what was most helpful, how the course might be improved, and any additional comments. A similar format is used for the instructor evaluation, (see Table 5 and Table 6).

Six months after the ATOM course, participants are asked to complete another self-efficacy instrument and course evaluation. The 6-month course evaluation has seven items using the 5-point Likert scale described above. There are three questions that request written comments. Participants are asked if they have used the knowledge and techniques taught in ATOM and if they are better able to perform the essential skills to identify and repair traumatic injuries. They are also asked if they would recommend the course to colleagues and how the course has been helpful to them. In addition, participants are asked how ATOM might be improved, (see Table 7).

Conclusion

The evaluation tools for ATOM have been designed to provide comprehensive assessment of student performance and evaluation of the course itself. Evaluation of ATOM participants assesses performance in the cognitive, affective, and psychomotor domains. Assessments include knowledge, self-efficacy for surgical performance and laboratory skill to identify injuries, and ability to develop appropriate treatment plans and repair the injuries. Students' evaluations of the course and the instructor are also essential components the ATOM course.

Table 1. Ways to Increase Students' Self-Efficacy for Successful Performance

1. Performance Accomplishment	Create ample opportunity for the student to practice the techniques. Point out previous success. Allow repetition until student is successful.
2. Vicarious Experience	Have student observe others performing the tasks successfully. Use CD-ROM and laboratory to demonstrate.
3. Verbal Persuasion	Act as a cheerleader. Offer your confidence that the student can be successful. "You can do it."
4. Physiologic Cues	Help student control physiology. Redirect negative physiology to achieve a calm state. Use stress management. Break task into smaller tasks. Point out previous success.

Adapted from Bandura, 1986.

Table 2. Evaluation of Surgical Self-Efficacy

Name:_____ Age: _____ Sex:_____

Level of Residency Training: PG4 ____ PG5 ____ Fellow ____

Attending (Years in Practice): 1 ____ 2 ____ 3 ____ 4 ____ 5 ____ 6-10 ____ 11-15 ____
16-20 ____ 21-25 ____ >25 ____

Type of Practice: Exclusively Trauma ___   Trauma and General Surgery ___   General Surgery ___

Please circle the number that represents the level of confidence you have in performing each of the following procedures.

	1	2	③	4	5
EXAMPLE	Very little confidence		Quite a lot of confidence		

Resection and ligation for small bowel enterotomies	1	2	3	4	5
Two-layer closure for gastrotomies	1	2	3	4	5
Running locked-stitch closure for gastrotomies	1	2	3	4	5
Pyloric exclusion for gastrotomies	1	2	3	4	5
Repair with simple interrupted stitches for diaphragm	1	2	3	4	5
Check for pneumostasis in diaphragm laceration	1	2	3	4	5
Pledgeted horizontal mattress repair for splenic laceration	1	2	3	4	5
Splenectomy for splenic laceration	1	2	3	4	5
Distal pancreatectomy for pancreatic laceration	1	2	3	4	5
Ligation of splenic artery and vein for pancreatic laceration	1	2	3	4	5
Control of renal artery and vein for renal laceration	1	2	3	4	5
Pledgeted repair for renal laceration	1	2	3	4	5
Nephrectomy for renal laceration	1	2	3	4	5
Repair with running Prolene stitch for inferior vena cava laceration	1	2	3	4	5
Kocher maneuver for duodenal injury	1	2	3	4	5
Two-layer repair for duodenal injury	1	2	3	4	5
Primary repair with stent for ureteral laceration	1	2	3	4	5
Finger-fracture technique for hepatic laceration	1	2	3	4	5
Cautery and suture repair for hepatic laceration	1	2	3	4	5
Median sternotomy for cardiac injury	1	2	3	4	5
Proximal inflow control for cardiac injury	1	2	3	4	5
Fingertip control of hemorrhage for right ventricular stab wound	1	2	3	4	5
Foley catheter insertion for right ventricular stab wound	1	2	3	4	5
Pledgeted suture repair/staple repair for right ventricular stab wound	1	2	3	4	5
Control with vascular clamp for right atrial stab wound	1	2	3	4	5

Table 3. Laboratory Evaluation: ATOM Part 1 – Injuries Requiring Repair

Name:_____ Age:_____ Sex: _____

Level of Residency Training: PG4 ____ PG5 ____ Fellow ____

Attending (Years in Practice):   1 ___   2 ___   3 ___   4 ___   5 ___   6-10 ___   11-15 ___
16-20 ___   21-25 ___   >25 ___

Type of Practice: Exclusively Trauma __   Trauma and General Surgery __   General Surgery ___

Example:
1 ☐ Unable   2 ■ With Help   3 ☐ Independent

TRAUMATIC INJURY	PROCEDURE	SCORE 1	SCORE 2	SCORE 3
Small bowel enterotomies	Resection & ligation (damage control)	☐	☐	☐
Gastrotomies:				
Anterior & posterior	Two-layer closure	☐	☐	☐
	Running locked-stitch closure	☐	☐	☐
	Pyloric exclusion	☐	☐	☐
Diaphragmatic laceration	Repair with simple interrupted sutures	☐	☐	☐
	Check for pneumostasis with saline irrigation	☐	☐	☐
Splenic laceration	Splenorrhaphy	☐	☐	☐
Inferior pole	Pledgeted horizontal mattress repair	☐	☐	☐
Laceration of hilum	Splenectomy	☐	☐	☐
Laceration to body of pancreas	Distal pancreatectomy	☐	☐	☐
	Ligation of pancreatic duct	☐	☐	☐
Renal laceration	Dissection/control of renal artery and vein	☐	☐	☐
Inferior pole	Nephorrhaphy	☐	☐	☐
	Pledgeted repair; inverting suture	☐	☐	☐
Laceration of hilum	Nephrectomy	☐	☐	☐
Ureteral laceration	Primary repair over IV tubing stent	☐	☐	☐
Inferior vena cava laceration	Repair with running suture	☐	☐	☐
Duodenal injury	Kocher maneuver	☐	☐	☐
	Two-layer repair	☐	☐	☐
Hepatic laceration	Finger-fracture technique	☐	☐	☐
	Cautery & pledgeted suture repair	☐	☐	☐
Bladder Laceration	Two-layered repair	☐	☐	☐
Cardiac injury	Median sternotomy	☐	☐	☐
	Proximal inflow control	☐	☐	☐
Ventricular stab wound	Fingertip control of hemorrhage	☐	☐	☐
	Foley insertion	☐	☐	☐
	Pledgeted repair	☐	☐	☐
Atrial stab wound	Control with vascular clamp	☐	☐	☐

Table 4. Laboratory Evaluation of Advanced Trauma Operative Management

Name:_____ Age:_____ Sex:_____

Level of Residency Training: PG4 ____ PG5 ____ Fellow ____

Attending (Years in Practice): 1 ____ 2 ____ 3 ____ 4 ____ 5 ____ 6-10 ____ 11-15 ____
16-20 ____ 21-25 ____ >25 ____

Type of Practice: Exclusively Trauma __   Trauma and General Surgery __   General Surgery __

Example:

| | 1 ☐ Unable | 2 ■ With Help | 3 ☐ Independent |

INJURY IDENTIFICATION

		Score		
		1	2	3
CASE I	Lower Abdomen – Penetrating injuries			
	Bladder	☐	☐	☐
	Small Bowel	☐	☐	☐
CASE II	Right Upper Quadrant Injuries			
	Kidney	☐	☐	☐
	Ureter	☐	☐	☐
	Duodenum	☐	☐	☐
CASE III	Left Upper Quadrant Injuries			
	Diaphragm	☐	☐	☐
	Spleen	☐	☐	☐
	Pancreas	☐	☐	☐
CASE IV	Heart Injury	☐	☐	☐

DEVELOPED CORRECT TREATMENT PLAN

		Score		
		1	2	3
CASE I	Lower Abdomen – Penetrating Injuries			
	Bladder	☐	☐	☐
	Small Bowel	☐	☐	☐
CASE II	Right Upper Quadrant Injuries			
	Kidney	☐	☐	☐
	Ureter	☐	☐	☐
	Duodenum	☐	☐	☐

Table 4. Laboratory Evaluation of Advanced Trauma Operative Management (Cont.)

DEVELOPED CORRECT TREATMENT PLAN (continued)

		Score		
		1	2	3
CASE III	Left Upper Quadrant Injuries			
	Diaphragm	☐	☐	☐
	Spleen	☐	☐	☐
	Pancreas	☐	☐	☐
CASE IV	Heart Injury	☐	☐	☐

PERFORMED REPAIR

		Score		
		1	2	3
CASE I	Lower Abdomen – Penetrating Injuries			
	Bladder	☐	☐	☐
	Small Bowel	☐	☐	☐
CASE II	Right Upper Quadrant Injuries			
	Kidney	☐	☐	☐
	Ureter	☐	☐	☐
	Duodenum	☐	☐	☐
CASE III	Left Upper Quadrant Injuries			
	Diaphragm	☐	☐	☐
	Spleen	☐	☐	☐
	Pancreas	☐	☐	☐
CASE IV	Heart Injury	☐	☐	☐

Table 5. ATOM Course Evaluation

Name:_____ Age:_____ Sex:_____

Course Date:_____ State:_____ Zip Code: _____

Course Location: _____

Level of Residency Training: PG4 ____   PG5 ____   Fellow ____

Attending (Years in Practice): 1 __ 2 __ 3 __ 4 __ 5 __ 6-10 __ 11-15 __ 16-20 __ 21-25 __ >25 __

Type of Practice: Exclusively Trauma __   Trauma and General Surgery __   General Surgery __

What percentage of your trauma practice is penetrating trauma?
       0-20 ____   21-40 ____   41-60 ____   61-80 ____   81-100 ____

What percentage of your practice is devoted to trauma?
       0-20 ____   21-40 ____   41-60 ____   61-80 ____   81-100____

Where do you perform your trauma surgery?
       Level I ____   Level II ____   Level III ____   Level IV ____   Non-Trauma Center ____

Hospital Bed Size: 100-200 ___   201-300 ___   301-400 ___   401-500 ___   501-600 ___   >600 ___
Location: Urban ___   Suburban ___   Rural ___
Type: Academic Center ___   Community Hospital ___

Please indicate how strongly you agree or disagree with the following statements. The scale is:
1 (strongly disagree)   2 (disagree)   3 (neither agree nor disagree)   4 (agree)   5 (strongly agree).

	Strongly Disagree				Strongly Agree
Example:	1	2	③	4	5

As a result of the ATOM course:

My psychomotor skills for managing trauma improved.	1	2	3	4	5
I gained new knowledge.	1	2	3	4	5
I learned new techniques.	1	2	3	4	5
I am better prepared to identify penetrating trauma.	1	2	3	4	5
I am better prepared to develop a treatment plan.	1	2	3	4	5
I am better prepared to repair penetrating injuries.	1	2	3	4	5
I am satisfied with what I learned.	1	2	3	4	5
I would recommend the course to colleagues.	1	2	3	4	5

Please state what part of the course was most helpful to you.

Please state how the course might be improved.

Please add any other comments.

Table 6. ATOM Instructor Evaluation

Name: _____ Age: _____ Sex: _____

Course Date: _____ State: _____ Zip Code: _____

Course Location: _____

Level of Residency Training: PG4 _____ PG5 _____ Fellow _____

Attending (Years in Practice): 1 __ 2 __ 3 __ 4 __ 5 __ 6-10 __ 11-15 __ 16-20 __ 21-25 __ >25 __

What percentage of your trauma practice is penetrating trauma?
    0-20 _____ 21-40 _____ 41-60 _____ 61-80 _____ 81-100 _____

What percentage of your practice is devoted to trauma?
    0-20 _____ 21-40 _____ 41-60 _____ 61-80 _____ 81-100 _____

Where do you perform your trauma surgery?
    Level I _____ Level II _____ Level III _____ Level IV _____ Non-Trauma Center _____

Hospital Bed Size: 100-200 _____ 201-300 _____ 301-400 _____ 401-500 _____ 501-600 _____ >600 _____

Location: Urban _____   Suburban _____   Rural _____
Type: Academic Center _____   Community Hospital _____

Please indicate how strongly you agree or disagree with the following statements. The scale is:
1 (strongly disagree)   2 (disagree)   3 (neither agree nor disagree)   4 (agree)   5 (strongly agree).

	Strongly Disagree				Strongly Agree
Example:	1	2	③	4	5

The ATOM instructor:

Was knowledgeable in the management of traumatic injuries.	1	2	3	4	5
Created a non-threatening learning environment.	1	2	3	4	5
Clearly explained new techniques.	1	2	3	4	5
Effectively demonstrated the necessary psychomotor skills.	1	2	3	4	5
Encouraged questions.	1	2	3	4	5
Provided appropriate feedback.	1	2	3	4	5
Evaluated learners' abilities fairly.	1	2	3	4	5

Please state how the instructor was most helpful to you.

_____
_____
_____
_____
_____
_____
_____
_____
_____
_____
_____
_____

Please state how the instructor was least helpful to you.

_____
_____
_____
_____
_____
_____
_____
_____
_____
_____
_____
_____

Please add any other comments.

_____
_____
_____
_____
_____
_____
_____
_____

Table 7. ATOM Post-Course Evaluation

Name:_____ Age:_____ Sex:_____

Course Date:_____ State:_____ Zip Code: _____

Course Location: _____

Level of Residency Training: PG4 ____ PG5 ____ Fellow ____

Attending (Years in Practice): 1 __ 2 __ 3 __ 4 __ 5 __ 6-10 __ 11-15 __ 16-20 __ 21-25 __ >25 __

Type of Practice: Exclusively Trauma ___ Trauma and General Surgery ___ General Surgery ___

What percentage of your trauma practice is penetrating trauma?
   0-20 ____ 21-40 ____ 41-60 ____ 61-80 ____ 81-100 ____

What percentage of your practice is devoted to trauma?
   0-20 ____ 21-40 ____ 41-60 ____ 61-80 ____ 81-100 ____

Where do you perform your trauma surgery?
   Level I ____ Level II ____ Level III ____ Level IV ____ Non-Trauma Center ____

Hospital Bed Size: 100-200 ___ 201-300 ___ 301-400 ___ 401-500 ___ 501-600 ___ >600 ___

Location: Urban ___ Suburban ___ Rural ___

Type: Academic Center ___ Community Hospital ___

Please indicate how strongly you agree or disagree with the following statements. The scale is:
1 (strongly disagree) 2 (disagree) 3 (neither agree nor disagree) 4 (agree) 5 (strongly agree).

	Strongly Disagree			Strongly Agree
Example:	1	2	③ 4	5

As a result of the ATOM course:

I am better able to identify traumatic injuries.	1	2	3	4	5
I am better able to repair traumatic injuries.	1	2	3	4	5
I have used the techniques I learned in the course.	1	2	3	4	5
I have used the knowledge that I gained from the course.	1	2	3	4	5
My practice is improved.	1	2	3	4	5
I am pleased that I took the course.	1	2	3	4	5
I would recommend the ATOM course to my colleagues.	1	2	3	4	5

In what ways has the ATOM course been most helpful to you?

_____

Please state how the course might be improved.

_____

Please add any other comments.

_____

REFERENCES

1.) Bandura A. *Social Foundations of Thought and Action: A Social Cognitive Theory*. Englewood Cliffs, NJ: Prentice Hall; 1986.

2.) Gable RK, Wolf MB. *Instrument Development in the Affective Domain: Measuring Attitudes and Values in Corporate and School Settings*. Boston: Kluwer Academic Publishers; 1993.

3.) Hertel JP, Millis BJ. *Using Simulations to Promote Learning in Higher Education*. Sterling, VA: Stylus Publishing, LLC; 2002.

4.) Jacobs LJ, Burns KJ, Kaban JM, Gross RI, Cortes V, Brautigam RT, Perdrizet GA, Besman A, Kirton O. Development and evaluation of the Advanced Trauma Operative Management course. *J Trauma*. 2003;55:471-479.

Index

A

AAST-OIS. *See American Association for the Surgery of Trauma-Organ Injury Scale*

Abdomen
  closure of
    Bogotá bag for, 22
    in damage control procedure, 28–29
    mesh for, 22
    towel clips for, 21, 37–38
    Vac Pack dressing for, 36
    Velcro dressings used with, 23
  intraabdominal pressure measurements, 58–59
  penetrating injuries of
    damage control of, 56–57
    description of, 17
    packing of, 212
    Wittman patch staged abdominal repair for, 30–33
  staged repair of
    artificial bur closure for, 30–31
    guidelines for, 33
    procedures for, 30–33
    Wittman patch, 30–33
  traumatic laparotomy preparations of, 3
  vascular injuries of, 307–309

Abdominal aorta
  control of, in vascular injuries, 308
  exposure of
    case study of, 303–304
    Mattox maneuver for, 13–14
  gunshot wounds to, 334
  infrarenal, laceration of, 335–336

Abdominal compartment syndrome, 24
Abdominal retractors, 4
Activated factor VII, 118
Advancing silo technique, for abdominal closure in damage control procedure, 19–21
Aird maneuver, 164–165
Allis clamps
  description of, 48, 98, 261, 318
  inferior vena cava laceration control using, 348–349

Aluminum silicate, 147

American Association for the Surgery of Trauma-Organ Injury Scale
  diaphragmatic injury grading, 89–90
  duodenal injury, 176, 178–179
  kidney injury grading, 229–231
  liver injury grading, 108–111
  pancreatic injury grading, 167–168
  splenic injury grading, 72

Ampulla of Vater, 167

Anastomoses
  biliary enteric, 219
  for cecal trauma repair, 40
  GIA stapled
    for gastrojejunostomy, 213
    for pulmonary tractotomy, 316–317
    for sigmoid colon laceration repair, 42
  jejuno-jejunal, 220
  pancreaticoenteric, 183

Antibiotics
  broad-spectrum, 258, 260
  in penetrating injuries, 17, 258, 260

Aorta
  abdominal. *See Abdominal aorta*
  control of
    supraceliac, 332–333
    through left chest, 330–331
  vascular repair of, 336

Aortic injuries
  abdominal aorta
    case study of, 303–304
    Mattox maneuver for, 13–14
  ascending aorta, 287
  blunt, 287
  complications of, 292
  diagnosis of, 288
  exploratory laparotomy of, 12–14
  interposition graft for, 290
  Mattox maneuver for, 13–14
  radiographs of, 288
  shunts for, 289
  surgical repair of, 288–291
  transection
    complications of, 292
    repair of, 290

Argon beam coagulator, 119
Arterial-portal venous fistulas, 133
Artery. *See specific artery*
Artery of Adamkiewicz, 289, 292
Artificial bur closure, for staged abdominal repair, 30–31
Ascending aorta injuries, 287
ATOM course
    affective learning assessments, 366
    cognitive learning assessments, 367
    evaluations of, 368, 374–376, 378–379
    instructor evaluations of, 376–377
    laboratory experience in, 365, 371–373
    learning assessments, 366
    participant evaluations, 366–367
    psychomotor learning assessments, 367
    results of, 367
    scoring scale, 367
    self-efficacy
        description of, 364
        educational activities for increasing, 364–365
        information sources for, 365
        instruments for assessing, 366
        methods of strengthening, 364, 369
        surgical, 370
    simulation uses of, 365–366
    theoretical framework for, 364
Atrial appendage, 318
Atrial caval shunt to superior vena cava, for vascular control in liver injuries, 127
Atrial laceration, 318–319
Autotransfuser, 2
Autotransfusion, 2, 5
Avitene, 65

B

Babcock clamps, 44, 48, 214
Balfour retractor, 216
Balloon catheter, 294
Balloon tamponade, for liver injuries, 142–144
Beck's triad, 279, 323
Bile duct, common
    exposure of, 190–191
    injury management, 218–220
    repair of, 218–220
Biliary enteric anastomosis, 219
Biliary fistula, 132–133, 155
Biliary tree, 8
Bladder
    anatomy of, 229
    cystogram of, 228, 245
    exposure of, 251
Bladder injuries
    diagnosis of, 229
    extraperitoneal, 245–246
    intraperitoneal
        description of, 246–247
        laceration, 256–258, 261
    laceration
        exposure and management of, 251
        intraperitoneal, 256–258, 261
        repair of, 262–263
    penetrating, 254–255, 258–260
    postoperative management of, 247
    repair of, 260
    treatment of, 246–247
    trigone, 256, 258–260
Bladder pressure, 56
Bleeding. *See also* Hemorrhage
    hemostatic agents for, 19
    of liver, 116–117
    tamponade of, 6–8
Blunt trauma
    aortic injuries secondary to, 287
    diaphragmatic injury caused by, 89, 97–98
    duodenal, 161–162
    liver injuries, 148
    pancreas, 159–160, 195–196
    in retroperitoneum, 11
Boari bladder flap, 242–243
Bogotá bag, for abdomen closure, 22
Bowel
    contamination control in, 9, 20
    enterotomies in, 20
    small
        lacerations of, incontinuity resection of, 46–47

stab wounds to, 48–51
stapled resection of, 46–47
sutured repair of, 50–51
Browner pelvic stabilizer, 60–61
Bulldog clamps, 352

C

Carbon dioxide insufflation, 314
Cardiac effusion, 280
Cardiac injuries
    atrial laceration, 318–319
    cardiac tamponade. See Cardiac tamponade
    complications of, 285
    diagnosis of, 277
    emergency department thoracotomy for, 278, 281–283, 358–360
    incidence of, 277
    management of, 278
    penetrating
        digital control for, 284
        Foley catheter for, 284
        thoracotomy for, 276, 284
    postoperative complications of, 285
    right ventricle
        laceration of, using Foley/staple/pledget technique, 320–322
        stab wound of, 323–324, 328–329
    signs and symptoms of, 279
    surgical approaches for, 281
    transesophageal echocardiography of, 285
    transthoracic echocardiography of, 285
    treatment of, 276
    types of, 279
Cardiac lacerations, stapled repair of, 325–327
Cardiac tamponade
    description of, 279
    diagnosis of, 280
    treatment of, 280
Cattel Braasch maneuver, 15, 164, 293
Cecum, stab wound to, 39–40
Celiac trunk
    anatomy of, 13–14
    exposure and repair of, 361–362
    injury of, 354–355, 361–362
Centromedian zone, of retroperitoneum, 11
Chevron-type incisions, 114
Cholecystocholangiography, fluoroscopic, 171, 174
Choledochojejunostomy, 193
Clamps
    Babcock, 44, 48, 214
    Bulldog, 352
    Kelly, 98
    Satinsky
        description of, 294, 318, 330
        double, for inferior vena cava repair, 339–341
    side-biting, 296
Closure. *See also* Sutures
    abdomen
        Bogotá bag for, 22
        in damage control procedure, 28–29
        mesh for, 22
        towel clips for, 21, 37–38
        Velcro dressings used with techniques for, 23
    Vac Pack dressing for, 36
Coagulation
    argon beam coagulator for, 119
    radiofrequency, 119
Coagulation sandwich, 62–63
Coagulopathy, 17
Colon
    distal colorectal irrigation, 52
    injuries of
        colostomy for, 16–17
        descending, 43
        exploratory laparotomy of, 16–17
        lacerations, 41–42, 44–45
        sigmoid, 41–42
    splenic flexure of, 189
Colorectal irrigation, distal, 52–53
Colostomy, diverting, 16–17, 54–55
Common bile duct
    exposure of, 190–191
    injury management, 218–220
    repair of, 218–220

Common iliac artery injury, 352–353
Common iliac vein injury, 298
Computed tomography
    of bladder injury, 245
    of duodenal injury, 162
    of genitourinary injuries, 228
    of pancreatic duct, 160
Contamination
    control of, 9, 19–20
    in damage control patients, 19
Cricothyroidotomy, 310
Cystogram, 228, 245

D

Damage control
    abdominal closure in, 28–29
    definition of, 18
    goals of, 18
    liver injuries, 124–125
    operating room considerations for, 18
    packing for, 124
    pancreaticoduodenectomy, 193–194
    penetrating abdomen injury, 56–57
    stapled resection for, 51
    supraceliac aortic control after, 332–333
    techniques for, 19–21
Descending colon, low velocity gunshot wound to, 43
Diaphragmatic injury
    American Association for the Surgery of Trauma-Organ
        Injury Scale grading of, 89–90
    blunt trauma-related, 89, 97–98
    burst wound of dome of diaphragm, 99–100
    characteristics of, 88
    complications of, 92
    diagnosis of, 88–89
    high-grade, 92
    laceration, 101–102
    laparoscopic repair of, 103–104
    penetrating trauma-related, 89
    prosthetic patch for, 92
    thoracostomy tube for, 91
    treatment of, 91–92
2,3-Diphosphoglycerate, 2
Distal colorectal irrigation, 52–53
Distal pancreatectomy, 169–171, 224–225
Diverting colostomy, 16–17, 54–55
Double Satinsky clamp technique, for inferior vena cava repair, 339–341
Dressings
    Esmarch rubberized, 22–23
    Vac Pack, for abdominal wall closure, 36
    Velcro, 23
Duodenal injuries
    Aird maneuver for, 164–165
    American Association for the Surgery of Trauma-Organ
        Injury Scale for, 176, 178–179
    blunt, 161–162
    Cattel Braasch maneuver for, 164
    decompressive techniques for, 180
    difficulties associated with, 158
    diversionary techniques for, 180–181
    duodenal lumen constriction considerations, 204
    Grade I, 176, 178
    Grade II, 176, 178
    Grade III, 176, 179
    Grade IV, 176, 179
    Grade V, 176
    Kocher maneuver for, 163, 202
    lacerations
        case study management of, 202–207
        grading of, 176
    mild, 179
    missed, 167
    operative strategy for
        description of, 176–177
        injury grading and, 178–179
    pancreatic injuries and, concomitant presentation of
        description of, 184
        operative management of, 199–201
    penetrating, 163, 211–212
    periduodenal drainage for, 216
    pyloric exclusion for
        description of, 181
        indications, 207

stapled, 216–217
technique for, 214–215
severe, 179–180
Snyder duodenal severity scale, 179–180
stab wounds, 179
surgical exposure techniques for, 164–165
tenuous complex, pyloric exclusion for, 213
three tube technique for, 180
Whipple for, 182–183
Duodenojejunal junction, 166
Duodenum
exploratory laparotomy of, 162
exposure of, 15, 190–191, 206
fourth portion of, 208
injury of, 8
ligament of Treitz, 166
second portion of
laceration of, 202–203
penetrating injury to, 211–212
third portion of
exposure of, 208
laceration of, 204–207

E

Electrocautery, 79, 147
Emergency department thoracotomy, 281–283, 358–360
Endoscopic retrograde cholangiopancreaticography, 132–133, 160, 172, 197
Enterotomy, 20
ERCP. *See Endoscopic retrograde cholangiopancreaticography*
Esmarch rubberized dressing, 22
Exploratory laparotomy. *See Laparotomy*
Extraperitoneal bladder injuries, 245–246

F

Factor VIIa, 118
Falciform ligament, 6
Fibrin glue, 65, 118, 146–147
Finochietto rib spreader, 282

Fistula
mucous, 53
pancreatic, 87
Flail chest, 311–312
FloSeal, 147
Fluoroscopic cholecystocholangiography, 171, 174
Focused abdominal sonogram in trauma examination, 66–68, 237, 323
Foley catheter
for bladder injuries, 247, 254
for cardiac injuries, 284
for cystogram, 245
for intraabdominal pressure measurement, 59
for right ventricle injury, 320
Foreign bodies, 241

G

Gastrocolic omentum, 166
Gastrojejunostomy, 200–201
Gelfoam, 63, 65, 268
Genitourinary injuries
anatomy of, 229
bladder. *See Bladder injuries*
computed tomography of, 228
diagnostic studies for, 228
hematuria, 227
incidence of, 227
intravenous pyelogram for, 228
ureter. *See Ureter*, injury of
Gerota's fascia, 77, 165, 239, 265, 268
GIA stapled anastomosis
for gastrojejunostomy, 213
for pulmonary tractotomy, 316–317
for sigmoid colon laceration repair, 42
Glisson's capsule, 122
Gunshot wounds
to abdominal aorta, 334
to descending colon, 43
to left common iliac artery, 352–353
to ureter, 273–274

H

Haemophilus influenzae vaccine, 85–86
Heaney maneuver, 141
Hematoma
    inframesocolic, 335
    intraparenchymal
        of liver, 109–110
        of spleen, 74
    retroperitoneal, 8, 11, 239, 264, 292–293, 298
    subcapsular
        of liver, 109, 155
        of spleen, 73
    supramesocolic, 355, 361–362
Hematuria, 227
Hemobilia, 132
Hemorrhage. *See also* Bleeding
    Avitene for, 65
    Browner pelvic stabilizer for, 60–61
    control of, 4–5, 65, 118, 294, 350–351
    hemostatic agents for, 118
    hepatic
        description of, 116–117, 145
        omental pack for, 122–123
        Pringle maneuver for, 112, 120, 126, 140–141, 155
        sutures for, 139
        techniques for controlling, 118–119
    inferior vena cava laceration-related, 5
    packing techniques for, 6–8
    pelvic, 11
    pulsatile, 5
    suturing techniques for, 317
Hemostasis
    argon beam coagulator for, 119
    radiofrequency coagulation for, 119
Hemostatic agents
    description of, 19, 64–65, 79
    fibrin glue, 65, 118, 146–147
    hemorrhage control using, 118
    for simple liver injuries, 116
Hemostatic coagulation sandwich, 62–63
Hemothorax, retained, 313–315

Hepatic arteries
    anatomy of, 113
    ligation of, 125
    variations in, 125
Hepatic injuries. *See* Liver injuries
Hepatic veins, 111–112
Hepatic venous exclusion
    case study of, 151–153
    limitations of, 128–129
    Pringle maneuver for, 129
    venovenous bypass and, 129–130, 141
Hepatotomy, 121
Hickman catheter, 201
Horizontal mattress suture, 319
Hyperpyrexia, 132
Hypothermia
    operating room precautions for, 2
    preincisional considerations, 2
    risks for, 2
Hypovolemia, 2

I

Ileocecetomy, for cecal trauma, 40
Incisions
    chevron-type, 114
    hypothermia precautions before, 2
    for liver injury management, 114
    midline laparotomy, 354
    right subcostal, 114
    staged abdominal repair, 30
    trapdoor, 281
Inferior mesenteric artery, 13–14
Inferior vena cava
    anatomy of, 337
    clamping of
        Allis, 348
        for hepatic vascular control, 126, 152
    compression of, 118
    dissection of, 342
    exposure of, 15, 293, 342
    hemorrhage secondary to laceration of, 5
    hepatic vein draining into, 112
    infradiaphragmatic, 126

infrahepatic injuries
    Cattel Braasch maneuver for, 293
    complications of, 298
    hemorrhage control in, 294
    lacerations, 348–351
    ligation of, 295
    management of, 293–294
    repair of, 295–297
    sutures for, 297
injuries of
    diagnosis of, 344
    double Satinsky clamp technique for, 339–341
    infrahepatic. *See Inferior vena cava, infrahepatic injuries*
    penetrating, 346–347
    repair of, 297, 344–345
    stab wound, 342–343
    suturing of, 343, 345
laceration of
    Allis clamp control of, 348–349
    description of, 5
    infrarenal portion of, 348–351
    two centimeters distal to the renal vessels, 356–357
    lumen of, 337
    penetrating injuries of, 346–347
    primary repair of, 297

Infrahepatic inferior vena cava injuries
    Cattel Braasch maneuver for, 293
    complications of, 298
    hemorrhage control in, 294
    lacerations
        Allis clamp control of, 348–349
        with hypotension and hemorrhage, 350–351
    ligation of, 295
    management of, 293–294
    repair of, 295–297
    sutures for, 297

Inframesocolic hematoma, 335
Infrarenal abdominal aorta laceration, 335–336
Injury. *See also specific injury*
    assessments of, 4
    blunt. *See Blunt trauma*
    identification of, 8
    penetrating. *See Penetrating injuries*

Intraabdominal abscess, 132
Intraabdominal pressure measurements, 58–59
Intraparenchymal hematoma
    of liver, 109–110
    of spleen, 74
Intraperitoneal bladder injuries, 246–247
Intravenous pyelogram, 228, 237
Intravesicular clots, 247
Irrigation, distal colorectal, 52–53

J

J stent, 240, 274
Jackson-Pratt drain, 122, 156, 201, 203, 212, 223, 240, 274
Jejuno-jejunal anastomosis, 220
Jejunostomy, 198

K

Kelly clamp, 98
Kidney(s)
    anatomy of, 229
    avascular, 162
    collecting system of, 266, 269–270
    contralateral, assessment of, 237–238
    exposure of, using Mattox maneuver, 232–233, 305–306
Kidney, ureter, and bladder x-rays, 161
Kidney injuries
    American Association for the Surgery of Trauma-Organ Injury Scale for, 229–231
    collecting system, 266, 269–270
    exposure for, 232–233
    Grade I
        characteristics of, 230
        treatment of, 233
    Grade II
        characteristics of, 230
        treatment of, 234–235
    Grade III
        characteristics of, 231
        treatment of, 234–235

Grade IV
    characteristics of, 231
    treatment of, 235–236
Grade V
    characteristics of, 231
    exposure of, 252–253
    management of, 252–253
    reimplantation for, 238
    renovascular disruption, 239
    treatment of, 235–236
laceration, of collecting system, 266, 269–270
lower pole, 266–268
open calyceal system secondary to, 235
operative scenarios for, 232
vascular pedicle control, 233

Kocher maneuver
for duodenal injuries, 163, 202
extended, 15, 308
for pancreatic injuries, 163, 189, 191
for retroperitoneal hematomas, 293

L

Lacerations
abdominal aorta, 335–336
atrial, 318–319
bladder
    exposure and management of, 251
    intraperitoneal, 256–258, 261
    repair of, 262–263
cardiac, stapled repair of, 325–327
colon, 44–45
diaphragm, 101–102
inferior vena cava
    Allis clamp control of, 348–349
    description of, 5
    infrarenal portion of, 348–351
    two centimeters distal to the renal vessels, 356–357
infrarenal abdominal aorta, 335–336
liver, 144–145
renal artery, 252–254, 264–265
right ventricle, 320–322
sigmoid colon, 41–42
small bowel, 46–47
spleen
    description of, 44–45
    grading of, 75–76

Laparoscopy, diaphragmatic injury repaired by, 103–104

Laparotomy, traumatic
abdomen preparations, 3
aortic injuries. *See* Aortic injuries
colonic injury assessments, 16–17
contamination control, 9
damage control
    abdominal closure in, 28–29
    definition of, 18
    goals of, 18
    operating room considerations for, 18
    supraceliac aortic control, 332
    techniques for, 19–21
duodenum, 162
elements of, 4
hemorrhage control, 4–5
inferior vena cava exposure, 15
injury
    assessment of, 4
    identification of, 8
operating room for, 2–4
packing techniques, 6–8, 34–36
preparations for, 46
reconstruction, 10–11
retroperitoneal hematoma, 11
in stable patient, 16
in unstable patients, 17

Left common iliac artery injury, 352–353
Left hepatic artery, 113
Left hepatic vein, 112
Left medial rotation. *See* Mattox maneuver
Left thoracotomy, for aortic injury assessments, 12
Levine-Penrose unit, 143
Lienophrenic ligament, 76, 164
Lienorenal ligament, 76, 164
Ligament of Treitz, 166, 191
Linea Alba, 191

Liver
    anatomy of, 111–113
    arteries of, 113
    exposure of, 115, 136–137
    ligaments of, 115
    mobilization of, 115
    veins of, 111–112

Liver injuries
    American Association for the Surgery of Trauma-Organ
        Injury Scale for, 108–111
    arterial-portal venous fistulas secondary to, 133
    balloon tamponade technique for, 142–144
    biliary fistula secondary to, 132–133
    blunt trauma, 148
    burst, 148–150, 155
    complex
        definition of, 120
        management of, 138–142
    complications of, 132–133
    damage control
        hepatic artery ligation for, 125
        packing for, 124
    damage control of, 124–125
    ductal injuries, 133
    Grade I, 108, 116
    Grade II, 109, 116
    Grade III, 109–110, 116
    Grade IV
        burst injury, 148–150, 155
        characteristics of, 110, 118, 136–137
        laceration, 144–145
        without active hemorrhage, 146–147
    Grade V, 111, 118
    Grade VI, 111, 125
    hemobilia secondary to, 132
    hemorrhage control in
        description of, 116–117, 145
        hepatotomy and intrahepatic balloon for, 124
        omental pack and drainage for, 122–123
        Pringle maneuver for, 112, 120, 126, 140–141, 155
        recurrence concerns, 132
        sutures for, 139
        techniques for controlling, 118–119
    hepatotomy for, 121
    hyperpyrexia secondary to, 132
    intraabdominal abscess secondary to, 132
    laceration, 144–145, 155
    lobular, 154–156
    operative management of
        exposure, 115, 136–137, 154–156
        goals for, 130
        hepatic artery ligation, 113
        incisions, 114
        intrinsic problems, 131
        lobectomy, 140
        mobilization, 115
        techniques for, 113
    packing/wrapping
        damage control uses of, 124
        decreased vascular return considerations, 117–118
        description of, 116–117
        indications for, 137
        PACHTER PACK, 136–137
    penetrating, 124–125
    portal triad occlusion, 120, 148
    Pringle maneuver for, 112, 120, 126, 140–141
    resectional debridement of, 123, 140
    simple, 116
    summary of, 133
    through and through, 142–143, 156
    vascular control of
        atrial caval shunt to superior vena cava, 127
        description of, 125
    vascular lesions, 125
    venous exclusion
        case study of, 151–153
        limitations of, 128–129
        Pringle maneuver for, 129
        venovenous bypass and, 129–130, 141

Liver replacement therapy, 133

Lobectomy, 140

M

Magnetic resonance cholangiopancreatography, for pancreatic duct injuries, 160–161
Major vein injury, 337–338
Mattox maneuver
    for aortic exposure, 13–14
    for kidney exposure, 232, 305–306
    technique of, 305–306
Median sternotomy, 281
Mesenteric window, 47
Mesh closure of abdomen, 22
Mesh wrap
    for hemorrhage control of liver, 117
    for splenorrhaphy, 80
Methylene blue
    contralateral kidney assessments, 238
    pancreatography using, 209–210
Metzenbaum scissors, 163, 165, 352
Middle hepatic artery, 113
Middle hepatic vein, 112
Mobilization of spleen, 10, 45, 76–78
Moore-Pilcher balloon caval shunt, 128
Morison's pouch, 67
Moss gastrojejunostomy, 194
Mucous fistula, 53

N

Nephrectomy, 236, 264–265
Nonabsorable sutures, 183, 235

O

Octreotide, 87
Omental pack, 122–123
Omental patch, 81
Operating room
    autotransfuser used in, 2
    damage control procedures, 18
    temperature of, 2
    transfusion device used in, 2
    for traumatic laparotomy, 2–4
OPSS. *See Overwhelming post-splenectomy*
Organ injury
    assessment of, 10
    reconstruction of, 10–11
Orthotopic liver transplantation, 133
Overwhelming postsplenectomy sepsis, 70, 86

P

PACHTER PACK, 136–137
Packing
    abdominal penetrating injuries, 212
    hemorrhage control using, 6–8, 116–117
    liver injuries
        damage control, 124
        decreased vascular return considerations, 117–118
        description of, 116–117
        indications, 137
        PACHTER PACK, 136–137
    techniques for, 6–8, 34–36
Pancreas
    exposure of, 15, 188–191
    inferior surface of, 188
    injuries of. *See Pancreatic injuries*
    lesser sac of, 159
    parenchymal resection of, 174
    partial transection of, 197–198
    superior border of, 188
    surgical exposure of, 165–166
    transected neck of, 159
Pancreatectomy
    distal, 169–171, 224–225
    spleen-saving, 225
Pancreatic duct
    computed tomography of, 160
    injuries of
        cholecystocholangiography for, 173
        diagnosis of, 171–173, 197
        endoscopic retrograde cholangiopancreatography of, 160, 172, 197
        intraoperative diagnosis of, 171–173
        magnetic resonance cholangiopancreatography of, 160–161
        stab wounds, 221–225
        treatment of, 174–175
Pancreatic fistula, 87

Pancreatic injuries
   American Association for the Surgery of Trauma-Organ
      Injury Scale for, 167–169
   blunt trauma, 159–160, 195–196
   difficulties associated with, 158
   duodenal injuries and, concomitant presentation of
      description of, 184
      operative management of, 199–201
   Grade I, 167, 169
   Grade II, 167, 169
   Grade III, 167, 169–170
   Grade IV, 167, 170
   Grade V, 167, 182
   intra-abdominal injuries associated with, 159
   Kocher maneuver for, 163, 189, 191
   lacerations, grading of, 168
   localization of, 168
   management algorithm for, 175
   methylene blue pancreatography for, 209–210
   missed, 167
   operative strategies for
      American Association for the Surgery of Trauma-Organ Injury Scale for guidance of, 169
      description of, 167
      distal pancreatectomy, 169–171, 224–225
   pancreaticoduodenectomy for. *see Pancreaticoduodenectomy*
   penetrating, 163
   surgical exposure techniques for, 165–166
   treatment of, 174–175
   Whipple for, 182–183, 197
Pancreatic insufficiency, 174
Pancreaticoduodenectomy
   for damage control, 193–194
   description of, 182
   reconstruction after, 195–196
   technique for, 192–194
Pancreaticoenteric anastomosis, 183
Pancreatograms, 172
Pancreatography, methylene blue, 209–210
Paraplegia, 289, 292
Partial splenectomy
   before splenorrhaphy, 82–83
   indications for, 82
   stapled, 83
PDS suture, 212
Pelvic retroperitoneum, 11
Pelvic stabilizer, Browner, 60–61
Penetrating injuries
   of abdomen
      damage control of, 56–57
      description of, 17
      packing for, 212
      Wittman patch staged abdominal repair for, 30–33
   antibiotics in, 17
   of bladder, 254–255
   to cecum, 39–40
   diaphragmatic, 89
   to duodenum, 211–212
   gunshot wounds. See Gunshot wounds
   of inferior vena cava, 346–347
Penrose drain, 142–143, 156, 199
Pericardial sac
   blood detection in, using focused abdominal sonogram in trauma examination, 67–68
   description of, 324
Pericardiocentesis, 323
Pericardium, 320, 322, 359
Pledgeted repair
   description of, 79
   of right ventricle laceration, 320–321
Pledgeted sutures, 282, 286, 327, 329
Pneumovax vaccine, 86
Porta hepatis, 112
Portal triad occlusion, 120, 148
Pouch of Douglas, 263
Pringle maneuver
   hemorrhage control using, 112, 120, 126, 140–141, 155
   hepatic venous exclusion using, 128
Pseudo Rommel tourniquet, 357
Psoas hitch, 242, 244
Pulmonary tractotomy, 316–317
Pulsus paradoxus, 279
Purse string suture, 54

Pyloric exclusion
    description of, 181
    indications, 207
    stapled, 216–217
    technique for, 214–215
    for tenuous complex duodenal injury, 213

R

Radiofrequency coagulation, 119
Renal artery
    anatomy of, 14
    laceration of, 252–254, 264–265
    thrombosis of, 239
Renal dysfunction, 59
Renal injuries. *See Kidney injuries*
Renal vein, 14
Renorrhaphy, 234
Renovascular disruption, 239
Resectional debridement, of liver injuries, 123, 140
Retroperitoneal hematoma, 8, 11, 239, 264, 292–293, 298
Retroperitoneum
    exploration of, 39–40
    zones of, 11
Right atrium, 286
Right hepatic artery, 113
Right ventricle
    laceration of, using Foley/staple/pledget technique, 320–322
    stab wound of, 323–324, 328–329
Right-sided visceral rotation, 308, 338
Roux-en-Y choledochojejunostomy, 219
Roux-en-Y hepaticojejunostomy, 133

S

Saphenous vein, 4
Satinsky clamps
    description of, 294, 318, 330
    double, for inferior vena cava repair, 339–341
Schrock shunt, 127
Self-efficacy
    description of, 364
    educational activities for increasing, 364–365
    information sources for, 365
    instruments for assessing, 366
    methods of strengthening, 364, 369
    surgical, 370
Shunts, for aortic injuries, 289
Side-biting clamp, 296
Sigmoid colon laceration, 41–42
Silo technique, for abdominal closure in damage control procedure, 19–21
Small bowel
    lacerations of, incontinuity resection of, 46–47
    stab wounds to, 48–51
    stapled resection of, 46–47
    sutured repair of, 50–51
Snyder duodenal severity scale, 179–180
Social cognitive theory, 364
Sphincter of Oddi, 171
Spleen
    blunt trauma injury of, 97–98
    exposure of, 95–96
    injury of
        blunt trauma, 97–98
        grading of, 72–73
        high-grade, 75–76
        low-grade, 73
        moderate-grade, 74–75
        splenectomy for. *See Splenectomy*
        stab wound, 105–106
        subcapsular hematoma, 73
    laceration of
        description of, 44–45
        grading of, 75–76
    lower pole of, stab wound to, 105–106
    mobilization of, 10, 45, 76–78
    nonoperative management of
        failure of, 71
        indications, 70
    operative management of
        intraoperative indications for, 72
        preoperative indications for, 71
    pancreatectomy with preservation of, 225
    salvage of, 70–71
    shattered, 95–96

stab wound to lower pole of, 105–106
Splenectomy
   complications of
      description of, 85
      overwhelming post-splenectomy, 86
      pancreatic fistula, 87
      sub-diaphragmatic abscess, 87
   indications for, 83–85
   partial
      before splenorrhaphy, 82–83
      indications for, 82
      stapled, 83
   procedure, 84–85
Splenic artery, anatomy of, 13–14
Splenorrhaphy
   indications for, 78
   mesh wrap for, 80
   omental patch during, 81
   partial splenectomy before
      indications for, 82
      stapled, 83
   pledgeted repair, 79
Sponge sticks, 294, 337, 340
Stab wounds
   anterior "mantel," 328
   to cecum, 39–40
   to duodenum, 179
   to inferior vena cava, 342–343
   multiple, 48–51
   to pancreas with ductal injury, 221–225
   to right ventricle, 323–324, 328–329
   to small bowel, 48–51
   to spleen, 105–106
Staged abdominal repair
   artificial bur closure for, 30–31
   guidelines for, 33
   procedures for, 30–33
   Wittman patch, 30–33
Stapled partial splenectomy, 83
Stapled pyloric exclusion, 216–217

Stapled repair
   of cardiac laceration, 325–327
   of small bowel stab wounds, 49
Stapled resection
   damage control, 51
   small bowel, 46–47
STAR. See Staged abdominal repair
Sternal fractures, 312
Streptococcus pneumoniae, 86
Subcapsular hematoma
   of liver, 109, 155
   of spleen, 73
Sub-diaphragmatic abscess, 87
Subxiphoid approach, 67
Suction catheter, 22
Superior mesenteric artery
   anatomy of, 13
   exposure and repair of, 361–362
Superior vena cava, atrial caval shunt to, 127
Supraceliac aortic control, 332–333
Supramesocolic hematoma, 355, 361–362
Suprapubic drain, 246, 260
Surgicel, 65
Sutures
   for abdominal aorta repair, 304
   for hepatic hemorrhage, 139
   horizontal mattress, 319
   for inferior vena cava repair, 343, 345
   for intrahepatic inferior vena cava injuries, 297
   nonabsorable, 183, 235
   PDS, 212
   pledgeted, 282, 286
   purse string, 54
   small bowel repair, 50–51

T

TA-55 stapler, 222
Teflon pledgets, 359
Thoracoabdominal injuries, focused abdominal sonogram in trauma examination for, 66–68
Thoracoscopy, for trapped lung syndrome, 313–315

Thoracotomy
    for cardiac injuries, 276, 278, 281–284
    emergency department, 281–283, 358–360
    left anterolateral, 283, 358
    technique for, 281–283
Three tube technique, for duodenal injuries, 180
Topical hemostatic agents, 64–65
Totally diverting loop colostomy with non-contaminating distal irrigation, 54–55
Towel clips, for abdomen closure, 21, 37–38
Tractotomy, pulmonary, 316–317
Transesophageal echocardiography, 285
Transfusion device, 2
Transfusions
    fluid warming before, 5
    risks associated with, 70
Transthoracic echocardiography, 285
Transureteroureterostomy, 242
Transurethral drainage, 260
Trapdoor incision, 281
Trapped lung syndrome, 313–315
Trauma. See Blunt trauma; Penetrating injuries
Trigone injuries, 256, 258–260
T-tube, 218–220

U

Unstable patients
    characteristics of, 17
    exploratory laparotomy in, 17
Ureter
    anatomy of, 13–14, 229
    exposure of, 15
    identification of, 273
    injury of
        closed-suction drain for, 240
        complete transection, 241
        exposure of, 239
        gunshot wound, 273–274
        repair of, 271–274
        transureteroureterostomy for, 242–243
        treatment of, 240
    lower
        anatomy of, 242
        Psoas hitch for, 242, 244
    middle
        anatomy of, 242
        Boari bladder flap, 242–243
        injuries to, 271
    proximal, transureteroureterostomy for, 242–243
    segments of, 242
    upper, 242
Ureterectomy, 236–237, 242
Ureterocalycostomy, 242
Urinary system injuries. See Urologic injuries
Urinary tract infection, 260
Urologic injuries
    anatomy of, 229
    computed tomography of, 228
    diagnostic studies for, 228
    hematuria, 227
    incidence of, 227
    intravenous pyelogram for, 228

V

Vac Pack dressing, for abdominal wall closure, 36
Vascular injuries
    abdominal, 307–309
    aorta. See Aortic injuries
    case study of, 337–338
    inferior vena cava. See Inferior vena cava
Velcro dressings, for abdomen closure, 23
Vena cava. See Inferior vena cava; **Superior vena cava**
Venous exclusion, hepatic
    case study of, 151–153
    limitations of, 128–129
    Pringle maneuver for, 129
    venovenous bypass and, 129–130, 141
Venovenous bypass, 129–130, 141
Ventricular injuries
    lacerations, 320–322
    stab wound, 323–324, 328–329
Ventricular septal defect, 328

W

Whipple procedure, 182–183, 197
Wittman patch staged abdominal repair, for penetrating abdominal trauma, 30–33

X

Xiphoid process, 190, 329

NOTES